New Approaches in Health Science

Gökhan Aba (ed.)

# New Approaches in Health Sciences

## New Methods and Developments in Health Sciences

**PETER LANG**

**Bibliographic Information published by the
Deutsche Nationalbibliothek**
The Deutsche Nationalbibliothek lists this publication in the Deutsche
Nationalbibliografie; detailed bibliographic data is available online at
http://dnb.d-nb.de.

**Library of Congress Cataloging-in-Publication Data**
A CIP catalog record for this book has been applied for at the
Library of Congress.

ISBN 978-3-631-80206-9 (Print)
E-ISBN 978-3-631-80228-1 (E-PDF)
E-ISBN 978-3-631-80229-8 (EPUB)
E-ISBN 978-3-631-80230-4 (MOBI)
DOI 10.3726/b16148

© Peter Lang GmbH
Internationaler Verlag der Wissenschaften
Berlin 2019
All rights reserved.

Peter Lang – Berlin · Bern · Bruxelles · New York · Oxford · Warszawa · Wien

This publication has been double-blind peer reviewed.

www.peterlang.com

# Preface and Acknowledgements

As a result of scientific and technological developments that have been experienced within the last twenty years, the increase of the global welfare level, the improvement of communication technologies, the development of new diagnosis and treatment methods, and developments in the pharmaceutical industry and the increased use of high-tech devices have been seen; the average global-level life expectancy has exceeded 70. It is estimated to increase to 80 in 2050. A long and healthy life brings along certain problems. Together with the increase of elderly population, there has been an increase in the prevalence of chronic diseases, need for qualified medical personnel and financial burden on the health system. As a result of new developments in health sciences, care services have become even more important. New methods, new approaches and advanced technologies have been used for patients to access less-costly and high-quality diagnosis and treatment services in a shorter time.

This book, which includes new approaches in health sciences, has been written by successful and expert researchers who work in different health disciplines of health sciences. The book consists of four sections. The first section includes recent developments in the area of nursing and midwifery. These developments are homeopathy in women's health, aromatherapy and other complementary and alternative medicine applications, complementary and alternative medicine applications in infertility, cognitive behavioral therapy in psychiatric nursing, current approaches in childbirth education, integrative pain management and telehealth practices in post-operative home care of elderly. The second section includes new developments and approaches in medicine. In addition to this, the place of robotic surgery in otorhinolaryngologic surgery, anti-mullerian hormone as a new indicator in determining the ovary reserve and new approaches in fetal aneuploidy scan are other topics in this section. The third section includes four chapters with new developments in health management. These chapters include doctor shopping as a new tendency of consumer behavior in healthcare services, innovation in the health sector and new health occupations that will direct health in the future. Finally, the fourth section includes developments in other health sciences. Telerehabilitation, basic body awareness therapy, new approaches in pharmacy and audiology are the topic titles in this section.

I would like to thank all the authors and reviewers who are experts in their field for their devotion and diligence and hope to help our readers. I also offer our endless gratitude to the families and children who are the source of the motivation for our authors with their patience and support during the conduct of these valuable works.

Sincerely yours,
Gökhan Aba
Editor

# Contents

# List of Authors

**Ayça Şolt Kırca**
Asst. Prof., PhD, Kırklareli University, aycasolt@klu.edu.tr

**Aysu Zekioğlu**
Asst. Prof., PhD, Trakya University, aysukurtuldu@trakya.edu.tr

**Berna Tunçer**
Dr., PhD, Trakya University, bernakuzuoglu@trakya.edu.tr

**Burcu Aracıoğlu**
Assoc. Prof., Ege University, burcu.aracioglu@ege.edu.tr

**Derya Kanza Gül**
Spec. Dr., MD, Private Nisa Hospital, deryakanza@yahoo.com

**Ebru Em Öztürk**
Spec. Dr., MD, İstanbul Bakırköy Dr. Sadi Konuk Training and Research Hospital, ebruem@yahoo.com

**Ebru Gözüyeşil**
Asst. Prof., PhD, Osmaniye Korkut Ata University, ebrugozuyesil@osmaniye.edu.tr

**Fatma Başar**
Asst., Prof., PhD, Kütahya Dumlupınar University, fatma.basar@dpu.edu.tr

**Figen Alp Yılmaz**
Asst. Prof., PhD, Bozok University, efigenden@gmail.com

**Figen Dığın**
Lecturer, Kırklareli University, figendigin@klu.edu.tr

**Filiz Süzer Özkan**
Asst., Prof., PhD, Düzce University, filizsuzer@duzce.edu.tr

**Gül Ergün**
Asst., Prof., PhD, Mehmet Akif Ersoy University, ergun@mehmetakif.edu.tr

**Gülbahtiyar Demirel**
Assoc. Prof., Sivas Cumhuriyet University, gdoganer@cumhuriyet.edu.tr

**Güliz Dirimen Arıkan**
Asst., Prof., PhD, Yeditepe University, guliz.dirimen@yeditepe.edu.tr

**Hamiyet Yüce**
Asst., Prof., PhD, Bandırma Onyedi Eylül University, hyuce@bandirma.edu.tr

**Işıl Işık**
Asst., Prof., PhD, Yeditepe University, isil.isik@yeditepe.edu.tr

**İnci Adalı**
Asst., Prof., PhD, İstanbul Aydın University, inciadali@aydin.edu.tr

**Mehmet Emin Bilge**
Prof. Dr., Ankara Sosyal Bilimler University, mehmetemin.bilge@asbu.edu.tr

**Meliha Güleryüz**
Dr., PhD, Başkent University Istanbul Health Application and Research Center, melihaguleryuz@yahoo.com

**Merve Ayşegül Kulular İbrahim**
Res. Assist., Ankara Sosyal Bilimler University, aysegul.kulular@asbu.edu.tr

**Mesut Sancar**
Prof. Dr., Marmara University, mesut.sancar@marmara.edu.tr

**Müge Seval**
Asst., Prof., PhD, Zonguldak Bülent Ecevit University, muge.uzun@beun.edu.tr

**Mümtaz Taner Torun**
Spec. Dr., MD, Bandırma State Hospital, mumtaztanertorun@gmail.com

**Münevver Sönmez**
Asst., Prof., PhD, Zonguldak Bülent Ecevit University, m.sonmez@beun.edu.tr

**Özgü İnal**
Asst. Prof., PhD, Trakya University, ozguinal@trakya.edu.tr

**Özlem Akgün**
Lecturer, Bozok University, ozlem.akgun@bozok.edu.tr

**Rauf Karasu**
Prof. Dr., Hacettepe University, raufkarasu@hacettepe.edu.tr

**Şirin Özkan**
Asst., Prof., PhD, Bandırma Onyedi Eylül University, sozkan@bandirma.edu.tr

**Yeliz Şahin**
Res. Assist., Marmara University, yeliz.sahin@marmara.edu.tr

**Yılda Arzu Aba**
Asst., Prof., PhD, Bandırma Onyedi Eylül University, yaba@bandirma.edu.tr

**Yılmaz Güzel**
Assoc. Prof., İstanbul Aydın University, yilmazguzel@aydin.edu.tr

# List of Reviewers

**Abdülkadir Kumbasar**
Prof. Dr., Sağlık Bilimleri University

**Ali Ünal**
Asst., Prof., PhD, Düzce University

**Arzu Uzuner**
Prof. Dr., Marmara University

**Aycan Çakmak Reyhan**
Asst., Prof., PhD, İstanbul Bilgi
University

**Ayça Şolt Kırca**
Asst. Prof., PhD, Kırklareli
University

**Aysu Zekioğlu**
Asst. Prof., PhD, Trakya University

**Ayşe Neriman Narin**
Asst., Prof., PhD, Bolu Abant İzzet
Baysal University

**Ayşegül Durmaz**
Asst., Prof., PhD, Kütahya
Dumlupınar University

**Ayten Arıöz Düzgün**
Asst., Prof., PhD, Ankara Yıldırım
Beyazıt University

**Azime Karakoç Kumsar**
Asst., Prof., PhD, Biruni University

**Berna Tunçer**
Dr., PhD, Trakya University

**Bulat Aytek Şık**
Asst. Prof., PhD, İstanbul Aydın
University

**Burçin Bayraktar**
Asst., Prof., PhD, Bandırma Onyedi
Eylül University

**Cemal Cingi**
Prof. Dr., Eskişehir Osmangazi
University

**Dilek Demirhan**
Assoc. Prof., Ege University

**Eda Aktaş**
Asst. Prof., PhD, İstanbul Sağlık
Bilimleri University

**Erhan Demirhan**
Assoc. Prof., Sağlık Bilimleri
University

**Eylem Toker**
Asst., Prof., PhD, Kahramanmaraş
Sütçü İmam University

**Fatma Başar**
Asst., Prof., PhD, Kütahya
Dumlupınar University

**Filiz Süzer Özkan**
Asst., Prof., PhD, Düzce University

**İlkay Keser**
Asst., Prof., PhD, Akdeniz University

**Kadriye Ağan Yıldırım**
Prof. Dr., Marmara University

**Mustafa Kemal Adalı**
Prof. Dr., Trakya University

**Mustafa Mete**
Asst. Prof., PhD, İstanbul Aydın University

**Nafiye Dutucu**
Asst., Prof., PhD, Kocaeli University

**Nilay Aksoy**
Asst., Prof., PhD, Altınbaş University

**Özlem Öztürk Şahin**
Asst. Prof., PhD, Karabük University

**Salih Kutay Demirkan**
Prof. Dr., Hacettepe University

**Semra Eyi**
Asst., Prof., PhD, Trakya University

**Serpil Abalı Çetin**
Asst., Prof., PhD, Yeditepe University

**Seyhan Alkan**
Prof. Dr., İstanbul Aydın University

**Süleyman Yılmaz**
Assoc. Prof., Ankara University,

**Şule Gökyıldız Sürücü**
Assoc. Prof., Çukurova University

**Yasemin Güllüoğlu**
Asst., Prof., PhD, Ankara Sosyal Bilimler University

**Yeliz Mercan**
Asst. Prof., PhD, Kırklareli University

**Yılda Arzu Aba**
Asst., Prof., PhD, Bandırma Onyedi Eylül University

**Yılmaz Gökşen**
Prof. Dr., Dokuz Eylül University

# SECTION 1: New Approaches in Nursing and Midwifery

Ayça Şolt Kırca

# 1: Women's Health and Homeopathy

## 1 Introduction

Homeopathy was developed 300 years ago by German Dr. Samuel Hahnemann. The related word is originated from the words homois (similar) and pathos (disease). Homeopathy is a treatment type that provides organisms to cope with acute or chronic diseases by strengthening human's immune system; it is also a holistic treatment type that has a personal approach and no side effect (Organon, 1842; Başar, 2014; Vithoulkas, 2017). It aims to treat the patient by handling him as a whole (physical, emotional and psychological).

Different medications are utilized for each patient and their diseases in homeopathy. The most important feature that makes homeopathy different from the modern medicine is the application of a personal treatment instead of massive treatment. Treatment mentality of homeopaths is to ensure a holistic recuperation via remedies by handling patient as a whole, not repressing the symptoms that disease generates in person. Homeopathy can contribute to arise a social order besides serving to personal health by this mentality. Homeopathy will be a leader treatment system that services to health by becoming popular in case of being supported in social order by this mentality and approach (Vithoulkas, 2017).

## 2 History of Homeopathy

Dr. Samuel Hahnemann, founder of homeopathy in the 18th century, developed a new approach which assumes that the materials formed specific symptoms in healthy people can be used as healing tools in individuals who have the same disease. Thus, Hahnemann revealed the theory of "similar" that is the main theory of homeopathy (Tedesco and Cicchetti, 2001; Geraghty, 2002; Merrell and Shalts, 2002; Vithoulkas, 2017; the Society of Homeopath, 2018).

Hahneman performed his first study about homeopathic treatment by deciding to experiment "chinchona" plant that causes malaria on himself. He repeated the same experiments by using plenty of different agents. He also named those experiments to determine the medical features of remedies as "persuasive experiments". He accepted the theory of "like cures like (similia similibus curentur)" as the fundamental principle of homeopathy based on the test results. With reference to the related hypothesis, the material (agent) that causes specific symptoms in healthy person treats the disease of a patient who has the same symptoms (Geraghty, 2002; Steinberg and Beal, 2003; Başar, 2014; Meran and Rafthish, 2016; Vithoulkas, 2017).

Homeopathic treatment started to sweep in the world after Hahneman. The first homeopathic medical faculty was established in America towards the end of the 1800s. Homeopathy began to be known also in England by being opened the first homeopathic hospital in London (Geraghty, 2002; Meran and Rafthish, 2016). Twenty two homeopathic medical schools, 100 homeopathic hospitals and more than 1000 pharmacies that sell homeopathic remedies were opened in America in the early 1900s. Moreover, many schools which give education of homeopathy were opened. Stanford and Boston Universities and New York Medical Faculty were among those schools. However, the number of institutions which give education of homeopathy gradually decreases by the establishment of the American Medical Association (AMA) and being launched it has become easy to use practical medications by drug companies in the 1920s. Organizations that give the education of homeopathy are few in number nowadays (Vithoulkas, 2017).

Homeopathy is a treatment method that is known and approved by the World Health Organization (WHO). For WHO estimations, 500 million people are treated with homeopathy at the present time (WHO, 2003). Furthermore, homeopathy is within the scope of health insurance in developed countries like England, France, Germany and the Netherlands (Vithoulkas, 2017). Fifty thousand physicians and 20,000 veterans and dentists took homeopathy education in Europe; 5,000 people have offered homeopathic consulting service. Twenty seven percent of practicing physicians prescribe homeopathic remedies; 18 % of them direct patients to a homeopath; 7 % of the same physicians offer homeopathic treatment to their patients as a choice (Başar, 2014).

## 3 Homeopathic Remedies

Medications in homeopathy are obtained by diluting minerals, metals, herbal essences and animal liquids in lactose, double distilled water or alcohol in certain proportions (1 cup of primary material and 99 cups of diluting agent) in private laboratories (Vithoulkas, 2017). This liquid solution is shaken at least 10 times. Name and dilution ratios are written in figures on each remedy. For example, being written 30 on aconite drug that is used for fear-based anxiety means that this remedy is diluted for 30 times (Geraghty, 2002; Merrell and Shalts, 2002; Kömürcü and Berkiten-Ergin, 2008; Vithoulkas, 2017).

Homeopathic remedies are at minimal dose. Related remedies contain too little of molecules in primary materials; on the other hand, some remedies contain none of the molecules in primary materials during dilution process; this is the reason they do not cause side effects (Smith, 2003; Vithoulkas, 2017). Homeopathic remedies are prescribed by a homeopath (certificated competent person who received an education of homeopathy) based on the symptoms and disease diagnosis in a person and the personal characteristics such as age, gender and mood (Geraghty, 2002; Vithoulkas, 2017).

Homeopathic remedies can be found in homeopathic pharmacies as being approved by the FDA (U.S. Food & Drug Administration) today. Homeopathic remedies are sold as granules, saccharose or sugar-coated pills and other shapes in stores which sell healthy life products and also in pharmacies as over the counter drug (Geraghty, 2002). Prices of homeopathic remedies are not so high in comparison with medications used in allopathic treatment (Başar, 2014).

## 4  Use Areas of Homeopathy

Much as studies about use and efficiency of homeopathy go back a long way, there can be seen a heavy increase in the early 19th century. It is determined when the studies are analyzed that homeopathy is used in treatments of several diseases such as chronic headache, allergic and bronchial asthma, gastritis and also the gynecologic diseases like pregnancy, birth/labor, postpartum period, mastitis, endometriosis, menopause, infertility, premenstrual syndrome and dysmenorrhea (Steinberg and Beal, 2003; Thomson, 2010; Danno et al., 2013; Vithoulkas, 2017).

### 4.1  Homeopathy Applications in Pregnancy, Birth and Postpartum Period

Women who are the key factor of each of the societies as from the beginning of humanity have maintained generations by being pregnant. Human body undergoes remarkable, physiological, anatomical and biochemical changes that start with fertilization to be adapted to pregnancy (Aydemir, 2014). Intervening in possible problems in this process of adaptation by non-pharmacological methods besides pharmacological techniques may create positive results in terms of both maternal and child health.

Homeopathy is frequently preferred for problems like herpex and pica, anemia and pain in the musculoskeletal system arising from posture change in pregnancy in many developed countries (Brennan, 1999). Homeopathic remedies that are used to minimize the most frequently encountered problems in pregnancy based on literature are as follows (Tab. 1.1):

**Tab. 1.1:** Homeopathic Remedies Used in Pregnancy Period (Created by the Author)

| Musculoskeletal pain | |
| --- | --- |
| Arnica-Bellis Perennis | Ferrum Metallicum-Ferrum Phosphoricum * |
| Calcarea Phosphorica | Natrum Muriaticum** |
| Kali Carbonica | Arsenicum*** |
| Magnesia Phosphorica | Ipecac-Nux Vomica-Colchicum-Pulsatilla-Sepia**** |
| Rhus Toxicodendron-Sepia | Calcarea C-Nitricum A***** |

*Anemia, **Genital and oral herpex, ***Food poisonings, ****Nausea, *****Pica

**Tab. 1.2:** Homeopathic Remedies Used in the First and Second Phase of the Birth (Meran and Rafthish, 2016)

| Fear of birth and labor or birth pain | Labor induction–fetus presentation changes | Prolonged and difficult labor |
| --- | --- | --- |
| Aconite | Caulophyllum** | Caulophyllum |
| Chammomilla | Cimicifuga** | Cimicifuga |
| Cimicifuga | Pulsatilla* | Aconite |
| | | Caulophyllum |
| | | Chammomilla |
| | | Pulsatilla |

*Only labor induction and fetus presentation changes, **Only labor induction

Labor is a natural process as well as there may occur problems with this process. Pharmacological methods that are used to solve related problems in the labor process cause birth to wander from the natural process. It is suggested to be used complementary and alternative methods that least affect the naturality of birth. One of these methods is homeopathy. Certificated homeopath midwives apply homeopathy in pregnancy, birth and postpartum period in many countries such as India, Europe and America where homeopathy use is legal (Geraghty, 2002; Smith, 2003; Baxter and Perrin, 2006; Steen and Calvert, 2007; Hall, McKenna and Griffiths, 2012; Foxell, 2013; ECH, 2018). Homeopathic remedies are utilized in the treatment of pain, breast and breastfeeding problems, problems on urinary system, depression and subinvolution or abnormal lochia in the postpartum period (Geraghty, 2002). Homeopathic remedies which are used in labor and postpartum period based on literature can be seen in tables below (Tab. 1.2; Tab. 1.3).

**Tab. 1.3:** Homeopathic Remedies Used in the Third and Fourth Phases of Birth (Created by the Author)

| Postpartum hemorrhage | Placental retention | Perineal laceration and episiotomy |
|---|---|---|
| Aconite Carboveg | Caulophyllum | Arnica |
| Caulophyllum Arnica | Cimicifuga | Hypericum |
| Cimicifuga Pulsatilla | Pulsatilla | Staphysagria |

Homeopathic remedies for pregnancy, birth and postpartum period need to be given to women by certificated homeopath by proper dose and frequency.

## 4.2 Homeopathy Applications in Infertility

Another factor that affects women's health is infertility that can be seen in one of the partners or both of them at the same time. Literature defines infertility as the absence of pregnancy in spite of unprotected ordered sex during a year (Barbieri, 2018). Infertility is seen at 30 % in developing countries all around the world (WHO, 2003). Infertility in women may be rooted in pelvic factors (endometriosis, infections and structural disorders), ovulation factor (ovulation and hormonal status), cervical and emotional factors (Taşkın, 2014). With reference to the results of the study that was performed on 67 infertile women by homeopathic remedies in Germany, pregnancy, as the result of increasing progesterone concentrations, occurring in positive ovulation is statistically higher when compared with women in the placebo group (Bergmann et al., 2000).

## 4.3 Homeopathy Applications in Menopause

Problems of menopause arise in women with symptoms such as hot flush, night sweating, vaginal dryness, change in psychology, sleeplessness, lack of energy, prostration, irritation, anxiety, depression and arthralgia because of increasing estrogen and progesterone levels (Borrelli and Ernst, 2010). These symptoms that are seen in 20%–25 % of women may continue at least for 5 years. First of all, hormone replacement therapy (HRT) is applied in menopause. The goal of the related therapy is to relieve the physical symptoms related to menopause and also avoid clinical results of estrogen deficiency. Using HRT for a long time especially increases paralysis, thromboembolism and breast cancer risk (Thomson, 2010; Zaw et al., 2018).

Homeopathy is an alternative and easy to use method for women who do not demand hormonal implementation used in menopause management. For observational study results, hot flush, prostration, anxiety and depression based on menopause can be reduced by homeopathic treatment (Weatherley-Jones et al., 2004; Thomson, 2010). Bordet et al. conducted a study with 438 women and pointed out that claims about hot flush diminished in intensity in group who took homeopathic medicines (Lachesis mutus, Belladonna, Sepia officinalis, Sulphur and Sanguinaria Canadensis) in comparison with the group which did not take related medicine (Bordet et al., 2008).

## 4.4 Homeopathy Applications in Dysmenorrhea and Premenstrual Syndrome

Homeopathy is used in the treatment of various gynecological diseases such as bleeding, kist, hemorrhage, vaginal secretion, dysmenorrhea and premenstrual syndrome (Oberbaum et al., 2005; Kassab et al., 2009; Crompton, 2012; Frass et al., 2015).

Dysmenorrhea is a common gynecologic disease that arises with a throbbing pain and cramps in pelvic and sub abdomen region in teenage girls (Ju et al., 2013). A related disease is seen in 50 % of women. Fifteen percent of those women express that their daily activities are restricted because of the pain (French, 2005; Kazama et al., 2015; Al-Jefou et al., 2015; Rani et al., 2015).

Much as the studies about homeopathy and dysmenorrhea are few in number, Witt et al., conducted a research on 57 female students and pointed out that there is a decrease in the pain of the experimental group who took homeopathic medicine in comparison with the pain of the control group (Witt et al., 2009). On the other hand, in the study conducted by Charandabi et al., it was determined that there was no change in the pain of the group that was administered homeopathic medicine, in comparison with the group that was not administered the relevant medicine (Charandi et al., 2016). Homeopathic remedies that are generally utilized in dysmenorrhea treatment are Phospor, Nat-M and Pulsatilla.

Premenstrual syndrome is seen in 3%–5 % of women in the reproductive age group (Brown et al., 2009). Symptoms (changes in mood and somatic problems) that arise in the luteal phase of the menstrual cycle disappear by starting menstrual bleeding (Halbreich et al., 2007). It was found in the study of Danno et al., on 34 women who have been diagnosed as a premenstrual syndrome that PMS syndromes considerably decreased in women who took a homeopathic remedy.

The most prescribed homeopathic remedy in PMS treatment is Folliculinum (Danno et al., 2013).

## 5 Status of Homeopathy Applications in the World and Role of Midwife

The use of homeopathy is pretty popular in the treatment of other gynecological diseases, notably pregnancy and birth by being legal homeopathy applications in many countries of Europe and America. Homeopathy applications can be given by physicians who take the education of homeopathy, pharmacologists, natural therapy specialists, midwives and nurses within the existing legal process (ECH, 2018).

Committees, associations and commissions have been established in Europe and America for homeopathy education as a common system for everyone. The first of related organizations is The Society of Homeopaths in England in 1978; The Accreditation Commission for Homeopathic Education in North America in 1982; Council for Homeopathic Certification in 1991 and The European Committee for Homeopathy in 1992 (ACHENA, 2018; CHC, 2018; ECH, 2018; the Society of Homeopaths, 2018).

Midwives and nurses need to successfully complete education or courses given by homeopathy schools to be able to apply homeopathic treatment (Baxter and Perrin, 2006; CHC, 2018). There is also a need for 500-hours theoretical lessons and homeopathic application for 10 cases under expert control for completing homeopathic training (CHC, 2018).

Homeopathy applications and use have shown a rapid increase across the world. Midwives who took the education of homeopathy need to fulfill several implementations like applying homeopathic remedies, taking required precautions, sending medical establishment when required and obeying ethical principles and legal procedures based on the situation of the individual in the treatment of dysmenorrhea, premenstrual syndrome and menopause in pregnancy, birth and postpartum period.

## 6 Conclusion

Homeopathy is a type of treatment peculiar to the individual. This is because it is a quite difficult and complex method. Receiving a first-class education is essential to learn and apply the issue. Establishing an effective homeopathy education system and legalizing this treatment method is of prime importance for women's, infant-children's and community health.

# References

Al-Jefout, M., Seham, A.F., Jameel, H., Randa, A.Q. & Luscombe, G. (2015). Dysmenorrhea: Prevalence and Impact on Quality of Life among Young Adult Jordanian Females, *Journal of Pediatric and Adolescent Gynecology*, 28(3), 173–185.

Aydemir, H. & Uyar Hazar, H. (2014). Düşük Riskli, Riskli, Yüksek Riskli Gebelik ve Ebenin Rolü, *Gümüşhane Üniversitesi Sağlık Bilimleri Dergisi*, 3(2), 815–833.

Barbieri, R.L. (2018). Female Infertility. *"Yen and Jaffe's Reproductive Endocrinology"*, 556–581, Elsevier, Philadelphia, USA.

Başar, G. (2014). Homeopati: Doğal, Yan Etkisiz ve Bütünsel Bir Tedavi Yöntemi. *Türkiye Klinikleri Journal of Family Medicine Special Topics*, 5(4), 41–45.

Baxter, J. & Perrin, C. (2006). Homeopathy as a Choice: The New Holistic Antenatal Clinic, *BJM*, 14(12), 718–721.

Bergmann, J., Luft, B., Boehmann, S., Runnebaum, B. & Gerhard, I. (2000). The Efficacy of the Complex Medication Phyto-Hypophyson L in Female, Hormone-Related Sterility. A Randomized, Placebo-Controlled Clinical Double-Blind Study. *Complementary and Natural Classical Medicine*, 7(4), 190–199.

Bordet, M.F., Colas, A., Marijnen, P., Masson, J.L. & Trichard, M. (2008). Treating Hot Flushes in Menopausal Women with Homeopathic Treatment – Results of an Observational Study, *Homeopathy*, 97(1), 10–15.

Borrelli, F. & Ernst, E. (2010). Alternative and Complementary Therapies for the Menopause, *Maturitas*, 66(4), 333–343.

Brennan, P. (1999). Homeopathic Remedies in Prenatal Care. *Journal of Nurse-Midwifery*, 44(3), 291–299.

Brown, J., O'Brien, P.M., Marjoribanks, J. & Wyatt, K. (2009). Selective Serotonin Reuptake Inhibitors for Premenstrual Syndrome, *Cochrane Database Systematic Reviews*, 15(2).

Charandabi, S.M.A., Biglu, M.H. & Rad, K.Y. (2016). Effect of Homeopathy on Pain Intensity and Quality of Life of Students with Primary Dysmenorrhea: A Randomized Controlled Trial, *Iranian Red Crescent Medical Journal*, 18(9).

Council for Homeopathic Certification (CHC). (2018). http://www.homeopathicdirectory.com/exam-process.html (accessed on 10.12.2018).

Crompton, R. (2012). Homeopathy for Common Complaints during Pregnancy and Childbirth, *Pract Midwife*, 15(8), 15–8.

Danno, K., Colas, A., Terzan, L. & Bordet, M.F. (2013). Homeopathic Treatment of Premenstrual Syndrome: A Case Series, *Homeopathy*, 102(1), 59–65.

Foxell, A. (2013). Homeopathy in Labour and Childbirth. Windsor Homeopathic Practice, *Information Sheet*, 4.

Frass, M., Friehs, H., Thallinger, C., Sohal, N.K., Marosi, C., Muchitsch, I., et al. (2015). Influence of Adjunctive Classical Homeopathy on Global Health Status and Subjective Wellbeing in Cancer Patients – A Pragmatic Randomized Randomized Controlled Trial, *Complement Therapies in Medicine*, 23(3), 309–317.

French, L. (2005). Dysmenorrhea, *American Family Physician*, 71(2), 285–291.

Geraghty, B. (Ed.) (2002). *"Homeopathy for Midwives"*. Churchill Livingstone Elsevier Science Limited, USA.

Halbreich, U., Backstrom, T., Eriksson, E., et al. (2007). Clinical Diagnostic Criteria for Premenstrual Syndrome and Guidelines for Their Quantification for Research Studies, *Gynecol Endocrinol*, 23, 123–130.

Hall, H.G., McKenna, L.G. & Griffiths, D.L. (2012). Complementary and Alternative Medicine for Induction of Labour, *Women Birth*, 25(3), 142–148.

Ju, H., Jones, M. & Mishra, G. (2013). The Prevalence and Risk Factors of Dysmenorrhea, *Epidemiologic Reviews*, 36(1), 104–113.

Kassab, S., Cummings, M., Berkovitz, S., Van Haselen, R. & Fisher, P. (2009). Homeopathic Medicines for Adverse Effects of Cancer Treatments, *Cochrane Database Systematic Reviews*, 15(2).

Kazama, M., Maruyama, K. & Nakamura, K. (2015). Prevalence of Dysmenorrhea and Its Correlating Lifestyle Factors in Japanese Female Junior High School Students, *The Tohoku Journal of Experimental Medicine*, 236(2), 107–113.

Kömürcü, N. & Berkiten-Ergin, A. (2008). Doğum Ağrısının Kontrolünde Nonfarmakolojik Yöntemler. Kömürcü, N., Berkiten- Ergin, A. (eds.), *"Doğum Ağrısı ve Yönetimi"*, 1. Baskı, Bedray Basın Yayıncılık Ltd. Şt., İstanbul.

Meran, H.E. & Rathfisch, G. (2016). Doğum Eyleminde Tamamlayıcı ve Alternatif Bir Yöntem Olan Homeopati Kullanımı, *Florence Nightingale Hemşirelik Dergisi*, 24(3), 191–199.

Merrell, W.C. & Shalts, E. (2002). Homeopathy. *Medical Clinics of North America*, 86(1), 47–62.

Oberbaum, M, Galoyan, N., Lerner-Geva, L., Singer, S.R., Grisaru, S., Shashar, D. & Samueloff, A. (2005). The Effect of the Homeopathic Remedies Arnica Montana and Bellis Perennis on Mild Postpartum Bleeding. A Randomized, Double-Blind, Placebo-Controlled Study –Preliminary Results. *Complementary Therapies in Medicine*, 13(2), 87–90.

Organon, S.H. (1842). *"İyileşme Sanatının Organon'u"*, 6. Baskı, Klasik Homeopati Derneği, İzmir.

Rani, A., Sharma, M.K. & Singh, A. (2016). Practices and Perceptions of Adolescent Girls Regarding the Impact of Dysmenorrhea on Their Routine Life: A Comparative Study in the Urban, Rural, and Slum Areas of Chandigarh. *International Journal of Adolescent Medicine and Health*, 28(1), 3–9.

Smith, C.A. (2003). Homoeopathy for Induction of Labour. *Cochrane Database Systematic Reviews*, 2003(4), 1–18.

Steen, M. & Calvert, J. (2007). Self-administered Homeopathy Part Two: A Follow-Up Study, *BJM*, 15(6), 359–365.

Steinberg, D. & Beal, M.W. (2003). Homeopathy and Women's Health Care, *Journal of Obstetric, Gynecologic, Neonatal Nursing*, 32(2), 207–214.

Taşkın, L. (2014). *"Doğum ve Kadın Sağlığı Hemşireliği"*, Genişletilmiş 7. Baskı, Akademisyen Tıp Kitabevi, İstanbul.

Tedesco, P. & Cicchetti, J. (2001). Like Cures Like: Homeopathy, *American Journal of Nursing*, 101(9), 43–49.

The Accreditation Commission for Homeopathic Education in North America (ACHENA). (2018). http://www.achena.org/ (accessed on 10.12.2018).

The European Committee for Homeopathy (ECH). (2018). http://homeopathyeurope.org/regulatory-status/ (accessed on 15.12.2018).

The Society of Homeopaths. (2018). http:// www.homeopathy-soh.org/about-homeopathy (accessed on 12.12.2018).

Thompson, E.A. (2010). Alternative and Complementary Therapies for the Menopause: A Homeopathic Approach, *Maturitas*, 66(4), 350–354.

Vithoulkas, G. (2017). *"Homeopatinin Temel İlkeleri"*, Günçe Yayın Evi, İstanbul.

Weatherley-Jones, E., Thompson, E.A. & Thomas, K.J. (2004). The Placebo-Controlled Trial as a Test of Complementary and Alternative Medicine: Observations from Research Experience of Individualised Homeopathic Treatment, *Homeopathy*, 93(4), 186–189.

Witt, C.M., Lüdtke, R. & Willich, S.N. (2009). Homeopathic Treatment of Patients with Dysmenorrhea: A Prospective Observational Study with 2 Years Follow-Up, *Archives of Gynecology and Obstetrics*, 280(4), 603–611.

World Health Organization (WHO). (2003). *"Progress Report in Reproductive Health Research"*. Geneva, Switzerland, 23.

Zaw, J.J.T., Howe, P.R.C. & Wong, R.H.X. (2018). Postmenopausal Health Interventions: Time to Move on from the Women's Health Initiative?, *Ageing Research Reviews*, 48, 79–86.

Gül Ergün and Işıl Işık

# 2: A Current Approach in Psychiatric Nursing: Cognitive Behavioral Therapy

## 1 Introduction

Psychotherapy is defined as a treatment process of psychological disorders by using psychological techniques and verbal and nonverbal dialogues in communication with counselee and consultant. In other words, it means creating an effect on thought, emotion, and behaviors of the individual; providing behaviors to replace with more acceptable behaviors and also improving the behaviors (Çam and Engin, 2015). The number of cognitive behavioral therapy (CBT) education has increased day by day all around the world. CBT is a treatment type that uses several techniques (e.g., theory of learning, improving problem-solving skills, and behavioral therapy techniques) to support individuals to cope with vital problems that they cannot solve or the possible problems in the later periods of life (Okanlı, 2016; Demiralp and Oflaz, 2007). This chapter aims to bring a new perspective to the principles, historical development, foundations, and use of CBT in nursing practices.

## 2 Cognitive Behavioral Therapy

Cognitive behavioral therapy is a treatment type that emerges by the integration of behavioral and cognitive theories and teaches people to cope with difficulties and daily problems via cognitive and behavioral techniques. It is frequently used in the treatment of depression, anxiety disorders, addiction disorders, coping with exam stress, domestic violence, and other psychopathologies, traumas, crisis situations, schizophrenia, and other psychotic disorders. Psychiatric nurses can use CBT techniques in several psychopathologies in case of receiving fundamental and advanced level CBT training.

CBT is a short-term, structured psychotherapy type that has a specific system. It is presented within a therapeutic approach that is built on 10 essential principles. These related principles submit a summary of the cognitive behavioral approach. Principles are as follows (Beck, 2011):

- A therapist in CBT acts based on a formulation that is established by cognitive concepts and continuously developed toward counselee and problems of the counselee.

- The therapist should establish a therapeutic relationship that includes respect, empathy, and intimacy with counselee for the therapy to be successful.
- The consultant should help counselee to understand that the related process is a teamwork and actively participating in this process is essential.
- CBT is goal-directional and problem-focused.
- First of all, CBT focuses on the present time.
- CBT is an approach that includes educations, which teach counselee to be the consultant of himself.
- CBT is short-dated and time-limited.
- Sessions are structured in CBT.
- In CBT, counselee needs to be taught to determine, evaluate and change the non-functional thoughts and beliefs.
- Different techniques are utilized in CBT to create change in thought, feeling, and behaviors of the counselor.

## 3  History of Cognitive Behavioral Therapy

### 3.1  Cognitive Approach

The general theory of cognitive approach is that emotional responses that disturb individuals are not rooted in the events which they directly experience, rooted in conception by the individual. 'Personal construct theory' that was developed by George Kelly (1905–1967) in terms of cognitive approach is essential for the reason of emphasizing the importance of cognitive processes that directly affect the behavior. Julian Rotter (1916–2014) pointed out that the general run of learnings of individuals is in social relations with other people. Besides, Albert Bandura significantly contributed to the cognitive approach by developing theories of social learning and self-efficacy. Bandura added a cognitive component to the theory of classical learning by expressing the importance of expectations and effects of internal processed in behavior training. Theory of learned helplessness that was developed by Martin Seligman defined the role of expectations in emerging behavior. Theory of learned helplessness has still been used as a remarkable cognitive theory that eases to understand the disease in depression treatment (Beck and Haigh, 2014; Türkçapar, 2007; Türkçapar and Sargın, 2012; Özdel, 2015).

### 3.2  Behavioral Approach

Behavioral approach or behavioral psychology argues that all the normal behaviors or the behaviors that wander from normal arise as the result of learning. Modern behavioral approach has its origins in the late 1800s by Ivan Petroviç Pavlov (1849–1936). Pavlov discovered classical conditioning that is the first big concept of a behavioral approach. In 1920, Watson proved that classical conditioning is valid in human learning. Watson conducted experiments in which phobia reactions are explained by classical conditioning. Skinner (1904–1990) systematized related approach as a holistic theory that clarifies human psychology (Türkçapar and Sargın, 2012; Özdel, 2015).

### 3.3  Cognitive Behavioral Therapy

Named after Aaron T. Beck and Albert Ellis; Cognitive Behavioral Therapy is encountered as an important integration especially in the field of psychotherapy, which has become popular since the 1980s. This is a frequently used method that is utilized in depression, anxiety disorders, personality disorders, somatoform disorders, and eating disorders (Lorenzo-Luaces, Keefe and DeRubeis, 2016).

## 4  Fundamentals of Cognitive Behavioral Therapy

CBT is a process that includes individuals to replace their automatic thought and evaluations, which arise in negative situations, with different alternative thoughts; CBT also includes restructuring-related thoughts. This approach argues that the perception and interpretation style of events is more important than how they are. Moreover, for this approach, when there is an emotional problem, the problem may be associated with the case and environment that person experienced and also the perception style of the person at the same time (Piştof and Şanlı, 2013; Türkçapar, 2007; Beck, 2011).

Emotion, thought, and behaviors of people do not arise as independent from each other. Ellis explains this issue by ABC model. A is the revealer event; B is the cognitive evaluation system, namely, evaluating and solving the event by the value systems of person; C is the results that emotionally and behaviorally emerge or the reaction of person. The reaction may be compatible with reality or inconsistent with reality. Cognitive status analyzes cognitions, which are considered in conceptualizing the cognitive status of the person under two main titles as automatic thoughts and schemas. Schemas are divided into two groups as intermediate beliefs and basic beliefs. In CBT sessions, the therapist supports counselor to be aware of the thoughts when he thought during events. The skills of specifying nonrealistic verbal cognition and visual images are developed in counselee. Afterward, it is aimed to bring in more realistic and functional thoughts substituted for nonrealistic and nonfunctional ones. In conclusion, there is an effort to notice to what extent the changes in counselee's life thanks to cognitive behavioral therapy are functional (Beck, 2011; Türkçapar, 2007).

**Automatic Thoughts:** Nonfunctional automatic thoughts that also are exaggerated and distortional have a basic role in the development of psychopathology in individuals. Automatic thoughts are spontaneous comments relating to an issue. Automatic thoughts emerge by themselves; they are not oriented or motivated ideas. Chief goal in CBT is to ensure counselee to take notice his automatic thoughts and replace them with more realistic, proper, and functional ones (Akkoyunlu and Türkçapar, 2013).

**Intermediate Beliefs:** There are intermediate beliefs just under automatic thoughts. Intermediate beliefs pave a proper way for occurring automatic thoughts. Related beliefs are absolute cognitions such as orders, rules, and things that must happen. For example, 'I am worthless if I am not loved', 'I must always succeed' and 'I must not ask for help from someone'. Intermediate beliefs are composed of person's rule, attitude, and assumptions on himself, other people, and his own personal world. Those beliefs are in the depths of the person and not expressed as verbal expressions (Türkçapar, 2007).

**Basic Beliefs:** A basic belief is the subgroup of the schemas. Basic beliefs are defined as the cognitive structures that include people's thoughts about themselves, other people, and the external world arising from previous experiences. Basic beliefs are doubled in all the people. For example, the following beliefs take place in the brain together; I am loved, I am not loved. The active one is the positive basic beliefs in a healthy person who has no certain personality disorder or psychiatric disease. Negative basic beliefs activate in healthy people when there are temporary negative emotions with an event or an adverse situation (Türkçapar, 2007).

**Cognitive Error:** For Beck, what causes a person to perceive themselves, their environment and their future negatively and consequently leads to stress and mental disorder symptoms are systematic errors made in information processing. Cognitive error is one of the essential concepts of cognitive and behavioral therapy. Since related errors are pretty consistent, they are also utilized as systematic errors. Cognitive errors are analyzed under eleven titles (Beck, 2011; Arkar, 1992).

• **Arbitrary inference:** Person makes a specific deduction from the circumstance despite the fact that there is no basis that supports the deduction.
• **Selective abstraction:** Person ignores the more important factors in the event; focuses only a single detail and interprets the event based on this detail.

- **Overgeneralization:** Person generalizes his deduction about an event to happenings that are related or not related to that event.
- **Magnification and minimizing:** Person underestimates the importance of positive events besides feeling negative events more magniloquently.
- **Personalization:** Person associates an external fact that is not about himself to himself.
- **Absolutistic, dichotomous thinking:** Person frequently uses one of two end poles while evaluating himself.
- **Labeling and mislabeling:** Person uses an extreme generalization or reacts to the event by misinterpreting.
- **Emotional reasoning:** Person evaluates the event by feelings more than tangible data.
- **Should statements:** Person's thoughts and expressions with have to/must that create pressure and stress in himself.
- **Mind reading:** Person assumes that other people think less of himself although there is no tangible evidence about their thoughts.
- **Fortunetelling:** Person accepts his negative estimations about the future as real.

Individuals may use only one or more than one of the cognitive errors above in daily life. Since cognitive errors rapidly and automatically pass through the mind of a person, related errors cannot be perceived most of the time. Therapy sessions aim to provide counselee to realize that his cognitive errors are unrealistic and fancy and develop a more realistic and functional point of view.

Techniques that are used in cognitive approach differs in literature. Some of the cognitive techniques are Socratic questioning and directed discovery, down arrows technique, evidence questioning, testing alternatives, stop catastrophizing, the record of nonfunctional thought, thought-stopping, refocus, and home works. Some of the behavioral techniques are confrontation with a fearsome stimulant, model-giving, self-monitoring, stimulant-response hierarchy, role-playing, and relaxation techniques (Türkçapar, 2013; Demiralp and Oflaz, 2007).

# 5  Use of Cognitive Behavioral Therapy in Psychiatric Nursing

There is the provision about psychotherapy services in mental health regulation bill as 'Psychotherapy services are conducted by member of mental health occupational groups who completed graduate study and application training under supervision about basic level training related to theoretical interventions; related services are performed on condition that staying loyal to authority, competencies, and limits of training received' (Turkey Psychiatric Association, 2019). For this regulation bill, a psychiatric nurse who receives related education can perform a psychotherapeutic intervention.

The psychiatric nurse uses CBT techniques in various applications. The psychiatric nurse who uses CBT can evaluate a person's thoughts, relevant emotions, and behavior patterns by asking questions. These questions are as follows:

• What is the problem?
• Where does the problem occur?
• When the problem occurs?
• What or who creates the problem?
• What is the scariest result of the problem?

The nurse should support counselee to find answers for questions. Moreover, there is a need for behavior analysis to collect more information by considering the time, frequency, and disturbance size of the problem. This information collecting process is composed of three stages (Demiralp ve Oflaz, 2007):

**The period before the behavior**: Determining the stimulant that actualizes before the behavior and causes the behavior to occur.

**Behavior stage:** This is the period in which things that person told or did not tell are specified in detail. Frequency and duration of the period are learned in this stage.

**Conclusion stage:** This is the period that learns the effect of behavior that a person thinks is positive, negative, or neutral.

The nurse selects the proper CBT methods toward supporting positive behaviors and restructuring negative behavior patterns after analyzing the behaviors.

## 6 Cognitive Behavioral Therapy Strategies

Cognitive Behavioral Therapies are quite proper for people in all age groups and applied as personal or group therapy. CBT aims to develop problem-solving skills and social skills and minimize undesirable behavior patterns. Psychiatric nursing literature analyzes CBT strategies under three groups (Demiralp and Oflaz, 2007):

**Therapy strategies that decrease anxiety:** Psychiatric nurses may frequently use familiarization techniques; teach relaxation exercises; and teach biofeedback method and systematic desensitization technique for an individual to cope with anxiety. Vestibular desensitization, response prevention, and eye movement desensitization are utilized less often.

**Cognitive restructuring strategies:** There can be created changes in cognitive schemas of the person by the techniques such as monitoring thoughts and feelings of the person, evidence questioning, evaluating alternatives, stopping catastrophizing, reorganizing-reframe, and thought-stopping.

**Strategies of learning new behaviors:** Psychiatric nurse can use learning strategies such as modeling, formalizing, token economy, role play, and training toward improving social skills, aversive therapy, and agreement in probability.

# 7 Literature's Studies in Which Psychiatric Nurses Used Cognitive Behavioral Therapy Techniques

It is seen in the literature that CBT has been used by psychiatric nurses in psychotherapeutic interventions for a long time. Some of the related studies can be seen below:

Kingdon and Turkington (1994) wrote a book on the use of CBT in the treatment of schizophrenia. CBT was introduced in psychotherapist nurses in the same book.

Cook (1998) used CBT method for elders to cope with pain. With reference to their findings, CBT is effective in pain.

Sensky et al. (2000) applied CBT-based therapy for 9 months via 2 experienced psychiatric nurses to heal symptoms of schizophrenic patients who have positive symptoms resistant to antipsychotics. An increase in accord to daily life and regression in symptoms were observed at the end of the research.

Turkington et al. (2002) used CBT methods in bringing schizophrenic patients in society during the rehabilitation process. They pointed out at the end of the research that community mental health nurses who receive psychotherapy training can apply effective CBT in schizophrenic patients.

Espie et al. (2007) applied CBT techniques on insomniac. For research findings, nurses who receive psychotherapy training at a sufficient level can accomplishedly use CBT techniques in insomnia treatment.

Moorey et al. (2009) researched the effect of CBT program that nurses applied in cancer patients with palliative care in the terminal period on depression. With reference to the findings, anxiety level in participants decreases; however, there is no significant decrease in depression scores.

Yavuzşen et al. (2012) conducted a group therapy by using CBT techniques like stress management, problem-solving, and cognitive restructuring via a

treatment team including a nurse for patients with breast cancer. They found
that anxiety and depression significantly made positive progress.

Meriç and Oflaz (2013) conducted a survey to research the effect on the cognitive approach-based nursing application on automatic thoughts of patients
with anxiety disorder about the treatment. They had 6 interviews whose each
session took 45 minutes. For the findings, the related model is a technique that
can be used in nursing applications.

Kelleci et al. (2014) used CBT techniques for anger management of high
school students. They divided students into two groups so as to be 12 students in
each group. Group came together for one day a week; each session took one and
half hour during 10 weeks. The research showed the efficiency of the program
applied.

Gümüş Şekerci et al. (2017) applied cognitive-behavioral approach-based
anger management program for middle school final year students. They completed anger management training in 7 weeks; sessions took 40–45 minutes.
Their research confirmed that education is effective.

Karaca et al. (2018) applied CBT for the experimental group that was composed of infertile couples for 11 weeks. For results, the experimental group's psychological symptoms such as depression and anxiety decrease.

## 8 Conclusion

CBT is a frequently used, short-dated, and goal-directional application that
continues based on an ever-growing formulation and structured sessions and
also purposes to create change in emotion, thoughts, and behaviors of the counselee. This therapy method that occurred as the integration of behavioral and
cognitive theories has been utilized for depression, anxiety disorders, personality disorder, somatoform disorders, and eating disorders. It is aimed in CBT
to ensure counselee to take notice his automatic thoughts and intermediate
and basic beliefs and replace them with more realistic, proper, and functional
thoughts. Psychiatric nurses who complete education programs and gain com-
petence frequently apply CBT in the world.

## References

Akkoyunlu, S. & Türkçapar, M.H. (2013). "A Technique: Exposure Therapy",
    *Journal of Cognitive-Behavioral Psychotherapy and Research*, 2(2), 121–128.
Arkar, H. (1992). "Beck'in Depresyon Modeli ve Bilişsel Terapisi", *Düşünen
    Adam: Psikiyatri ve Nörolojik Bilimler Dergisi*, 5(1–3), 37–40.

Beck, A.T. & Haigh, E.A. (2014). "Advances in Cognitive Theory and Therapy: The Generic Cognitive Model", *Annual Review of Clinical Psychology*, 10, 1–24.

Beck, J.S. (2011). "*Cognitive Behavior Therapy: Basics and Beyond*", 2nd Edition, Guilford Press, USA.

Çam, M.O. & Engin, E. (2015). Psikoterapi ve Hemşirelik, *Türkiye Klinikleri Journal of Psychiatric Nursing-Special Topics*, 1(1), 87–94.

Cook, A.J. (1998). Cognitive-Behavioral Pain Management for Elderly Nursing Home Residents, *The Journals of Gerontology Series B: Psychological Sciences and Social Sciences*, 53(1), 51–59.

Demiralp, M. & Oflaz, F. (2007). Bilişsel-Davranışçı Terapi Teknikleri Ve Psikiyatri Hemşireliği Uygulaması, *Anadolu Psikiyatri Dergisi*, 8, 132–139.

Espie, C.A., Macmahon, K.M., Kelly, H.L., Broomfield, N.M., Douglas, N.J., Engleman, H.M. & Wilson, P. (2007). Randomized Clinical Effectiveness Trial of Nurse-Administered Small-Group Cognitive Behavior Therapy for Persistent Insomnia in General Practice. *Sleep*, 30(5), 574–584.

Gümüş Şekerci, Y., Terz, H., Kitiş, Y. & Birimoğlu Okuyan, C. (2017). Sekizinci Sınıf Öğrencilerine Bilişsel Davranışçı Yaklaşıma Göre Uygulanan Öfke Kontrol Programının Etkinliği. *Dokuz Eylül Üniversitesi Hemşirelik Fakültesi Elektronik Dergisi*, 10(4), 201–207.

Karaca, A., Yavuzcan, A., Batmaz, S., Cangür, Ş. & Çalışkan, A. (2018). Effectiveness of Cognitive Behavioral Group Therapy with Improved Health Problems in Infertile Women: A Randomized Controlled Trial, *Journal of Psychiatric Nursing*, V. International, IX. National Psychiatric Nursing Congress, Supplements 1, 105.

Kelleci, M., Avcı, D., Erşan, E.E. & Doğan, S. (2014). Bilişsel Davranışçı Tekniklere Dayalı Öfke Yönetimi Programının Lise Öğrencilerinin Öfke Ve Atılganlık Düzeylerine Etkisi, *Anatolian Journal of Psychiatry*, 15(4), 296–303.

Kingdon, D.G. & Turkington, D. (1994). "*Cognitive-Behavioral Therapy of Schizophrenia*", The Guilford Press, New York.

Lorenzo-Luaces, L. Keefe, J.R. & DeRubeis, R.J. (2016). Cognitive-Behavioral Therapy: Nature and Relation to Non-Cognitive Behavioral Therapy, *Behavior Therapy*, 47(6), 785–803.

Meriç, M. & Oflaz, F. (2013). Anksiyete Bozukluğu Olan Hastalarda Bilişsel Yaklaşım Temelli Hemşirelik Uygulamasının Hastaların Tedaviyle İlgili Otomatik Düşünceleri Üzerine Etkisi, *Journal of Psychiatric Nursing*, 4(3), 109–118.

Moorey, S. & Cort, E., Kapari, M. et al. (2009). A Cluster Randomized Controlled Trial of Cognitive Behaviour Therapy for Common Mental

Disorders in Patients with Advanced Cancer, *Psychological Medicine*, 39, 713–723.

Okanlı, A. (2016). *"Psikiyatri Hemşireliğinde Tamamlayıcı ve Psikososyal Terapiler, Ruh Sağlığı ve Psikiyatri Hemşireliği"*, Nobel Tıp Kitabevi, Ankara.

Özdel, K. (2015). Dünden Bugüne Bilişsel Davranışçı Terapiler: Teori ve Uygulama, *Turkiye Klinikleri J Psychiatry-Special Topics*, 8(2), 10–20.

Piştof, S. & Şanlı, E. (2013). "Bilişsel Davranışçı Terapide Metafor Kullanımı", *Bilişsel Davranışçı Psikoterapi ve Araştırmalar Dergisi*, 2, 182–189.

Sensky, T., Turkington, D., Kingdon, D., Scott, J.L., Scott, J., Siddle, R. & Barnes, T.R. (2000). A Randomized Controlled Trial of Cognitive-Behavioral Therapy for Persistent Symptoms in Schizophrenia Resistant to Medication, *Archives of General Psychiatry*, 57(2), 165–172.

Turkey Psychiatric Association. (2019). http://www.psikiyatri.org.tr/uploadFiles/2811201717434-Ruh-Sagligi-Yasa-Taslagi.pdf (accessed on 01.01.2019).

Türkçapar, H. (2007), *"Bilişsel Terapi: Temel İlkeler ve Uygulama"*, 3. Baskı, HYB Yayıncılık, Ankara.

Türkçapar, M.H. & Sargın, A.E. (2012). Bilişsel Davranışçı Psikoterapiler: Tarihçe ve Gelişim, *Bilişsel Davranışçı Psikoterapi ve Araştırmalar Dergisi*, 1, 7–14.

Turkington, D., Kingdon, D. & Turner, T. (2002). Effectiveness of a Brief Cognitive–behavioural Therapy Intervention in the Treatment of Schizophrenia, *The British Journal of Psychiatry*, 180(6), 523–527.

Yavuzşen, T, Karadibak, D., Cehreli, R. & Dirioz, M. (2012). Effect of Group Therapy on Psychological Symptoms and Quality of Life in Turkish Patients with Breast Cancer, *Asian Pacific Journal of Cancer Prevention*, 13(11), 5593–5597.

Figen Dığın

# 3: Tele-Health Practices in Postoperative Home Care of Elderly

## 1 Introduction

The elderly population in all over the world shows a rapid increase. The most important reason for increasing the elderly population is the prolongation of life. While 962.3 million elderly people live in 2017, this number is expected to rise to 2.1 billion in 2050 (United Nations, 2017). In the last century, the elderly population is more common in developing countries. Therefore, the importance of health services for elderly people is increasing in these countries (Ceylan, 2015). The increase in the workload of health institutions and employees due to increasing life expectancy and increasing chronic diseases in the workload cause an increase in the economic burden of countries (Tezcan, 2016).

While aging is a normal and inevitable physiological process, World Health Organization (WHO) has defined aging as a "continuous reduction of vital functions, a general reduction in the efficiency of the whole organism, and a reduced ability to adapt to environmental factors" (WHO, 2015). With age, the functional capacity and abilities of individuals are lost or decreased. Therefore, the daily activities of the elderly are decreasing and the elderly individuals become semi-dependent or fully dependent. This situation causes elderly people to be perceived as "dependency period" in developed countries (Çilingiroğlu and Demirel, 2004). Chronic diseases in old age result in physical and mental regression, which leads to continuous supervision and the need for health and social care centers. For this reason, health and care services for the elderly should be aimed at increasing the functional capacity of the elderly, supporting the activities of daily life and increasing the level of independence. In this way, the quality of life of the elderly will be increased (Kutsal, 2003).

## 2 Surgery in Elderly

The increasing number of aging societies has led to the updating of the concept of healthy and successful aging. Definition of healthy and successful aging process: The fact that the person's health, physical condition, social and spiritual well-being are at the highest level, while the individual being able to support their quality of life by means of their functional independence (Aslan and Başar, 2010).

Elderly individuals are hospitalized and operated upon for different reasons (Mayir et al., 2010). In most elderly patients, elective surgery is performed with very low complication and mortality rates. However, in older patients undergoing emergency surgery, more complications are seen and the mortality rate increases (Aygin, 2017). In the literature, the rate of mortality in elective surgery was 2.6 % in elderly patients while the mortality rate in emergency surgery was 13.9 % (Mayir et al., 2010). In order to decrease the mortality rate in elderly surgical patients, a good preoperative preparation should be done and functional disorders, mental disabilities, chronic diseases, nutritional status, physical activity and geriatric syndromes should be considered in the physical evaluation of patients. In order to reduce the postoperative complication risk and the rate of mortality in elderly patients, the surgical nurse must perform a comprehensive evaluation before, during and after the surgery (Akbuğa ve Bahçeli, 2017: http:// www.ucdenver.edu/academics/colleges/medicalschool/departments/surgery/ education/GrandRounds/Pages/default.aspx).

## 2.1 Post-operative Period in the Elderly

The most critical period of treatment of elderly patients undergoing surgery is the postoperative period. In this period, quality care should be given to minimize post-operative complications in patients and to prevent these complications from reaching life-threatening dimensions (Akbuğa and Bahçeli, 2017).

In the early postoperative period, the existing system insufficiency in elderly patients suggests the need for additional support. Therefore, it is important to determine the risk factors that threaten the functional independence of elderly patients such as hypotension, hypoxia, hypothermia, fluid-electrolyte imbalance, cognitive dysfunction, postoperative delirium, pain, malnutrition and surgical wound infection by monitoring them in the early postoperative period and taking the necessary precautions (Karadakovan, 2014; Griffiths et al., 2016).

Elderly patients need comprehensive information to maintain their self-care after surgery. Nowadays, the most common approach is to discharge the elderly patient after helping them grow the power, courage and skill to maintain their self-care as soon as possible (Aslan, 2011). Discharge planning is a process that begins with the hospitalization of the patient and ends with the separation from the hospital. In order to maintain the patient's treatment and care at home, discharge training should be done by nurses with a good planning (Tuna, 2012).

Elderly patients are expected to perform many applications at home, including wound care, drug use, exercise, hygienic care, diet and medical device use. For this reason, discharge training (including these subjects) should cover many topics such as pain management, rest, sexual activity, mood changes and smoking (Özcan, 2008; Demirkıran, 2011; Dal, Bulut and Demir, 2012). Along with all these, elderly patients need to cope with the problems of aging simultaneously, so the improvement and maintenance periods in the home are more complicated. (Ouellet et al., 2003).

## 2.2 Postoperative Home Care of Elderly

In parallel with the innovations and changes in technology, elderly patients can also be operated. The need for home care is increasing due to the early discharge of elderly patients with accelerated care protocols (Jerant et al., 2002).

Home care services, in general, are to deliver health care and social services by the professional or family members in an individual's own home or living environment in order to protect, promote and recover the health of the individual (Karahan and Güven, 2002). The elderly and their families experience varying problems in the post-operative home care processes (Weaver and Doran, 2001). Postoperative care for elderly patients can continue for weeks, even months. Therefore, the patient who is sent home with a good discharge education should be supported with home care services (Dal, Bulut and Demir, 2012). Physiological changes related to age, surgical methods applied, anesthesia applications, duration and technique of surgery, postoperative intensive care unit stay and developing complications affect the healing process of patients. In addition, the presence of social support systems in the elderly patients' home after discharge contributes to the recovery of the patient (Tuna, 2012). Discharge education should be trained by considering the patients' self-care process who are sent home postoperatively.

Demographic, sociological, social and economic differences lead to major changes in lifestyle. With these changes in the lifestyle, women began to take part in the business life and this led the need for "home care services" for the elderly to increase. This increase in the demand for home care has enabled home care services to be supported by different technologies (Giraldo-Rodríguez et al., 2013). In recent years, the support of home care services with technology has led to widespread use of home care services (Tezcan, 2016).

It is stated that elderly patients have problems in wound care, pain management, sleep, drug use, nutrition, exercise, excretion, hygienic care and daily life activities during the home care process. Patients and their families need professional support to cope with these problems (Yılmaz and Çiftçi, 2010). It is thought that the necessary professional support can be provided thanks to the well planned and personalized discharge training and home care services given to the operated elderly patients. In this way, the elderly patients will have fewer problems with the home care process after surgery, the complications due to surgery will decrease and the quality of life of the patients will increase. In elderly patients, the mortality rates associated with the operation after discharge will decrease.

## 2.3 Tele-Health Practices in Home Care

Tele-health practices were first used in 1920 in Norway to provide health services to ships in the sea through radio connection. In the literature, it is stated that tele health practices are becoming more common with the developments in technology and communication after 1960 (Acar and Pınar, 2013). However, the concept of tele-health was first defined by Kenneth Bird in 1975 and the American Telemedicine Association was established in 1994. Telemedicine, which is used synonymously with e-health and tele-care, is to provide healthcare services through established networks to individuals who are far away from health institutions. Tele-health includes preventive, supportive and curative practices and includes regulation of clinical practice, education, patient information records and transmission of this information in electronic form (Ertek, 2011).

Tele-health is the sharing of interactive health-related information for healthcare practices, diagnostics, counseling and treatment using audiovisual tools. In other words, tele-health is the provision of information exchange between professional health professionals and patients in health care through the use of various technological communication tools (telephone, computer, television, teleconference, etc.) (Opot, 2011). While providing information exchange with tele-health applications, patient care and education can also be performed (Opot, 2011; Dixon, Hook and Mcgowan, 2008). Tele-health practices are categorized under different sub-titles as teleconsultation, storage and transmission and remote monitoring. Technologies such as video conferencing and telephony are used for teleconsultation. The transmission and transmission of patient data for evaluation at a later time is included in the storage and transmission process. Monitoring of the physiological findings of patients who need home care via devices is a remote monitoring process (Miskelly, 2014).

Tele-health practices in health services have begun with video conferences. In this way, health professionals have started to transfer information about health to individuals in remote areas (Merrell, 2015). Although different technological methods have been tried for tele health applications, developments in telecommunication services have reached its current use with the expansion of mobile phone, internet access, fiber optic connections and wireless communication.

Home care with tele-health is offered to:

- the patients who cannot move,
- the patients living in distance places,
- the patients with chronic diseases,
- the patients in need of care (Schlachta, 2009; Westra, 2009).

The benefits of tele-health include:

- access to care by advanced method,
- improving health quality,
- effective use of time in healthcare delivery,
- health service adapted to the needs of the patient,
- fewer health costs (Schlachta, 2009).

Around the world, tele-radiology practices are the most common among tele-health practices. More than half of the WHO member states have a telemedicine strategy, and over half of them are using tele-pathology, remote patient monitoring and tele dermatology practice. According to WHO data, in Finland, France, Germany and Greece, triage and health education counseling services are provided on a seven-day, twenty-four-hour basis. In addition to this, it was stated that nurse counseling was provided free of charge in England and Scotland (WHO, 2011).

In Turkey, tele-health applications have accelerated via the "Health Transformation Program" launched in 2003 by the Ministry of Health. With this program, Turkey has aimed to establish Health Information System. About the tele-health applications in Turkey, it has been stated that drug follow-up systems, e-prescription application, Organ Transplant Information System, Family Medicine System, Central Hospital Appointment System, Core Resource Management System, Online Health Servers (MEDULA) and Health-Net Platform are included (www.itadvisor.com; Toygar, 2018). In addition, comprehensive projects are being carried out by mobile communication companies in the field of telemedicine. In addition to this, telemedicine practices, which are made in cooperation with the public and private sector, are becoming more common, and more elderly patients are provided with services.

In parallel with the technological advances in medical applications, the use of technological applications in home care services is becoming more common, and the quality and effectiveness of home care services is increasing. The tele-health practices used in the provision of home care services are changing and developing day by day (Jerant et al., 2002). The "home care services" carry out several tasks in Turkey; one of them is measuring data from the elderly patients: blood pressure, blood sugar, heart and respiratory rate, health facilities, etc. These collective packs of information are also reported to physicians and/or health facilities through technological devices. Within the scope of Tele Health practices, elderly patients are provided with video and voice communication with physicians and remote monitoring and diagnosis is provided. In addition, devices are used to inform health facilities and emergency units for elderly patients in emergencies (www.itadvisor.com). With the use of tele health applications, elderly patients can be monitored and maintained at low costs.

Day by day, with the expansion and development of tele health practices, nursing practices change and develop. For this reason, nurses have many roles in tele health practices. These roles of nurses include collecting data about the patient, monitoring the patient's vital signs, planning and fulfilling the care of the patient according to the information he collects, training the patient and advising on public health issues (Westra, 2009). In addition to these, Tele health nurses are involved in research, consultancy, education, community and public health, hospital services, intensive care and ambulatory care. In a study comparing classical care with nurse counseling, it was found that nurse counseling by phone rather than classical care reduced the hospitalization rate of patients (Jerant et al., 2002), while in a similar study, it was emphasized that patient follow-up by phone at home supported positive self-care process (Furuya et al, 2013).

Studies have shown that tele-health practices support the functional independence of the elderly, improve the quality of life (Giraldo-Rodríguez et al., 2013) and contribute to family well-being (Sävenstedt, Zingmark and Sandman, 2003; Giraldo-Rodríguez et al., 2013). In the literature, it was found that hospitalization rates of patients followed by home tele-monitoring method decreased (Jerant et al., 2002), and post-operative patients were provided with symptom management at home care (Kleinpell and Avitall, 2007), while the rate of hospitalization of patients (Weaver and Doran, 2001; Armstrong et al., 2007), the total cost is reported to decrease (Bernstein, 2000). It was also emphasized that the burden of caregivers of patients can be reduced by the use of tele health practices (Temizer, 2009). In the literature, it is emphasized that tele health practices can be used to support the functional independence of the elderly and to ensure the maintenance and maintenance of care (Bernstein, 2000; Hintistan and Çilingir, 2012). Additionally, it is stated that the use of technology in the health services for the elderly is very beneficial for patients (Giraldo-Rodríguez et al., 2013).

Although many studies have shown that telemedicine practices have contributed positively to the home care process of elderly patients, it is known that there are some disadvantages. The fact that elderly people have the ability to reach and use technological means reduces the effectiveness of tele health practices.

Also, some factors like how some of the elderly are technophobic, and/or they do not know how to use technological devices, and/or they do not believe in the usefulness of using technology, are among the disadvantages (Arnaert and Delesie, 2001).

## 3 Conclusion

With the use of tele-health practices in elderly patients during the post-operative home care process, the healing process at home will be supported positively. With the provided tele-health services, the self-care capability of the elderly patients will be supported and their functional independence will be increased. In terms of the risks of surgical operations, "tele health practices" will be offered to the elderly (of who are in a more risky group compared to other age groups), postoperative hospitalization rates will be reduced, and cost efficiency will be ensured. In addition, after an uncomplicated surgery with lesser problems, the quality of life and comfort of the elderly will be increased in the home care process. For this reason, it is necessary to follow the improvements in the home care process of elderly patients and give more attention to "tele health practices" in home care services, to provide counseling services to their physiological problems, to determine and prevent the complications early, to increase the overall quality of life.

## References

Acar, B.G. & Pınar, G. (2013). Tele Tıp Uygulamaları ve Hemşireliğe Yansımaları. *Yıldırım Beyazıt Üniversitesi Sağlık Bilimleri Fakültesi Hemşirelik E Dergisi*, 1(1), 47–54.

Akbuğa, G.A. & Bahçeli, A. (2017). Kalp Cerrahisi Girişimi Uygulanan Bireylere Yönelik Bakım, *Bozok Tıp Dergisi*, 7(2), 71–6.

Armstrong, A.W., Dorer, D.J., Lugn, N.E. & Kvedar, J.C. (2007). Economic Evaluation of Interactive Teledermatology Compared with Conventional Care, *Telemedicine Journal and e-Health*, 13(2), 91–9.

Arnaert, A. & Delesie, L. (2001). Telenursing for the Elderly. The Case for Care via Video-Telephony, *Journal of Telemedicine and Telecare*, 7(6), 311–6.

Aslan, D. & Başar, M.M. (2010). Konuşma metinleri, 4. Ulusal Yaşlı Sağlığı Kongresi: 1–4 Nisan 2010, İzmir.

Aslan, F.E. (2011). Ameliyat Sonrası Bakım. Karadakovan, A. & Aslan, F.E. (eds.), *Dâhili ve Cerrahi Hastalıklarda Bakım*, Adana: Nobel Kitabevi., 367–72.

Aygin, D. (2017). Yaşlı Cerrahisinde Bakım. Aslan, F.E. (eds.), *Cerrahi Bakım Vaka Analizleri İle Birlikte*, Ankara: Akademisyen Tıp Kitabevi, 181-247.

Bernstein, M. (2000). Low-Tech Personal Emergency Response Systems Reduce Costs and Improve Outcomes, *Manag Care Quaterly*, 8(1), 38–43.

Ceylan, H. (2015). Yaşlanan Türkiye'de Yaşlı Bakım Personeline Duyulan İhtiyaç ve Yaşlı Bakım Programlarının Önemi, *Electronic Journal of Vocational Colleges*, 4, 61–68.

Çilingiroğlu, N. & Demirel, S. (2004). Yaşlılık ve Yaşlı Ayrımcılığı, *Turkish Journal of Geriatrics*, 7(4), 225–230.

Dal, Ü., Bulut, H. & Demir, S.G. (2012). Cerrahi Girişim Sonrası Hastaların Evde Yaşadıkları Sorunlar, *Bakırköy Tıp Dergisi*, 8(1), 34–40.

Demirkıran, G. (2011). Koroner Arter Bypass Greft Ameliyatı Geçiren Hastaların Taburculuk Sonrası Öğrenim Gereksinimlerinin Belirlenmesi dissertation, İnönü Üniversitesi-Malatya.

Dixon, B.E., Hook, J.M. & McGowan, J.J. (2008). *Using Telehealth to Improve Quality and Safety Findings from the AHRQ Health IT Portfolio.* U.S. Department of Health and Human Services AHRQ Publication. https:// healthit.ahrq.gov/sites/default/files/docs/page/Telehealth_Issue_Paper_ Final_0.pdf (accessed on 19.03.2018).

Ertek, S. (2011). Endokrinolojide Tele-Sağlık ve Tele-Tıp Uygulamaları, *Acıbadem Üniversitesi Sağlık Bilimleri Dergisi*, 2(3), 126–30.

Furuya, R.K., Mata, L.R., Veras, V.S., Appoloni, A.H., Dantas, R.A., Silveira, R.C. & Rossi, L.A. (2013). Original research: telephone follow-up for patients after myocardial revascularization: a systematic review. *American Journal of Nursing*, 113(5), 28–31.

Giraldo-Rodríguez, L., Torres-Castro, S., Martínez-Ramírez, D., Gutiérrez-Robledo, L.M. & Pérez-Cuevas, R. (2013). Tele-Care and Tele-Alarms for the Elderly: Preliminary Experiences in Mexico, *Revista Saúde Pública*, 47(4), 1–6.

Griffiths, R., Beech, F., Brown, A., Dhesi, J., Foo, I., Goodall, J., et al. (2016). Guidelines Peri-Operative Care of the Elderly, *Anaesthesia*, 69(1), 81–98.

Hintistan, S. & Çilingir, D. (2012). Hemşirelik Uygulamalarında Güncel Bir Yaklaşım: Telefon Kullanımı, *Hemşirelikte Eğitim ve Araştırma Dergisi*, 9(1), 30–5.

Jerant, A.F., Azari, R., Martinez, C. & Nesbitt, T.S. (2002). A Randomized Trial of Telenursing to Reduce Hospitalization for Heart Failure: Patient-Centered Outcomes and Nursing Indicators, *Home Health Care Services Quarterly*, 22(1), 1–20.

Karadakova, A. (2014). Yaşlıda İlaç Kullanımı. Karadakovan, A. (eds.), *Yaşlı Sağlığı ve Bakım*, Ankara: Akademisyen Tıp Kitabevi.

Karahan, A. & Güven, S. (2002). Yaşlılıkta Evde Bakım, *Geriatri*, 5(4), 155–9.

Kleinpell, R.M. & Avitall, B. (2007). Integrating Telehealth as a Strategy for Patient Management after Discharge for Cardiac Surgery, *Journal of Cardiovascular Nursing*, 22(1), 38–42.

Kutsal, G.Y. (2003). Yaşlanan Dünya, Yaşlanan Toplum, Yaşlanan İnsan, *Hacettepe Toplum Hekimliği Bülteni*, 24, 1–6.

Mayir, B., Altınel, Ö., Özerhan, İ.H., Ersöz, N., Harlak, A., Kılbaş, Z., et al. (2010). Yaşlı Hastalarda Cerrahi Sonrası Mortaliteye Etki Eden Faktörler, *Anatolian Journal of Clinical Investigation*, 4(1), 32–5.

Merrell, R.C. (2015). Geriatric Telemedicine: Background and Evidence for Telemedicine as a Way to Address the Challenges of Geriatrics. *Healthcare Informatics Research*, 21(4), 223–9.

Miskelly, F. (2014). What Role Can Technologies Play in Supporting and Sustaining Independent and Healthy Living in Individuals 65 and Above? A Systematic Review of the Literature. Future of Ageing: Evidence Review. *British Geriatrics Society*, 1–24. http://www.bgs.org.uk/pdfs/telecare_ review_2014.pdf (accessed on 25.12.2018).

Opot, R. (2011). Application of Telenursing in the Rehabilitation of Elderly Hip Fracture Patients at Home: A Literature Review, Laurea University of Applied Sciences-Vantaa.

Ouellet, L.L., Hodgins, M.H., Pond, S., Knorr, S.P. & Geldart, G. (2003). Post-discharge Telephone Follow-Up for Orthopaedic Surgical Patients: A Pilot Study, *Journal of Orthopaedic Nursing*, 7, 87–93.

Özcan, H. (2008). *Açık Kalp Ameliyatı Sonrası Hemşireler Tarafından Verilen Taburculuk Eğitiminin Hastalar Tarafından Kullanılma Oranları* (Master dissertation), Trakya Üniversitesi-Edirne.

Sävenstedt, S., Zingmark, K. & Sandman, P.O. (2003). Video-phone Communication with Cognitively Impaired Elderly Patients, *Journal of Telemedicine and Telecare*, 9(2), 52–4.

Schlachta, L. (2009). Telehealth and Telenursing: Looking Toward the Future, *AACN Hot Issues Conference*. http://www.aacn.nche.edu/membership/ members-only/presentations/2009/09hotissues/satschlachtafairchild.pdf (accessed on 26.12.2017).

Temizer, H. (2009). *İnmeli Hastalara Evde Bakan Aile Üyelerine Verilen Hemşirelik Girişimlerinin Bilgi Düzeylerine Ve Bakım Yükünü Algılamalarına Etkisi* (Doctoral dissertation), Atatürk Üniversitesi-Erzurum.

Tezcan, C. (2016). "*Sağlığa Yenilikçi Bir Bakış Açısı: Mobil Sağlık*", Dicle, E, Çelik, E & Karataş, D. (eds.), İstanbul: Sis Matbaacılık.

Toygar, Ş.A. (2018). E-Sağlık Uygulamaları. *Yasama Dergisi*, 37, 101–23.

46                                      Figen Dığın

Tuna, Z. (2012). *Koroner Arter Bypass Greft Ameliyatı Olan Yaşlı Hastalara Fonksiyonel Bağımsızlık Düzeyleri Doğrultusunda Verilen Taburculuk Eğitiminin Hastaların Fonksiyonel Bağımsızlıklarına Etkisi* (Master Dissertation), Hacettepe Üniversitesi-Ankara.

United Nations. *United Nations Demographic Yearbook 2009–2010*. http:// unstats. un.org/unsd/demographic/products/dyb/dybsets/2009-2010.pdf. August 13, 2012 (accessed on 22.12.2018).

United Nations. (2017). *World Population Prospects: the 2017 Revision*. https:// esa.un.org/unpd/wpp/publications/files/wpp2017_keyfindings.pdf (accessed on 10.12.2018).

Weaver, L.A. & Doran, K.A. (2001). Telephone Follow-up after Cardiac Surgery: Facilitating the Transition from Hospital to Home, *The American Journal of Nursing*, 101(5), 84–96.

Westra, B. (2009). Telehealth Nursing Practice Essentials. American Academy of Ambulatory Care Nursing 2009. http://www. aacn.nche.edu/ qsen-informatics/2012- workshop/presentations/westra/Telehealth.pdf (11.01.2018).

World Health Organisation. (2011). *mHealth: New Horizons for Health through Mobile Technologies: Second Global Survey on eHealth*. https://www.who.int/ goe/publications/goe_mhealth_web.pdf (accessed on 05.01.2018).

World Health Organisation. (2015). *World report on Ageing and Health 2015*. http://www.who.int/ageing/events/world-report-2015-launch/en/ (accessed on 05.01.2018).

www.itadvisor.com (accessed on 08.03.2018).

http://www.ucdenver.edu/academics/colleges/medicalschool/departments/ surgery/education/GrandRounds/Pages/default.aspx (accessed on 07.03.2018).

Yılmaz, M. & Çifçi, E.S. (2010). Açık Kalp Ameliyatı Geçirmiş Bireylerin Evde Bakım Gereksinimlerinin Belirlenmesinde Bir Model: Fonksiyonel Sağlık Örüntüleri, *Türk Göğüs Kalp Damar Cerrahisi Dergisi*, 18(3), 183–9.

Gülbahtiyar Demirel and Özlem Akgün

# 4: An Approach in Women's Health: Aromatherapy

## 1 Introduction

Aromatherapy is one of the major complementary and alternative therapy methods commonly used in the world and is a branch of phytotherapy. In phytotherapy, some or all of the plant is used for medical purposes, while in aromatherapy only essential oils obtained by distillation and squeezing method are used (Başer and Taşcı, 2015; Bunckle, 2015). High concentration essential oils distilled from plants used in aromatherapy are extracted from the flowers, shells, roots, leaves, fruits and other parts of the plant by various methods (Esposito et al., 2014; Ali et al., 2015; Pirak et al., 2015; Bilgic, 2017; Tiran, 2018). Majority of the essential plants used for this purpose in aromatherapy are rose, lavender, jasmine, clove, sage, geranium, orange flower, pike, cinnamon leaf, bergamot and lemon (Ebcioglu, 2009; Sayowan, 2013; Kömürcü, 2014; Kheirkhah et al., 2014; Marzouk et al., 2015; Ali et al., 2015; Rashidi Fakari et al., 2015; Hergenç, 2015; Esmaelzadeh-Saeieh et al., 2018; Makvandi et al., 2018).

While the use of alternative and complementary therapies in the world is gaining momentum, one of the main reasons for these practices is the side effects of pharmacological agents on human health, particularly women and children's health. Along with the benefits provided by aromatherapy, the low number of side effects of it is one of the reasons of its widespread use (Tillett and Ames, 2010; Esposito et al., 2014; Kheirkhah et al., 2014; Kömürcü, 2014; Buckle, 2015; Ali et al., 2015; Pirak et al., 2015; Lakhan et al., 2016; Bilgiç, 2017; Makvandi et al., 2018). Among the benefits of aromatherapy, causing relaxation by increasing the neurotransmitter antispasmodically, reducing anxiety and pain by reducing the amount of epinephrine and norepinephrine in the blood, encouraging, being antiinflammatory, antiviral and antifungal, and having antibacterial effect in skin infections can be counted (Kheirkhah et al., 2014; Kömürcü, 2014; Buckle, 2015; Ali et al., 2015; Pirak et al., 2015; Lakhan et al., 2016; Bilgic, 2017; Chen et al., 2017; Chen et al., 2018; Makvandi et al. 2018).

Aromatherapy has a wide range of applications in the field of women's health. In addition to health problems such as premenstrual syndrome (PMS), vaginal infections, menopausal symptoms, cystitis, infertility and lichen sclerosis, it can be used as an example for the reduction of labor pain (Tillett and Ames, 2010;

48     Demirel and Akgün

Karabulut, 2014; Kömürcü, 2014; Kheirkhah et al., 2014; Baser and Tasci, 2015; Lakhan et al., 2016; Dimitriou et al., 2017; Ghiasi et al., 2017; Makvandi et al., 2018). Healthcare workers can contribute to raising women's health by ensuring that aromatherapy is used effectively and accurately in all these areas of application (Karabulut, 2014; Bilgiç, 2017).

## 2 Plants Used in Aromatherapy

In aromatherapy, various plants (rose, lavender, jasmine, clove, sage, geranium, orange flower, pine cone, cinnamon leaf, bergamot, lemon, etc.) and essential oils accompanied by various methods (from a candle-heated container by evaporating, massage, inhalation after dropping into hot water, direct inhalation, adding into the hot water used for bathing) can be used for treatment (Başer, 2009; Kömürcü, 2014; Kheirkhah et al., 2014; Marzouk et al., 2015; Ali et al., 2015; Rashidi Fakari et al., 2015; Hergenç, 2015; Esmaelzadeh-Saeieh et al., 2018; Makvandi et al., 2018). Major plants used in aromatherapy are as follows:

**Rose:** One of the basic plants used in aromatherapy is rose. The smell of rose is effective on the central nervous system. The two materials in the rose, sytrinol and 2-phenyl ethyl alcohol, work as an anticancer agent while being an antidepressant and acts as an uterotonic, providing deep and calm breathing (Ebcioğlu, 2009; Kömürcü, 2014; Kheirkhah et al., 2014). It has been stated that rose water and oil prove an analgesic, providing physiological relaxation and psychological relief, working as an anti-depressant, as well as providing improvement against sexual dysfunction, anti-aging, and anti-anxiety effects (Mohebitabar et al., 2017; Şentürk and Dogan, 2017). Studies have shown that rose oil is effective in reducing the severity of primary dysmenorrhea pain (Shahr et al., 2015; Uysal et al., 2016). In a study comparing the effect of rose oil and warm foot bath on anxiety in Nullipar women, it was found that both rose oil and warm foot bath decreased anxiety (Kheirkhah et al., 2014).

**Pelargonium:** Pelargonium is a 40–100 cm height, herbaceous plant with a scent similar to that of roses (Rashidi Fakari et al., 2015). Fakari et al. reported that inhalation of essential oil aroma in nulliparous women reduced anxiety and diastolic blood pressure in the first stage of labor. In the study by Rafsanjani et al. (2018), it was found that essential oil obtained from sardine decreases the physical and mental symptoms of premenstrual syndrome.

**Geranium:** The Geranium, which belongs to the Geraniaceae family, is used for dermatitis, eczema, aging skin, some fungal infections, anxiety and stress-related problems, and is also anti-inflammatory and anti-hemorrhagic (Kömürcü, 2014; Ali et al., 2015).

**Jasmine:** Jasmine, one of the major plants of aromatherapy, has been scientifically labeled as Jasminum sambac. Jasmine oil is useful in the treatment of severe depression, calming the nerves, invigorating and restoring energy, improving memory, relaxing, trust, optimism and euphoria feeling, strengthening contraction in labor, while it is known to also have analgesic and antispasmodic effects (Sayowan, 2013; Kömürcü, 2014; Hergenç, 2015). In one study, it was concluded that the application of jasmine with incense to nulliparous women was effective in decreasing the birth pain, and that the baby did not adversely affect APGAR score (Kaviani et al., 2014).

**Boswellia Carteria (BC):** Boswellia carteria, one of the plants used in aromatherapy is characterized by its analgesic effect. Esmaelzadeh-Saeieh et al. (2018) found out in a study conducted with nulliparous women, that Boswellia carteria essential oil inhalation aromatherapy was effective in reducing the birth pain in the first stage of labor.

**Clove Bud Oil:** Eugenol, the main volatile component of clove, which itself is the dried flower buds of the Syzgium aromaticum tree, has effects on anti-inflammatory and immune system. Clove oil prevents cell proliferation, protects against cancer, and prevents tooth decay by suppressing microorganisms that cause it. Clove oil, which also has stimulant and antispasmodic effects, is often used to relieve pain during delivery (Kömürcü, 2014; Hergenç, 2015).

**Clary Sage:** The sage oil of the Lamiaceae family, with large hairy green leaves including purple color, is often used in aromatherapy (Ali et al., 2015; Hergenç, 2015). Sage essential oil has various therapeutic properties. Oil helps to control the uterine problems, to regulate menstrual periods, to remove hot flashes in menopause and to have an aphrodisiac activity, to control the production of sebum (acne, wrinkles and cellulite control). In a study, an increase was observed in oxytocin level and uterine contractions after inhalation of sage essential oil odor in single pregnancies between 38 and 40 weeks of gestation (Tadokoro et al., 2017).

**Orange Flower (Neroli):** It is one of the plants used in aromatherapy, which can calm fear and excitement by being poured on a napkin and sniffed for 2 minutes. The orange flower is antispasmodic, moderately hypnotic and stimulant, a tonic for the cardiovascular system. It also supports deep, calm and rhythmic breathing, facilitates delivery by softening the uterus (Kömürcü, 2014; Hergenç, 2015).

**Lavender:** Lavender oil, one of the essential oils of aromatherapy, has various therapeutic and curative properties, including anti-bacterial, anti-fungal, sedative and anti-depressive properties. Also effective for burns and insect bites, lavender oil reduces the feeling of panic and strengthens contractions and is used in the treatment of dysmenorrhea (Kömürcü, 2014; Marzouk et al., 2015; Ali et al.,

2015). Marzouk et al. (2015) supported the improvement of lavage-thymol-treated episiotomy; lavender oil was effective in episiotomy recovery, and women in the placebo-treated group had worse redness, edema and ecchymosis scores. In the study by Pirak et al. (2015), it was found that massage aromatherapy with Lavender oil decreased the birth pain, while a similar study conducted by Makvandi et al. stated that inhaling the essential oil also had the same effect.

**Ylang-ylang**: Ylang-ylang is a small tree belonging to the Annonaceae family, specific to Madagascar, Indonesia and the Philippines. The best feature of this tree is its use in shock and trauma: With excellent application, it can delay/slow the heartbeat and rapid breathing. Ylang-ylang essential oil is obtained based on a fractionation related to distillation times. Aromatherapy with Ylang-ylang oil is used in depression, anxiety, hypertension, frigidity, stress, palpitation and improvement of self-esteem. It can also be used in various infectious skin diseases, insect bites, high blood pressure and antidepressant conditions (Groot and Schmidt, 2017). In the pilot study of 34 professional nurses from a nursing group in Portugal, there was clear evidence that the use of this plant increased self-esteem (Gnatta et al., 2014).

**Cinnamon Leaf**: Cinnamon leaf is one of the essential oils of aromatherapy. Eugenol, cinnamaldehyde and camphor were found in the main component of it is the bark and root essential oils; In addition, alpha ylangen, methyl and ethyl cinnamate were found in its leaf oil, while 4-terpinen-1-ol was found in its shell oil. Cinnamon leaf oil is a stimulant that stimulates the circulatory and respiratory system. Jaafarpour et al. (2015) reported that the duration and severity of dysmenorrhea pain decreased in women given cinnamon capsule (containing 420 mg).

**Bergamot**: Bergamot, one of the aromatherapy plants, is a painkiller, antiseptic, antidepressant and a refreshing agent for the user. It is also helpful in the problem of cystitis frequently encountered during pregnancy (Amanak et al., 2013; Hergenç, 2015).

**Lemon**: Lemon, which is one of the indispensable plants of aromatherapy, is an antiseptic, antibacterial and antifungal, and is useful and stimulating in circulatory problems, preventing varicose veins and relaxing in morning sickness (Amanak et al., 2013; Hergenç, 2015). Studies on pregnant women have shown that the lemon applied by inhalation is effective in reducing the severity of nausea and vomiting (Yavari Kia et al., 2014; Kustriyanti and Purti, 2019).

## 3 Benefits of Aromatherapy

Aromatherapy is one of the complementary and alternative therapy methods frequently used for women's health benefits. Essential oils reduce anxiety and pain, are anti-inflammatory, antiviral, antifungal or antibacterial, while having have encouraging effects for the user (Tillett and Ames, 2010; Kömürcü, 2014; Kheirkhah et al., 2014; Buckle, 2015; Lakhan et al., 2016).

Premenstrual syndrome (PMS), vaginal infections, insomnia, nausea-vomiting, inflammation, menopausal symptoms, cystitis, infertility, lichen sclerosis and birth pain are among the main health problems of women that can be treated with essential oils. Aromatherapy can also be used in cases such as stress management, cardiological problems, aged care, dermatological, endocrinological, immunological, oncological, pediatric, end of life care, psychiatric care, respiratory system and intensive care problems (Kheirkhah et al., 2014; Başer and Taşcı, 2015; Lakhan et al., 2016; Makvandi et al., 2018).

PMS is one of the problems that women often encounter and where essential oils are used to alleviate the pain and the side effects. Women during PMS can benefit from the juniper or lavender applied in the bath for fluid retention of the body; neroli, ylang ylang or sage for the symptoms of stress and tension (applied to the abdomen or chest massager); and can take advantage of geranium, juniper, evening primrose oil and vitamin E oil for breast sensitivity (applied by massage) (Kheirkhah et al., 2014; Lakhan et al., 2016; Makvandi et al., 2018).

Essential oils in aromatherapy are also used to reduce menstrual symptoms. The oils used for menstrual cramps include chamomile, mint, black pepper, rosemary, sweet marjoram and ylang ylang (Tillett and Diane, 2010). These oils applied by massage or inhalation can significantly reduce dysmenorrhea pain (Sut and Kahyaoğlu, 2017).

Labor pain is one of the areas where essential oils are used. The most commonly used aromatherapy methods to minimize pain during childbirth are massage, bath and inhalation (Tillett and Ames, 2010; Kömürcü, 2014; Kheirkhah et al., 2014; Lakhan et al., 2016; Makvandi et al., 2018). In the meta-analysis of randomized controlled trials, it was determined that aromatherapy had a positive effect on the elimination of labor pain and was reliable for mothers (Ghiasi et al., 2017; Chen et al., 2018). In another study conducted in this area, aromatherapy decreased the anxiety and anxiety levels of the woman, increased pain threshold and confidence and the duration of the delivery was found to be reduced while no maternal and fetal side effects related to aromatherapy were reported (Karabulut, 2014). Aromatherapy is also an effective and inexpensive method of relieving postoperative pain (Dimitriou et al., 2017).

Essential oils are used to relieve menopausal symptoms. Sage, fennel and Sardinia, which are some of the essential oils that provide estrogenic support, can be applied by massage while lavender can be applied by inhalation. Studies have shown that inhalation of essential oils and massage can significantly reduce menopausal symptoms (Rafsanjani et al., 2015; Kazemzadeh et al., 2016; Babakhanian et al., 2018; Nikjou et al., 2018).

## 4 Responsibilities of Health Professionals in Aromatherapy

People believe in the healing properties of plants for thousands of years and have practiced aromatherapy. Health professionals, especially midwives and nurses, should be aware of the pharmacological and nonpharmacological methods, their effects and limitations in the health problems of women and should be able to assist the person in the effective application of these methods. Aromatherapy, when used with in-service trainings and scientific studies in every phase of women's life, when used by health professionals, such as midwives and nurses, by integrating them with standard care and treatment, increase the job satisfaction while providing significant benefits to women's health (Karabulut, 2014; Tiran, 2016; Johnson et al., 2016; Bilgiç, 2017).

## 5 Conclusion

Aromatherapy, one of the most frequently used complementary and alternative therapies, is now popular due to its economic aspect, low side effects and various benefits. The use of aromatherapy in women's health should be further enhanced by supporting evidence-based studies. Evidence based on valid information will avoid the wrong practices and contribute to the development of women's, family and community health in general.

## References

Ali, B., Al-Wabel, N.A., Shams, S., Ahamad, A., Khan, S.A. & Anwar, F. (2015). Essential Oils Used in Aromatherapy: A Systemic Review, *Asian Pacific Journal of Tropical Biomedicine*, 5(8), 601–611.

Amanak, K., Karaöz, B. & Sevil, Ü. (2013). Alternatif/Tamamlayıcı Tıp ve Kadın Sağlığı, *TAF Preventive Medicine Bulletin*, 12(4), 441–448.

Babakhanian, M., Ghazanfarpour, M., Kargarfard, L., Roozbeh, N., Darvish, L., Khadivzadeh, T. & Dizavandi, F.R. (2018). Effect of Aromatherapy on the Treatment of Psychological Symptoms in Postmenopausal and Elderly Women: A Systematic Review and Meta-Analysis, *Journal of Menopausal Medicine*, 24(2), 127–132.

Başer, H.C. (2009). Uçucu Yağlar ve Aromaterapi, *Fitomed*, 7, 8–25.

Başer, M. & Taşcı, S. (2015). "*Kanıta Dayalı Rehberleriyle Tamamlayıcı ve Destekleyici Uygulamalar*", Akademisyen Kitabevi, Ankara.

Bilgic, Ş. (2017). Hemşirelikte Holistik Bir Uygulama; Aromaterapi, *Namık Kemal Tıp Dergisi*, 5(3), 134–141.

Bunckle, J. (2015). *"Clinical Aromatherapy Essential Oils in Healthcare"*, Third Edition, Elsevier Inc, London.

Chen, P., Chou, C., Yang, L., Tsai, Y., Chang, Y. & Liaw, J. (2017). Effects of Aromatherapy Massage on Pregnant Women's Stress and Immune Function: A Longitudinal, Prospective, Randomized Controlled Trial, *The Journal of Alternative and Complementary Medicine*, 23(10), 778–786.

Chen, S., Wang, C., Chan, P., Chiang, H., Hu, T., Tam, K. & Loh, E. (2018). Labor Pain Control by Aromatherapy: A Meta-Analysis of Randomized Controlled Trials, *Women and Birth*, 884, 1–9.

Dimitriou, V., Mavridou, P., Manataki, A. & Damigos, D. (2017). The Use of Aromatherapy for Postoperative Pain Management: A Systematic Review of Randomized Controlled Trials, *Journal of PeriAnesthesia Nursing*, 32(6), 530–541.

Ebcioğlu, N. (2009). *"Şifalı, Tıbbi ve Yararlı Bitkiler"*, İnkılap Kitabevi, İstanbul.

Esmaelzadeh-Saeieh, S., Rahimzadeh, M., Khosravi-Dehaghi, N. & Torkashvand, S. (2018). The Effects of Inhalation Aromatherapy with Boswellia Carterii Essential Oil on the Intensity of Labor Pain among Nulliparous Women, *Nursing and Midwifery Studies*, 7(2), 45–49.

Esposito, E.R., Bystrek, M.V. & Klein, J.S. (2014). An Elective Course in Aromatherapy Science, *American Journal of Pharmaceutical Education*, 78(4), 79.

Ghiasi, A., Hasani, M., Mollaahmadi, L., Hashemzadeh, M. & Haseli, A. (2017). The Effect of Aromatherapy on Labor Pain Relief: A Systematic Review of Clinical Trials, *Iranian Journal of Obstetrics, Gynecology and Infertility*, 20(2), 89–105.

Gnatta, J.R., Piason, P.P., Lopes, C.L., Rogenski, N.M. & Silva, M.J. (2014). Aromatherapy with Ylang Ylang for Anxiety and Self-Esteem: A Pilot Study, *Revista da Escola de Enfermagem da USP*, 48(3), 492–499.

Groot, A.C. & Schmidt, E. (2017). Essential Oils, Part V1: Sandalwood Oil, Ylang-Ylang Oil, and Jasmine Absolute. *Dermatitis*, 28(1), 14–21.

Hergenç, G. (2015). *"En Son Bilimsel Verilerin Işığında Beslenme, Sağlık ve Hastalıkta Bitkiler"*, Nobel Tıp Kitabevleri, İstanbul.

Jaafarpour, M., Hatefi, M., Khani, A. & Khajavikhan, J. (2015). Comparative Effect of Cinnamon and Ibuprofen for Treatment of Primary Dysmenorrhea: A Randomized Doubleblind Clinical Trial. *Journal of Clinical and Diagnostic Research*, 9(4), 4–7.

Johnson, K., West, T., Diana, S., Todd, J., Haynes, B., Bernhardt, J. & Johnson, R. (2016). Use of Aromatherapy to Promote a Therapeutic Nurse Environment. *Intensive and Critical Care Nursing*, 40, 18–25.

Karabulut, H. (2014). *Doğum Eyleminde Aromaterapinin Etkileri* (Master dissertation), İstanbul Üniversitesi Sağlık Bilimleri Enstitüsü-İstanbul.

Kaviani, M., Maghbool, S., Azima, S. & Tabaei, M.H. (2014). Comparison of the Effect of Aromatherapy with *Jasminum officinale* and *Salvia officinale* on Pain Severity and Labor Outcome in Nulliparous Women, *Iranian Journal of Nursing and Midwifery Research*, 19(6), 666–672.

Kazemzadeh, R., Nikjou, R., Rostamnegad, M. & Norouzi, H. (2016). Effect of Lavender Aromatherapy on Menopause Hot Flushing: A Crossover Randomized Clinical Trial, *Journal of the Chinese Medical Association*, 79(9), 489–492.

Kheirkhah, M., Pour, N.S.V., Nisani, L., & Haghani, H. (2014). Comparing the Effects of Aromatherapy with Rose Oils and Warm Foot Bath on Anxiety in the First Stage of Labor in Nulliparous Women, *Iranian Red Crescent Medical Journal*, 16(9), 144–155.

Kömürcü, N. (2014). *"Doğum Ağrısı ve Yönetimi"*, Nobel Kitabevi, İstanbul.

Kustriyanti, D. & Putri, A.A. (2019). The Effect of Ginger and Lemon Aromatherapy on Nausea and Vomiting among Pregnant Women, *Journal Keperawatan Soedirman*, 14(1), 15–22.

Lakhan, S.E., Sheafer, H. & Tepper, D. (2016). The Effectiveness of Aromatherapy in Reducing Pain: A Systematic Review and Meta-analysis, *Pain Research and Treatment*, 1–13.

Makvandi, S., Mirzaiinajmabadi, K., Mirteimoori, M. & Sadeghi, R. (2018). An Update on the Effect of Massage and Inhalation Aromatherapy with Lavender on Labor Pain Relief: A Systematic Review and Meta-analysis, *Journal of Obstetrics, Gynecology and Cancer Research*, 3(1): 29–37.

Marzouk, T., Barakat, R., Ragap, A., Badria, F. & Badawy, A. (2015). Lavender-Thymol as a New Topical Aromatherapy Preparation for Episiotomy: A Randomised Clinical Trial, *Journal of Obstetrics and Gynaecology*, 35(5), 472–475.

Mohebitabar, S., Shirazi, M., Bioos, S., Rahimi, R., Malekshahi, F. & Nejatbakhsh, F. (2017). Therapeutic Efficacy of Rose Oil: A Comprehensive Review of Clinical Evidence, *AJP*, 7(3), 206–213.

Nikjou, R., Kazemzadeh, R., Asadzadeh, F., Fathi, R. & Mostafazadeh, F. (2018). The Effect of Lavender Aromatherapy on the Symptoms of Menopause. *Journal of the National Medical Association*, 10(3), 265–269.

Pirak, A., Salehian, T., Yazdkhasti, M., Didehvar, M. & Arzani, A. (2015). The Effect of Lavender Essence on Labor Pain and Length of Delivery Time in Nulliparous Women. *Journal of Ilam University of Medical Sciences*, 23(6), 175–184.

Rafsanjani, S.M.L., Vazirinejad, S., Ismailzadeh, S., Jaberi, A.A., Bekhradi, R., Ravari, A. & Akbari, J. (2015). Comparison of the Efficacy of Massage and Aromatherapy Massage with Geranium on Depression in Postmenopausal Women: A Clinical Trial, *Zahedan Journal of Research in Medical Science*, 17(4), 970–75.

Rafsanjani, S.M.L., Ravari, A., Ghorashi, Z., Haji-Maghsoudi, S., Akbarinasab, J. & Bekhradi, R. (2018). Effects of Geranium Aromatherapy Massage on Premenstrual Syndrome: A Clinical Trial, *International Journal of Preventive Medicine*, 9(1), 98.

Rashidi Fakari, F., Tabatabaeichehr, M., Kamali, H., Rashidi Fakari, F. & Naseri, M. (2015). Effect of Inhalation of Aroma of Geranium Essence on Anxiety and Physiological Parameters during First Stage of Labor in Nulliparous Women: A Randomized Clinical Trial, *Journal of Caring Sciences*, 4(2), 135–141.

Sayowan, W., Siripornpanich, V., Hongratanaworakit, T., Kotchabhakdi, N. & Ruangrungsi, N. (2013). The Effects of Jasmine Oil Inhalation on Brain Wave Activities and Emotions, *Journal of Health Research*, 27(2), 73–77.

Shahr, H.S.A., Saadat, M., Kheirkhah, M. & Saadat, E. (2015). The Effect of Self-Aromatherapy Massage of the Abdomen on the Primary Dysmenorrhoea, *Journal of Obstetrics and Gynaecology*, 35, 382–385.

Sut, N. & Kahyaoğlu, H. (2017). Effect of Aromatherapy Massage on Pain in Primary Dysmenorrhea: A Meta-analysis, *Complementary Therapies in Clinical Practice*, 27, 5–10.

Şentürk, S. & Doğan, N. (2017). Geçmişten Günümüze Tıbbi Bir Bitki Olarak Gül, *Göller Bölgesi Aylık Hakemli Ekonomi ve Kültür Dergisi*, 54, 11–15.

Tadokoro, Y., Horiuchi, S., Takahata, K., Shuo, T., Sawano, E. & Shinohara, K. (2017). Changes in Salivary Oxytocin after Inhalation of Clary Sage Essential Oil Scent in Term-Pregnant Women: A Feasibility Pilot Study, *BMC*, 10, 717.

Tillett, J. & Ames, D. (2010). The Uses of Aromatherapy in Women's Health, *Journal of Perinatal & Neonatal Nursing*, 24(3), 238–245.

Tiran, D. (2016). "*Aromatherapy in Midwifery Practice*", Singing Dragon, London.

Tiran, D. (2018). "*Complementary Therapies in Maternity Care: An Evidence-Based Approach*", Singing Dragon, Philadelphia.

Uysal, M., Doğru, H.Y., Sapmaz, E., Tas, U., Çakmak, B., Özsoy, A.Z., Şahin, F., Ayan, S. & Esen, M. (2016). Investigating the Effect of Rose Essential Oil in Patients with Primary Dysmenorrhea, *Complementary Therapies in Clinical Practice*, 24, 45–49.

Yavari Kia, P., Safajou, F., Shahnazi, M. & Nazemiyeh, H. (2014). The Effect of Lemon Inhalation Aromatherapy on Nausea and Vomiting of Pregnancy: A Double-Blinded, Randomized, Controlled Clinical Trial, *Iranian Red Crescent Medical Journal*, 16(3), 143–160.

Figen Alp Yılmaz and Ebru Gözüyeşil

# 5: The Use of Complementary and Alternative Medicine (CAM) Applications in Women's Health

## 1 Introduction

Traditional, complementary and alternative medicine applications are widely used in the prevention, diagnosis and treatment of a wide range of diseases in the world (Çağlayan et al., 2018). According to the World Health Organization (WHO), traditional medicine is defined as "knowledge, skills and practices based on different cultures, beliefs and experiences that are used for the protection, improvement or maintenance of health" (WHO, 2014). Complementary medicine, on the other hand, is a group of applications that are parallel to traditional medicine, aimed at supporting and strengthening the treatment and/or alleviating the side effects of the treatment (Somer and Vatanoglu-Lutz, 2017). Lastly, the concept of alternative medicine consists mostly of unproven therapies used in place of modern medicine and are used in some countries as a synonym for complementary medicine or traditional medicine (WHO, 2014; Oral et al., 2016).

Today, many individuals in the society refer to both Traditional and Complementary Medicine (TCM) methods for treatment, protective and cultural purposes. It is also mentioned that TCM applications are being used in increasing amounts. According to the WHO, 80 % in Africa, 70 % in Canada, 48 % in Australia and 42 % of the population in the United States refer to traditional practices (WHO, 2000). The prevalence of TCM use was reported to be 9.8–76.0 % in Europe (WHO, 2014). In Turkey, TCM has become very popular in health care. Although there are a limited number of studies on TCM in Turkey, the frequency of the use of the application is found to be in the range of 42 % to 70 % (Sönmez et al., 2018).

TCM Practices Regulations were published in Turkey in the Official Gazette (No. 29158, dated October 27, 2014). There are 15 TCM applications defined in the regulation. They are 1. Acupuncture, 2. Apitherapy, 3. Phytotherapy, 4. Hypnosis, 5. Hirudotherapy, 6. Homeopathy, 7. Chiropractic treatment, 8. Cup treatment, 9. Larva treatment, 10. Mesotherapy, 11. Prolotherapy, 12. Osteopathy, 13. Ozone, 14. Reflexology, 15. Music therapy (Çaglayan et al., 2018).

The personnel, indications, contraindications, the materials that should be included in the application center, etc. are explained in the related regulation (Şahin, 2017). The Regulation only authorized certified physicians in terms of TCM applications. Applications can be made by physicians who have an "application certificate" in the relevant field and only by dentists who are in the field of dentistry (Somer and Vatanoğlu-Lutz, 2017). The regulation also prevents other healthcare professionals from practicing these applications unless they are practiced within the scope of supervision of certified physicians or dentists.

Changes in the roles and responsibilities of nurses have occurred with the increase in the scientific developments in the field of health. In this respect, nurses are expected to develop nursing practices related to the use of traditional and complementary therapies, determine effective strategies and enable healthy/patient individuals to use these therapies effectively and correctly. When the literature is examined, it can be seen that TCM therapies can be applied as a nursing intervention (Turan, 2010; Lindquist et al., 2014). In this context, it can be thought that these therapies can be applied within the scope of independent nursing roles of nurses for the protection and development of women's health. It is stated that there are shortcomings within the TCM Regulations in Turkey, like the limited number of applications, and the fact that only physicians are authorized to practice them (Somer and Vatanoğlu-Lutz, 2017).

In this chapter, it is aimed to discuss the effectiveness of acupuncture, phytotherapy, hypnosis, homeopathy, reflexology and music therapy methods in the light of evidence-based scientific research.

## 2 Acupuncture

Acupuncture is one of the oldest forms of complementary medicine therapies that have been applied over 5000 years and are still widely used in the world. Acupuncture is a scientific treatment method based on the principle of stimulating energy sources. The stimulation is performed electrically and by pricking with the needle, by manual pressure, with low power laser, and by ultrasound. Acupuncture is most commonly used in pain (Taşçı and Sevil, 2007; Mucuk and Ceyhan, 2011). Acupuncture prevents pain in the central nervous system by stimulating endogenous opioid release and modulating the hypothalamic-limbic system. The majority of studies have focused on the analgesic effect of acupuncture and the role of endogenous opioids (Mucuk and Ceyhan, 2011).

Acupuncture is widely used in obstetrics and gynecology. It can be applied in various complaints related with pregnancy or menopausal period, especially the labor pain (Taşçı and Sevil, 2007). As for the birth, acupuncture has been reported to have a positive effect on initiating contractions (Lim et al., 2009). According to the results of a Cochrane Review, it has been reported to be useful in developing cervical maturation (Smith and Cochrane, 2009). In addition, in studies on the effects of acupuncture on the onset, duration and pain of labor, conflicting results have been reported partly due to the heterogeneity of methodology and control group procedures (Smith and Cochrane, 2009; Cho et al.,2010; Gaudet et al., 2008; Modlock et al., 2010).

There is growing evidence that acupuncture may be useful in the treatment of pregnancy-related complaints such as nausea, vomiting, back/low back pain and depressive symptoms (Smith and Cochrane, 2009; Soliday and Hapke, 2013; Chen et al., 2014).

In a randomized controlled study examining the effect of acupuncture on post-partum depression, it was found that after an eight-week manual acupuncture treatment in pregnant women with major depressive disorder, more positive results were obtained compared to the control group and the post-partum depression was completely cured in majority of women after delivery (Chung et al., 2012).

Acupuncture is recommended as a treatment option for women with sexual dysfunctions, especially women with low sexual desire. It has been reported that when acupuncture is applied to women with sexual desire disorder in the premenopausal period, a significant improvement has been observed (Oakley et al., 2016). There are many studies on the effect of acupuncture on reducing the frequency and severity of hot flashes during menopause and improving the quality of life (Painovic et al., 2012; Kim et al., 2011; Avis et al., 2008; Borud et al., 2009). In the randomized controlled studies of Alraek and Malterud (2009), acupuncture treatment has been found to reduce the intensity and frequency of hot flashes in women day and night (Alraek and Malterud, 2009). According to the results of a Cochrane review, it is reported that more research is needed in order to obtain more accurate results in decreasing hot flashes (Dodin et al., 2013). In addition, the need for high-quality clinical studies on the effect of acupuncture on reducing sleep problems has been stated (Cheuk et al., 2012).

## 3 Phytotherapy

Phytotherapy is simply defined as the use of plants in the prevention or treatment of diseases (Şentürk, 2015). 21,000 plant species have been found suitable by WHO for therapeutic use. In order to be used in pharmacotherapy, a product – prepared from an herbal source – must be prepared from an effective and standardized extract, while the stability of the product, pharmacological and clinical findings as well as toxicological data should be determined (Çankaya, 2014). A variety of plants, in Turkey as well as in the entire world, has been used among the people for the purpose of treatment (Şentürk, 2015).

Various studies have reported that 7 % to 56 % of pregnant women use herbal treatments (Hepner et al., 2002; Holst et al., 2011). The most common cause of herbal treatment usage during pregnancy were specified as nausea in the morning, fatigue, indigestion and heartburn, colds and constipation. In their study on the safety and efficacy of phytotherapy, it was found that 57.8 % of pregnant women used herbal treatment at least once or more. The most commonly used herbs during pregnancy are ginger, cranberry, raspberry leaf, chamomile, mint and echinacea. Morning sickness, urinary tract infection and easy birth were reported as the most common cause of use (Holst et al., 2011).

Phytoestrogens (Black cohosh, red clover, etc.) are the most preferred herbal products used by menopausal women. According to the results of a compilation by Posadzki et al. (2013), black cohosh and red clover appear to be marginally effective in reducing menopausal symptoms. It has been reported that soybean may be effective in reducing the frequency and severity of hot flashes. There are Cochrane reviews present on the efficacy and safety of some herbs used in phytotherapy. According to the results of a Cochrane review, there is no conclusive evidence showing that phytoestrogen supplements effectively reduce the frequency or severity of hot flashes and night sweats (Lethaby et al., 2013).

The National Center for Complementary and Integrative Health (NIH) in the United States reported their views on phytoestrogens used in the menopausal period. According to NIH; many natural products have been studied for menopausal symptoms (phytoestrogens, black cohosh, etc.). However, none have been shown to be beneficial. There is little information about the long-term safety of natural products, and some may cause harmful side effects, or may interact with drugs. Short-term use of phytoestrogens can be labeled 'safe'; however, long-term safety has not been ensured (NIH, 2019).

## 4 Hypnosis

Hypnosis, which means "sleeping" in ancient Greek, is a state of deep physical relaxation that suspends significant abilities and can reach the subconscious. During hypnosis, it is easier to affect or influence individuals. It is known that hypnosis is used in analgesic, anesthetic and psychological treatment all over the world (Mamuk and Davas, 2010). The areas of application in women's health are primarily pain of birth, reduction of fear and stress at birth, experience of a positive birth, menopause (Elkins et al., 2013) and dysmenorrhea (Shah et al., 2014).

Hypnosis therapies can also be used in the treatment of psychosexual problems (Taştan and Işık, 2015; Mamuk and Davas, 2010; Altuntuğ, 2015).

According to a study by Atis and Rathfisch (2018) related to the effect of hypnosis in the the fear of birth and the labor pain, the experimental group experienced less labor pain and fear, the second and third stages of labor were shorter and breastfeeding has been reported to occur earlier.

According to the results reported in Cochrane, hypnosis may reduce the use of pain medication in general during labor, but it seems to reduce the use of epidurals. There is insufficient evidence for the effect of hypnosis on reducing the pain of birth or in dealing with labor pain. Higher quality research is needed (Madden et al., 2016).

According to the results of Al-Sughayir (2005), in the treatment of vaginismus, it is reported that hypnotherapy has better results than behavioral therapy in reducing sex anxiety of women and improving sexual satisfaction of their spouses. However, it is reported that there is not enough research in Cochrane (Melnik et al., 2012).

# 5 Reflexology

According to the Reflexology Institute, Reflexology is defined as a technique that is used manually (by hands) in the hands, feet and ears to reflex points, which helps normalize the body functions, and is associated with all the glands, organs and body parts (Tabur and Basaran, 2009). Reflexology is one of the most commonly used methods of complementary medicine (Lee et al., 2011).

Reflexology method can be applied in every period of women's health. It enables women to experience dysmenorrhea and Premenstrual Syndrome (which affect their quality of life at an early age) more positively while increasing overall their quality of life. In this study, reflexology was found to be effective in reducing PMS and dysmenorrhea (Lee, 2011).

Reflexology is used to treat various physiological conditions in pregnancy, including nausea and vomiting, constipation, headache, back pain, low back pain, pelvic pain and carpal tunnel syndrome (Mcneil et al., 2006; Tabur and Basaran, 2009; Poorghazneyn and Ghafari, 2006). It is reported that reflexology is effective in regulating contractions during delivery, loosening during contractions and reducing the experienced pain level (Mcneil et al., 2006). There are studies about the application of the reflexology method in the birth process and its effectiveness. In a study by Valiani et al. (2010), it has been observed that reflexology reduced the labor pain and shortened the active-phase of labor; while in the study conducted by Yılar Erkek (2018), it was determined that reflexology decreased the labor pain and accelerated the second phase of the event. Hanjani et al. (2015) found that reflexology was effective in reducing the level of anxiety and in pain management, and Mathew and Francis (2016) found that reflexology reduced the pain of labor.

Reflexology is stated to help to relax the body, rebalance of the nerve and endocrine system, reducing the symptoms of menopause, and that it is a treatment method which can help to create a smooth transition to menopause (Pinto, 2012). In studies conducted on this subject, reflexology application during menopause is reported to be effective in improving the quality of life of women (Pinto, 2012), improving sleep disorder (Asltoghiri and Ghodsi, 2012) and reducing vasomotor problems in this period (Gözüyeşil and Başer, 2016).

## 6 Homeopathy

The word origin of homeopathy comes from Greek. The word is consisted of Homoios – "like/familiar" and Pathos – "suffering". Although it is stated that the origins of the philosophy of Homeopathy are based on Hippocrates, it is stated that the basic philosophy extends to the ancient Egyptian scientists. In the 18th century, German physician Samuel Hahnemann found the principle of Homeopathy on the basis of the concept of "Familiar Suffering" (the Society of Homeopaths, 2014). Homeopathy enables the patient to be treated with the diluted concentration of the substance produced by similar symptoms. The basis of homeopathy is to mobilize our life energies and enable our body's instinct to survive, and to instill health through the instincts of being healthy (Sezer, 2015).

Homeopathy application is used during pregnancy, postpartum period, infertility treatment and menopause period. Homeopathy is practiced to alleviate the commonly experienced symptoms during pregnancy like back pain, carpal tunnel syndrome, constipation, muscle cramps, diarrhea, dizziness and fainting, frequent urination, gestational hypertension, hemorrhoids, heartburn, sleep problems, sciatica pain, sexual problems, varicose in legs and vulva, nausea, vomiting, vaginal bleeding and discharge problem. In addition to that, in postpartum period, it is used to reduce pain, breast and breastfeeding problems, problems related to urination, depression, subinvolution and abnormal lochia (Geraghty, 2002).

In a pilot study of 45 patients treated with homeopathic medication prescribed for 10.3 months in infertile men, general health status, hormone values and sperm count were evaluated. Significant results were obtained especially in oligospermia cases, sperm density, sperm percentage and sperm motility (Gerhard and Wallis, 2002).

During a research conducted by Borud et al. (2009), homeopathic medication was given to 438 women in eight countries in the menopausal period and homeopathy was found to be effective in reducing hot flashes in 90 % of the women the research was conducted upon.

## 7 Music Therapy

Music therapy is defined as the method of treatment performed under a regular method by adjusting the physiological and psychological effects of musical sounds and melodies according to various mental disorders (Gencel, 2006).

Music therapy is one of the complementary alternative therapies used in normal delivery (Cepeda et al., 2013). In studies, it was reported that music significantly decreased labor pain and anxiety at normal birth (Surucu et al., 2018), and increased the satisfaction after postnatal cesarean delivery (Chang and Chen, 2005).

Today, music therapy has been found to be effective and effective in removing anxiety in normal physiological pregnancies, in in-risk pregnant women with bed rest, in pregnant women with transvaginal ultrasonography, in pregnant women with transvaginal trauma and in removing anxiety seen in pregnant women who underwent "Non-Stress Test" (Chang et al., 2008; Yang et al., 2009; Shin and Kim, 2011; Kafali et al., 2011).

## 8 Conclusion

Traditional, complementary and alternative medicine applications contribute to solving many problems in women's health. Although these practices are becoming increasingly widespread, the number of well-designed, randomized controlled trials with sufficient power is limited. In particular, randomized controlled trials and extensive populations are needed. In addition, increasing the number of studies to be carried out on the subject is important in terms of demonstrating the effectiveness of traditional, complementary and alternative medicine applications.

Traditional, complementary and alternative medicine applications are considered as natural, complementary and alternative methods that provide holistic care. Changes in the roles and responsibilities of healthcare personnel have occurred with the increase in the scientific developments in the field of health. Healthcare workers should inform and advice women about these practices, which are generally preferred by women.

# References

Alraek, T. & Malterud, K. (2009). Acupuncture for Menopausal Hot Flashes: A Qualitative Study about Patient Experiences, *The Journal of Alternative and Complementary Medicine*, 15(2), 153–158.

Al-Sughayir, M. (2005). Vaginismus Treatment Hypnotherapy versus Behavior Therapy, *Neurosciences*, 10(2), 163–167.

Altuntuğ, K. (2015). Hipnoz ve Hipnoterapi. Başer, M. & Taşçı, S (eds.), *Kanıta Dayalı Rehberleriyle Tamamlayıcı ve Destekleyici Uygulamalar*, (pp. 3–7), Ankara: Akademisyen Kitabevi.

Asltoghiri, M. & Ghodsi, Z. (2012). The Effects of Reflexology on Sleep Disorder in Menopausal Women. *Procedia-Social and Behavioral Sciences*, 31, 242–246.

Atis, F.Y. & Rathfischb, G. (2018). The Effect of Hypnobirthing Training Given in the Antenatal Period on Birth Pain and Fear. *Complementary Therapies in Clinical Practice*, 33, 77–84. doi: 10.1016/j.ctcp.2018.08.004

Avis, N.E., Legault, C., Coeytaux, R.R., Pian-Smith, M., Shifren, J.L., Chen, W. & Valaskatgis, P. (2008). A Randomized, Controlled Pilot Study of Acupuncture Treatment for Menopausal Hot Flashes. *Menopause*, 15, 1070–1078. doi: 10.1097/gme.0b013e31816d5b03

Bordet, M., Colas, A., Marijnen, P., Masson, J. & Trichad, M. (2008). Treating Hot Flushes in Menopausal Women with Homeopathic Treatment – Result of Observational Study. *Homeopathy*, 97(1), 10–15.

Borud, E.K., Alreak, T., White, A., Fonnebo, V., Eggen, A.E. & Grimsgaard, S. (2009). The Acupuncture on Hot Flushes among Menopausal Women (ACUFLASH) Study. A Randomized Controlled Trial. *Menopause*, 16(3), 484–493. doi: 10.1097/gme.0b013e31818c02ad

Çağlayan, H.Z.B., Ataoğlu, E.E. & Kibaroğlu, S. (2018). Nörolojide Geleneksel ve Tamamlayıcı Tıp Uygulamalarının Etkinliğinin Değerlendirilmesi. *Turkish Journal of Neurology*, 24, 111–116.

Çankaya, İ.T. (2014). Fitoterapi'ye Genel Yaklaşım. Kalaycı, M.Z., *Geleneksel, Tamamlayıcı ve Alternatif Tıp Uygulamalarına Uluslararası Bakış Konferans Bildirisi*, T.C. Sağlık Bakanlığı Yayınları, Pozitif Matbaa: İstanbul.

Cepeda, M.S., Carr, D.P., Lau, J. & Alvarez, H. (2013). Music for Pain Labor (Review). *Cochrane Database of Systematic Reviews*, doi: 10.1002/14651858. CD004843.pub3

Chang, M.Y., Chen, C.H. & Huang, K.F. (2008). Effects of Music Therapy on Psychological Health of Women during Pregnancy. *Journal of Clinical Nursing*, 17(19), 2580–2587.

Chang, S.C. & Chen, C.H. (2005). Effects of Music Therapy on Women's Physiologic Measures, Anxiety and Satisfaction during Cesarean Delivery, *Research in Nursing and Health*, 28, 453–461.

Chen, Y., Zhang, X., Fang, Y. & Yang, J. (2014). Analyzing the Study of Using Acupuncture in Delivery in the Past Ten Years in China. *Evidence Based Complementary Alternative Medicine*, 2014, 1–8. doi: 10.1155/2014/672508

Cheuk, D.K.L., Yeung, W.F., Chung, K.F. & Wong, V. (2012). Acupuncture for Insomnia (Review). *Cochrane Database of Systematic Reviews*, 9, CD005472.

Cho, S.H., Lee, H. & Ernst, E. (2010). Acupuncture for Pain Relief in Labour: A Systematic Review and Meta-analysis. *BJOG*, 117, 907–920. doi:10.1111/j.1471-0528.2010.02570.x

Chung, K.F., Yeung, W.F., Zhang, Z.J., Yung, K.P., Man, S.C. & Taam Wong, V. (2012). Randomized Non-invasive Sham-Controlled Pilot Trial of Electroacupuncture for Postpartum Depression. *Journal of Affective Disorder*, 142, 115–121. doi: 10.1016/j.jad.2012.04.008

Dodin, S., Blanchet, C., Marc, I., Ernst, E., Wu, T. & Maunsell, E. (2013). Acupuncture for Menopausal Hot Flushes, *Cochrane Database of Systematic Reviews*, 1–87.

Elkins, G.R., Fisher, W.I., Johnson, A.K., Carpenter, J.S. & Keith, T.Z. (2013). Clinical Hypnosis in the Treatment of Post-menopausal Hot Flashes: A Randomized Controlled Trial. *Menopause*, 20(3), 1–16.

Gaudet, L.M., Dyzak, R., Aung, S.K. & Smith, G.N. (2008). Effectiveness of Acupuncture for the Initiation of Labour at Term: A Pilot Randomized Controlled Trial. *Journal of Obstetrics and Gynaecology Canada*, 30, 1118–1123.

Gençel, Ö. (2006). Müzikle Tedavi. *Kastamonu Eğitim Dergisi*, 14(2), 697–706.

Geraghty, B. (Ed.) (2002). *Homeopathy for Midwives*, 2nd ed., Churchill Livingstone Elsevier Science Limited, USA.

Gerhard, I. & Wallis, E. (2002). Individualized Homeopathic Therapy for Male Infertility. *Homeopathy*, 91(3), 133–44.

Gözüyeşil, E. & Başer, M. (2016). The Effect of Foot Reflexology Applied to Women Aged Between 40 And 60 on Vasomotor Complaints and Quality of Life. *Complementary Therapies in Clinical Practice*, 24, 78–85.

Hanjani, S., Tourzani, Z. & Shoghi, M. (2015). The Effect of Foot Reflexology on Anxiety, Pain and Outcomes of the Labor in Primigravida Women. *Acta Medica Iranica*, 53(8): 507–511.

Hepner, D.L., Harnett, M., Segal, S., Camann, W., Bader, A.M. & Tsen, L.C. (2002). Herbal Medicine Use in Parturients. *Anesthesia & Analgesia*, 94(3), 690–693.

Holst, L., Wright, D., Haavik, S. & Nordeng, H. (2011). Safety and Efficacy of Herbal Remedies in Obstetrics-Review and Clinical Implications. *Midwifery*, 27(1), 80–86.

Kafali, H., Derbent, A, Keskin, E., Simavli, S. & Gözdemir, E. (2011). Effect of Maternal Anxiety and Music on Fetal Movements and Fetal Heart Rate Patterns. *Journal of Maternal-Fetal and Neonatal Medicine*, 24(3), 461–464.

Kim, D., Jong, J.C., Kim, K.H., Rho, J.J., Choi, M.S. & Lee, M.S. (2011). Acupuncture for Hot Flushes in Perimenopausal and Postmenopausal Women: A Randomised, Shamcontrolled Trial. *Acupuncture in Medicine*, 29, 249–256.

Lee, J., Han, M., Chung, Y., Kim, J. & Choi, J. (2011). Effects of Foot Reflexology on Fatigue, Sleep and Pain: A Systematic Review and Meta-analysis. *Journal of Korean Academy of Nursing*, 41(6), 821–833.

Lee, Y.M. (2011). Effects of Aroma-Foot-Reflexology on Premenstrual Syndrome, Dysmenorrhea and Lower Abdominal Skin Temperature of Nursing Students. *Korean Journal of Adult Nursing*, 23(5), 472–481.

Lethaby, A., Marjoribanks, J., Kronenberk, F., Roberts, H., Eden, J. & Brown, J. (2013) Phytoestrogens for Menopausal Vasomotor Symptoms, *Cochrane Database Systematic Reviews*, 12, 1–130.

Lim, C.E.D., Wilkinson, J.M., Wong, W.S.F. & Cheng, N.C.L. (2009). Effect of Acupuncture on Induction of Labor. *The Journal of Alternative and Complementary Medicine*, 15(11), 1209–1214.

Lindquist, R., Snyder, M., & Tracy, M. F. (2014). Complementary and Alternative Therapies in Nursing (7th ed.). New York: Springer Publishing Company, LLC.

Madden, K., Middleton, P., Cyna, A.M., Matthewson, M. & Jones, L. (2016). Hypnosis for Pain Management during Labour and Childbirth. *Cochrane Database of Systematic Reviews*, 5, 1–4.

Mamuk, R. & Davas, N.İ. (2010). Doğum Ağrısının Kontrolünde Kullanılan Nonfarmakolojik Gevşeme ve Tensel Uyarılma Yöntemleri. *Şişli Etfal Hastanesi Tıp Bülteni*, 44(3), 137–144.

Mathew, A. & Francis. F. (2016). Effectiveness of Foot Reflexology in Reduction of Labour Pain among Mothers in Labour Admitted at PSG Hospital, Coimbatore. *International Journal of Nursing Education*, 8(3), 11–16.

Mcneill, J.A., Alderdice, F.A. & Mcmurray, F.A. (2006). Retrospective Cohort Study Exploring the Relationship between Antenatal Reflexology and Complementary Therapies in Clinical Intranatal Outcomes. *Practice*, 12, 119–122.

Melnik, T., Howton, K. & McGuire, H. (2012). Interventions for Vaginismus Cochrane Systematic Review. *Intervention Version Published*, 12, 1–3.

Modlock, J., Nielsen, B.B. & Uldbjerg, N. (2010). Acupuncture for the Induction of Labour: A Double-Blind Randomised Controlled Study. *BJOG*, 117, 1255–1261.

Mucuk, S. & Ceyhan, Ö. (2011). Akupres. Başer, M., & Taşçı, S. (eds.), *Kanıta Dayalı Rehberleriyle Tamamlayıcı ve Destekleyici Uygulamalar*, Ankara: Akademisyen Kitabevi.

NIH. *Menopausal Symptoms: In Depth*. https://nccih.nih.gov/health/menopause/menopausesymptoms (accessed on 01.01.2019).

Oakley, S.H., Liu, J.W., Crisp, C.C. & Pauls, R.N. (2016). Acupuncture in Premenopausal Women with Hypoactive Sexual Desire Disorder: A Prospective Chort Pilot Study. *Sexual Medicine*, 4, 176–181.

Oral, B., Öztürk, A., Balcı, E. & Sevinç, N. (2016). Aile Sağlığı Merkezine Başvuranların Geleneksel /Alternatif Tıpla İlgili Görüşleri Ve Kullanım Durumu. *TAF Preventive Medicine Bulletin*, 15(2), 75–82.

Painovich, J.M., Shufelt, C.L., Azziz, R., Yang, Y. et al. (2012). Pilot Randomized, Single-Blind, Placebo-Controlled Trial of Traditional Acupuncture for Vasomotor Symptoms and Mechanistic Pathways of Menopause. *Menopause*, 19(1), 54–61.

Pınto, P.C. & Paul, S. (2012). Effect of Foot Reflexology on the Quality of Life among Menopausal Women in Selected Schools in Mangalore. *National Junior Honor Society*, 2(3), 75–79.

Poorghazneyn, T. & Ghafarı, F. (2006). The Effect of Reflexology on the Intensity of Fatigue on Pregnant Women Referred to Health Center of Ramsar City. *Nursing and Midwifery Journal*, 12, 5–11.

Posadzki, P., Lee, M.S., Moon, T.V., Choi, T.Y., Park, T.Y. & Ernst, E. (2013). Prevalence of Complementary and Alternative Medicine (Cam) Use by Menopausal Women: A Systematic Review of Surveys. *Maturitas*, 75(1), 34–43.

Şahin, S. (2017). Geleneksel, Tamamlayıcı, Alternatif Tıp Uygulamalarına Genel Bir Bakış, *Türk Aile Hek Derg*, 21(4), 159–162.

Şentürk, S. (2015). Fitoterapi. Başer M, Taşçı S (eds.), *Kanıta Dayalı Rehberleriyle Tamamlayıcı ve Destekleyici Uygulamalar*, Ankara: Akademisyen Kitabevi.

Sezer, Ö. (2015). Türkiye'de Yeni Parlayan Bir Integratif Tıp Yöntemi: Homeopati. *Eurasian Journal of Family Medicine*, 4(1), 1–6.

Shah, M., Monga, A., Patel, S., Shah, M. & Bakshi, H. (2014). The Effect of Hypnosis on Dysmenorrhea. *International Journal of Clinical Experimental Hypnosis*, 62(2), 164–178.

Shin, H.S. & Kim, J.H. (2011). Music Therapy on Anxiety, Stress and Maternal-Fetal Attachment in Pregnant Women during Transvaginal Ultrasound. *Asian Nursing Research*, 5(1), 19–27.

Smith, C.A. & Cochrane, S. (2009). Does Acupuncture Have a Place as an Adjunct Treatment during Pregnancy? A Review of Randomized Controlled Trials and Systematic Reviews. *Birth*, 36, 246–253.

Soliday, E. & Hapke, P. (2013). Research on Acupuncture in Pregnancy and Childbirth: The U.S. Contribution. *Medical Acupuncture*, 25, 252–260.

Somer, P. & Vatanoğlu-Lutz, E.E. (2017). Geleneksel ve Tamamlayıcı Tıp Uygulamaları Yönetmeliği'nin Hukuki ve Etik Açıdan Değerlendirilmesi. *Anadolu Kliniği*, 22(1), 58–65.

Sönmez, C.I., Başer, D.A., Küçükdağ, H.N., Kayar, O., Acar, İ. & Güner, P.D. (2018). Tıp Fakültesi Öğrencilerinin Geleneksel Ve Tamamlayıcı Tıp İle İlgili Bilgi Durumlarının ve Davranışlarının Değerlendirilmesi. *Konuralp Tıp Dergisi*, 10(3), 276–281.

Surucu, Ş.G., Oztürk, M., Vurgeç, A.B., Alan, S. & Akbaş, M. (2018). The Effect of Music on Pain and Anxiety of Women during Labour on First Time Pregnancy: A Study from Turkey. *Complementary Therapies in Clinical Practice*, 30, 96–102.

Tabur, H. & Başaran, E.B.Z. (2009). *Refleksolojiye Giriş*, İstanbul: Ezgi Matbaacılık.

Taşçı, E. & Sevil, Ü. (2007). Doğum Ağrısına Yönelik Farmakolojik Olmayan Yaklaşımlar. *Genel Tıp Dergisi*, 17(3), 81–86.

Taştan, K. & Işık, M. (2015). Vajinusmus Tedavisinde Hipnoterapi: Bir Olgu Sunumu. *Ankara Medical Journal*, 15(1), 35–7.

The Society of Homeopaths. (2014). About Homeopathy. http://www.homeopathy-soh.org/about-homeopathy (accessed on 21.01.2019).

Turan, N., Öztürk, A. & Kaya, N. (2010). Hemşirelikte Yeni Bir Sorumluluk Alanı: Tamamlayıcı Terapi. *Maltepe Üniversitesi Hemşirelik Bilim ve Sanatı Dergisi*, 3, 94–97.

Valiani, M., Shiran, E. & Hasanpour, M. (2010). Reviewing the Effect of Reflexology on the Pain and Certain Features and Outcomes of the Labor on the Primiparous Women. *Iranian Journal of Nursing and Midwifery Research*, 15, 302–310.

WHO. (2000). *General Guidelines for Methodologies on Research and Evaluation of Traditional Medicine*, Geneva.

WHO. (2014). *Traditional Medicine Strategy 2014-2023*. www.who.int/topics/traditional_medicine/en/ (accessed on 01.01.2019).

Yang, M., Li, L., Zhu, H., Alexander, I.M, Liu, S., Zhou, W. & Ren, X. (2009). Music Therapy to Relieve Anxiety in Pregnant Women on Bedrest: A Randomized, Controlled Trial MCN. *American Journal of Maternal/Child Nursing*, 34(5), 316-323.

Yılar Erkek, Z. & Pasinlioğlu, T. (2018). Ayak Refleksolojisinin Doğum Ağrısına ve Doğum Eyleminin Süresine Etkisi. Uluslararası *Hakemli Kadın Hastalıkları ve Anne Çocuk Sağlığı Dergisi*, 12, 1-24.

Fatma Başar

# 6: Complementary and Alternative Medicine Applications in Infertility[1]

## 1 Introduction

Fertility is one of the key factors of reproductive health; infertility is accepted as a global public health concern by the World Health Organization (WHO). Infertility is defined as the absence of pregnancy in spite of having sexual intercourse during at least one year by couples at reproduction age. The frequency of infertility varies from region to region and country to country. From 2010 data of the World Health Organization, 15 % of couples at reproductive age are affected by infertility. The frequency of infertility in our country is 10 %–20 %. Infertility that is an important health problem is a situational crisis which threatens the psychosocial state and is hard to be managed; it also affects both family and society. Moreover, infertility causes psychosocial, economic and sexual problems on couples.

Patients are in the tendency to use complementary and alternative medicine applications to increase the change to be pregnant. National Complementary and Alternative Medical Center defined complementary and alternative medicine as various medical attention, products or disciplines that are not accepted as a part of conventional medicine. Use of complementary and supportive care applications have increased during the infertility process in recent years. A part of couples appeal to complementary medicine applications before and during infertility treatment and also after unsuccessful treatments. Moreover, since patients actualize these applications under their own control, the anxiety level of patients decreases; this situation positively contributes to the treatment. More than 50 % of the population in Europe, North America and other industrial countries used complementary medicine applications at least once. Edirne et al. (2010) conducted a study on infertile women and pointed out that 82 % of related women used Complementary Alternative Medicine (CAM) application at least once. Healthcare professionals have serious responsibilities such as informing patients and healthy individuals about effective use of complementary and supportive care applications; giving psychosocial support; providing and maintaining effective team communication. It was aimed to express the areas of

---

1 This chapter was presented at the 4th International Scientific Research Congress as an oral presentation (February 14–17, 2019, Yalova, Turkey).

usage and efficiency of complementary and alternative medicine applications in this chapter.

## 2 Complementary and Alternative Medicine Applications in Infertility

### 2.1 Nutrition and Life Style Change

Having a normal body mass index (BMI) and keeping a balanced diet positively contribute to the success of the treatment of infertile patients. With reference to the study of Barbieri (2001), infertility risk increases when BMI is higher than 27 kg/m$^2$ or lower than 17 kg/m$^2$. Martini et al. (2010) conducted a research on 794 male patients and found a negative relationship between BMI and sperm motility with sperm rate.

The goal of a healthy life is not only for avoiding any disease or disorder but also improving the general state of health and wellbeing. Improving healthy lifestyle and the general state of health have a remarkable place in avoiding infertility and bringing fertility skill to an ideal level. It is extremely important to avoid changeable habits, behaviors or situations (smoking and alcohol abuse, caffeine, drug addiction, obesity, weakness, exercise, environmentally hazardous substances/occupation, stress) that negatively affect fertility, taking required precautions and getting individuals adopt positive health habits.

### 2.2 Vitamins and Minerals

Vitamins and Minerals (Fe, Folic acid) are required for a healthy pregnancy period and becoming pregnant. Nalavade et al. (2016) analyzed the effect of diet and food consumption on fertility. For research findings, infertile women take less iron, zinc, folic acid, calories and protein in comparison with fertile women.

There are sources about Selenium, Zinc and Indian ginseng use and also antioxidant-rich food consumption like vitamin E and coenzyme to improve semen parameters with malefactors. Twenty six studies including infertile male patients were analyzed; research results show that the treatment of antioxidant (vitamin E, vitamin C, carnitines, N-acetyl cysteine, co-enzyme Q10, zinc, selenium, folic acid and lycopene) has a significant positive effect on basic semen parameters, advanced sperm functions, assisted reproductive therapy results and live birth ratio.

### 2.3 Herbal Methods

Sis Çelik and Kırca (2018) analyzed complementary and supportive care applications that are used by infertile women and they also expressed that the majority of women (65 %) eat or drink a herbal mix (including foalfoot, horse-tail, Urtica urens, onion juice, royal jelly, propolis and locust pekmez). In the same research, 37.9 % of women expressed that the commonly used herbal mix is onion juice cure. For the related research's results, 95.7 % of women who apply complementary or supportive care applications do not tell the physician about this cure; 51.8 % of the same women use the herbal mixes with medications given by the physician.

A systematic review was performed by Tan et al. (2012) to scrutinize the effect and reliability of China herbal medicine. For research findings, China herbal medicine significantly increases pregnancy ratios. Besides, there was seen an increase in ovulation, decrease in a number of aborts and a recovery in cervical mucus.

In Turkey, Ayaz and Efe (2010) made research on infertile women and found that 27,3 % of related women have tried a traditional application. Those traditional applications are the intravaginal applications (i.e wool, garlic and olive oil) such as herbal mixtures (67,8 %), pulling the dorsi (41 %), herbal ovules and sitting on the herbal mixture (dead nettle, daisy, mint, etc.) (16,9 %).

## 2.4 Acupuncture

Turkish Language Society defines acupuncture as 'the treatment that is administered by pricking in specific points of the body' (Edirne et al., 2010). Acupuncture use in infertility treatment has increased in the last 15 years (Majzoub and Agarwal, 2018). It is applied on meridian points consonant with the energy flow throughout the body. Acupuncture points are selected based on the traditional Chinese medicine by diagnosis and symptoms peculiar to the patient.

Zhu et al. (2018) applied acupuncture to a couple of women and men once a week for three months. It is pointed out in a related study that acupuncture is a successful treatment in regaining the fertility by balancing the endocrine system and hormones also by improving the quality of sperm and ovarian function. The effect of acupuncture on the pregnancy ratio in patients who receive assisted reproductive therapy was scrutinized by Paulus et al. (2002). While there was found clinical pregnancy in 34 (42.5 %) of 80 patients in the group who received acupuncture treatment, pregnancy ratio was only 26.3 % (21 of 80 patients) in the control group.

## 2.5 Mind-Body-Energy Medicine and Aromatherapy

Mind-body medicine focuses on brain, mind, body and behaviors besides emotional, social and mental factors that directly affect human health. They are relaxation, hypnosis, yoga, meditation, cognitive-behavioral therapies, group supports, autogenic training, spirituality, biofeedback and escapism strategies. Domar et al. (2011) had a study on 143 women; they found that pregnancy ratios in women who were applied mind-body therapy with IVF treatment were higher. While the pregnancy ratio in women who were only applied IVF treatment was 20 %, this same ratio was found as 43 % in the group who received IVF treatment with mind/body therapy.

## 2.6 Hypnosis

Hypnosis is to create changes in emotions, thoughts and memories of individuals via techniques like suggestions. Using hypnosis for medical purpose is hypnotherapy. Hypnosis is utilized in popular medicine and psychotherapy. Moreover, it has also been used in the infertility treatment process. Levitas et al. (2006) reviewed the pregnancy and implantation ratio of hypnosis that is implemented during embryo transfer and found pregnancy and implantation ratios are higher in patients who were applied hypnotherapy (D:53 %, K:30 %).

## 2.7 Yoga

This is an aerobics that includes breath techniques, meditation, relaxation and exercises, which provide flexibility for muscles. Yoga also provides infertile couples to mentally relax, steer away from the stressful event by decreasing anxiety and also be more patient. Kırca and Pasinlioğlu (2019) emphasized that yoga increased the success of treatment by reducing stress in infertile women. It is seen in research of Darbandi et al. (2017) that yoga increases the success rate of assisted reproductive techniques. However, there is a need for more studies on this issue.

## 2.8 Massage

Massage is one of the commonly used methods in infertility treatment. It reduces the fluidity of blood, blood pressure and level of stress. Fourteen infertile women in the 25–44 age group were applied an intense pelvic massage treatment by physiotherapists in the research by Wurn et al. (2004). There was earned 70 % of success in infertility treatment arising from cohesion.

## 2.9 Energy Medicine

Voice, music, prayer, electromagnetic power and rays are used in this application as well as the application manners may vary by culture to culture. It is called as discharging, external energy, life force and life energy. Voice and music that are utilized to minimize the stressful situations interfere with mind-body medicine field; studies in this domain remain incapable.

## 2.10 Aromatherapy

It is known as aromatic compounds obtained from volatile oils and plants. This method that was first used in cancer and palliative care increases the life quality and decreases the psychological distress. Aromatherapy provides relaxation and is used with other treatments.

## 2.11 Homeopathy

Homeopathy is a method that activates the body's own resilience. It is a scientific system that was developed by Dr. Samuel Hahnemann in Germany in the 18th century and it helps the body to heal itself naturally. 'Cure the similar by the similar' is the basic principle of homeopathy. There are more than 300 types of medicine in homeopathy; while almost 200 of them is used for infertility, 179 of the same medications are utilized for abort treatment. It is seen that the activities of homeopathy can be more effective when it is used with other adjuvant therapies.

## 2.12 Reflexology

Reflexology is an old and noninvasive method that is used in a widespread manner. It is defined as a holistic recovery technique that compounds body, mind and soul. The goal in reflexology is to ensure more food and oxygen pass to the cells as a result of increased blood flow and relaxation by using pressure techniques to foot, hand and ear. Holt et al. (2009) conducted a survey on 49 infertile patients and found that while pregnancy ratio was 15 % in patients who were applied reflexology, pregnancy ratio of the placebo group was found as 9 %. However, there is a need for more studies on this topic because of the lack of sufficient samples and available restrictions in blinding the groups.

# 3 Conclusion

It is essential for the physician, nurse and midwives in health facilities with beds to be informed about CAM methods and consult for patient and patient's relatives on these methods. Medical personnel need to know the advantages and disadvantages of CAM methods. They should observe whether possible adverse effects arise. In addition to all these, also healthy people use these methods today. Therefore, this issue is among the topics that need to be considered in terms of community health care; healthcare professionals have remarkable responsibilities here.

The use of complementary and supportive care applications has increased in infertility treatment day by day. Complementary and supportive care implementations may vary from country to country and from society to society. It is observed that people whose educational level is low and who live in a rural region prefer related applications more. Medical personnel have serious duties in terms of informing healthy individuals and patients about effective use of complementary and supportive care applications; giving psychosocial support and providing and maintaining effective team communication. Moreover, individuals who use these techniques should be encouraged about sharing their methods with the health care providers.

## References

Ayaz, S. & Yaman Efe, S. (2010). Traditional Practices Used by Infertile Women in Turkey, *International Nursing Review*, 57(3), 383–387.

Darbandi, S., Darbandi, M., Khorram Khorshid, H.R. & Sadeghi, M.R. (2017). Yoga Can Improve Assisted Reproduction Technology Outcomes in Couples with Infertility, *Alternative Therapies in Health and Medicine*, 24(4), 50–55.

Domar, A.D., Rooney, K.L., Wiegand, B., Orav, E.J., Alper, M.M., Berger, B.M. & Nikolovski, J. (2011). Impact of a Group Mind/Body Intervention on Pregnancy Rates in IVF Patients, *Fertility and Sterility*, 95(7), 2269–2273.

Edirne, T., Gunher Arica, S., Gucuk, S., Yildizhan, R., Kolusari, A., Adali, E. & Can, M. (2010). Use of Complementary and Alternative Medicines by a Sample of Turkish Women for Infertility Enhancement: A Descriptive Study, *Complementary and Alternative Medicine*, 10(11), 1–7.

Holt, J., Lord, J., Acharya, U., White, A., O'Neill, N., Shaw, S., et al. (2009). The Effectiveness of Foot Reflexology in Inducing Ovulation: A Sham-Controlled Randomized Trial, *Fertility and Sterility*, 91(6), 2514–2519.

Kırca, N. & Pasinlioğlu, T. (2019). The Effect of Yoga on Stress Level in Infertile Women, *Perspectives in Psychiatric Care*, 55(2), 319–327.

Levitas, E., Parmet, A., Lunenfeld, E., Bentov, Y., Burstein, E., Friger, M., et al. (2006). Impact of Hypnosis during Embryo Transfer on the Out Come of In Vitro Fertilization-Embryo Transfer: A Case-Control Study, *Fertility and Sterility*, 85(5), 1404–1408.

Majzoub, A. & Agarwal, A. (2018). Systematic Review of Antioxidant Types and Doses in Male Infertility: Benefits on Semen Parameters, Advanced Sperm Function, Assisted Reproduction and Live-Birth Rate, *Arab Journal of Urology*, 16, 113–124.

Martini, A.C., Tissera, A., Estofán, D., Molina, R.I., Mangeaud, A., de Cuneo, M.F. & Ruiz, R.D. (2010). Overweight and Seminal Quality: A Study of 794 Patients, *Fertility and Sterility*, 94(5), 1739–1743.

Nalavade, D., Shekar, A. & Shah, K. (2016). Effect of Diet and Nutrient Intake on Women Who Have Problems of Fertility, *International Journal of Pure & Applied Bioscience*, 4(4), 198–204.

Paulus, W.E., Zhang, M., Strehler, E., El-Danasouri, I. & Sterzik, K. (2002). Influence of Acupuncture on the Pregnancy Rate in Patients Who Undergo Assisted Reproduction Therapy, *Fertility and Sterility*, 77(4), 721–724.

Robert, L. & Barbieri, M.D. (2001). The Initial Fertility Consultation: Recommendations Concerning Cigarette Smoking, Body Mass Index, and Alcohol and Caffeine Consumption, *American Journal of Obstetrics and Gynecology*, 185(5), 1168–1173.

Sis Çelik, A. & Kırca, N. (2018). İnfertil Kadınların Uyguladıkları Tamamlayıcı ve Destekleyici Bakım Uygulamaları, *Anadolu Hemşirelik ve Sağlık Bilimleri Dergisi*, 21(3), 178–188.

Tan, L., Tong, Y., Sze, C.W., Xu, M., Shi, Y., Song, X.Y. & Zhang, T.T. (2012). Chinese Herbal Medicine for Infertility with Anovulation: A Systematic Review, *The Journal of Alternative and Complementary Medicine*, 18(12), 1087–1100.

Wurn, B.F., Wurn, L.J., King, C.R., Heuer, M.A., Roscow, A.S., Scharf, E.S. & Shuster, J.J. (2004). Treating Female Infertility and Improving IVF Pregnancy Rates with a Manual Physical Therapy Technique, *Medscape General Medicine*, 6(2), 51.

Zhu, J., Arsovska, B. & Kozovska, K. (2018). Acupuncture Treatment for Fertility, *Journal of Medical Science*, 6(9), 1685–1687.

Filiz Süzer Özkan

# 7: Methods Used in Childbirth Education and Current Approaches

## 1 Introduction

Birth as a normal, natural and healthy action, it is a very special experience for the new born (baby), the mother and her spouse. The aim of antenatal education given during pregnancy is to protect the health of the mother and the baby by giving specific information about pregnancy, birth, postpartum and neonatal period (İşbir et al., 2015). At birth, the goal (independent of the form of birth) is the birth of a healthy baby, a healthy mother and an exuberant birth moment. The aim of childbirth education is to inform the mother and father through the trainings before birth, to reveal their expectations from birth, to ease and relieve the birth pain with relaxation and breathing exercises, to provide the information, support and care needed in this process to determine their preferences about the method of delivery, and to ensure their active participation in delivery (Buran, 2015; İşbir et al., 2015). The foundation of the methods used in childbirth education was taken by Grantly Dick Read in the 1930s to discover the importance of fear at birth and to create the circle of Fear-Tension-Pain (Mongan, 2016). The most well-known and applied methods in the world are "Lamaze", "Bradley", "HypnoBirthing-Mongan Method" and "Active Birth" method (Onat Bayram and Şahin, 2010; Buran, 2015; Serçekuş and Yenal, 2015). "Mindfulness-Based Birth and Parenthood" and "Birthing from Within" are the other methods that are preferred and used in recent years (Onat Bayram and Şahin, 2010; Buran, 2015). Apart from these methods being implemented the "Birth with No Regret Model" that's been implemented in Turkey since 2011 (Coker et al., 2015) will be described in detail below in conjunction with other methods.

## 2 "Birth with No Regret" Model and Team

"Birth with No Regret" model that has been implemented since 2011 in Turkey was created by considering multidisciplinary approach; it is a method that is led by physician-midwife-birth psychotherapist.

"Birth with No Regret" is defined as a method of birth where the families were given childbirth education, the birth starts spontaneously as long as there was no medical obstacle, the natural hormones are actively secreted, no intervention is made as much as possible and where no one who witnessed the occasion (mother, father, baby, midwife, physician and other people) would leave it with a "no regret" feeling or any sort of regret. The aim of the method, regardless of the method of delivery, is for every mother to receive uninterrupted support before and during the childbirth, and become stronger afterwards. "Birth with No Regret" is more of an approach than a technique (Coker et al., 2015).

With "Birth with No Regret" model, during the preparation of the mother and/or the family for the childbirth:

- The whole team (physician, midwife, birth psychologist) works together and everyone has a backup when necessary,
- Family participates in 18 hours of preparation for childbirth based on physical preparation and mental purification,
- The mother makes the necessary sessions with the birth psychologist (at least 4). Father and grandmothers must work with a birth psychologist,
- Mother's birth preferences are always at the forefront. With education, active participation of families is ensured,
- Except for the emergencies, decisions are taken together by the team and the family,
- If there is no medical obstacle, birth starts spontaneously,
- Women act freely in the course of the action, not hungry unless they are necessary,
- They give active birth in any position including water birth,
- Fathers take an active role in childbirth,
- Time is taken at birth. Non-drug relaxing techniques are used during contractions,
- The babies meet the mothers' arms as soon as they are born. The first treatments are done in the mother's chest. Time is given for first breastfeeding,
- Other than the mother and father, relatives do not come to the hospital until the birth, even if they do, they do not visit the delivery unit of the hospital.
- If necessary with the consent of the family, "Birth with No Regret" method does not reject interventions and epidural analgesia,
- If cesarean section is required, the "Mother/Father/Baby Friendly Cesarean section" can be applied. During the surgery, the father can be present if they wish to do so. The baby always stays in the mother's arms during and after the surgery (Coker et al., 2015).

The "Birth with No Regret" team consists of:

**Physician**: protects the health of the mother and the baby in accordance with the information based on evidence-based medicine.

**Midwife**: the midwife – who has already met the family – makes home visits. According to the family's preference, when the birth starts, she comes back to home. She gives medical and physical support in the latent phase of labor. During the active period of labor, she helps the family to safely transfer to the hospital. Basic follow-up and one-to-one support during the birth is done by the midwife. She uses all non-drug relaxing techniques during support. If the harmony between the mother and her spouse is good, she supports the father to take an active role. She observes the needs of both. The midwife also informs the physician about the medical issues. The second day after birth, she makes home visits. If there are any shortcomings in breastfeeding and baby care, she resolves them while observing the general satisfaction of the mother about the birth.

**Birth Psychologist**: gives psychological support to the family and to the birth team during pregnancy and delivery. The goal is to resolve all the anxiety and questions of the expectant mother during pregnancy and to make her feel fearless. For this purpose, individual sessions are performed and traumas in the history of the mother and father are examined. Individual interviews are made with granny, grandmother or even other family members if necessary. If any subconscious process that stops or slows down at birth occurs, the Birth Psychologist performs the necessary therapeutic intervention during delivery, provides psychological support to the family members waiting in the hospital and balances the team's compliance with other health personnel in the hospital. Regardless of the type of childbirth, the Birth Psychologist allows the whole team to leave without regret or the feeling of "If Only" for any reason. This support eases the work of the team, especially in difficult situations (Coker et al., 2015).

Birth-with-No-Regret service is given today in six different provinces in Turkey (Istanbul, Manisa, İzmir, Denizli, Aydın and Antalya), and in eleven centers. To be a "Birth with No Regret Center"; 200 hours of theoretical and practical applications are taken, which consists of "Childbirth Educator" training and a "Doula" training. During the training, a group consisting of at least 6 couples should give childbirth. While providing prenatal training, one-to-one supervision is received from the founders of Istanbul Delivery Academy (IDA) regarding the two deliveries attended after the training for four times. When they want to become a Birth with No Regret Center, they should prepare and work together through 4 births together with IDA founders. After becoming Birth with No Regret Centers, while they continue helping families (who demand) with standard childbirth procedures, they help families who demand "Birth with No Regret" method to be practiced during childbirth as midwife/doula and Birth Psychologists alongside teams consisted of IDA graduates (Keşkesiz Doğum Merkezleri, 2019).

## 3 HypnoBirthing-Mongan Method

HypnoBirthing-Mongan Method was developed by Marie Mongan and was defined in her first book, "HypnoBirthing: A Life of Celebration" (1989) (Varner, 2015). HypnoBirthing® Institute, founded by Marie Mongan at the same year, is still active.

Mongan, who dreams of having a safe and satisfactory birth for each woman and her baby, began by applying the HypnoBirthing method on her own daughter for the first time after adding the title of hypnotherapist to her experiences of childbirth. Her grandson Kyle, born in 1990, was the first to be born through the HypnoBirthing method (Onat Bayram and Şahin, 2010; Varner, 2015; Mongan 2016).

HypnoBirthing: The method is actually a birth philosophy as well as a technique that believes that birth is a normal, natural and healthy action for women (Walker et al., 2009; Onat Bayram and Şahin, 2010; Mongan 2016; HypnoBirthing Institute, 2019). HypnoBirthing philosophy believes that "women's bodies are created to conceive, to develop and give birth to their babies" and it aims to help mothers to give birth gently and comfortably (Onat Bayram ve Şahin, 2010; Varner, 2015; Mongan, 2016). The method has been developed as a training process that includes breathing, relaxation, visualization, meditative practice, attention to nutrition and using positive language (Mongan, 2016; HypnoBirthing Institute, 2019). "Relaxation Breath" and "Wave Breath" techniques are the most important elements of the method (Mongan, 2016). In training, the woman is taught how to release fear, thoughts and feelings that cause pain and strained muscles at birth. With HypnoBirthing, the mother is awake, aware and fully under control when she is giving birth – not in trance or sleep, but in deep relaxation (HypnoBirthing Institute, 2019).

HypnoBirthing practitioners are available in 45 countries worldwide (HypnoBirthing Institute, 2019). Courses consist of five weeks, textures, relaxation CD and everything you need to experience a wonderful birth experience (Walker, 2009; HypnoBirthing Institute 2019).

Mongan method led to the recognition in Turkey by Hakan Çoker, an obstetrician, in 2009, when he organized the Hypnobirthing course with the international participation of HypnoBirthing® Institute, after his participation in training in Scotland (Serçekuş and Yenal, 2015; Mongan, 2016).

## 4 Lamaze Method

Lamaze Method was started in 1951 by French obstetrician Fernand Lamaze. Dr. Lamaze was influenced by Ivan Pavlov, known for his scientific work on

Conditional Reflexes. Lamaze method consists of childbirth education, relaxation and breathing techniques. After reading the book of Dick-Read in the late 1950s, Marjorie Karmel was influenced by Lamaze at her childbirth and, later on, wrote a book called *Thank You Dr. Lamaze*. This book helped to recognize the Lamaze method in the United States and helped fathers to participate in birth. In 1958, Elisabeth Bing and Karmel, who worked together to teach the Lamaze method to as many women as possible founded the American Society for Psychoprophylaxis in Obstetrics (ASPO) in 1960 (Walker et al. 2009; Onat Bayram and Şahin, 2010; Lamaze International, 2019). Now known as Lamaze International, it is one of the most widespread childbirth education institutions in the world.

Lamaze International's mission is to promote, support and protect natural, safe and healthy births with the support and trainings of professional childbirth educators and their families (Walker et al., 2009; Lamaze International, 2019).

Lamaze training and applications are based on the best, most current medical evidence. "Lamaze Healthy Birth Practices" forms the foundation of the organization. Evidence-based practices adapted from the World Health Organization are as follows:

• Birth should begin spontaneously and on its own.
• Women should be allowed to move during the birth.
• During the birth, women should be given physical and emotional support.
• Interventions – that are not medically necessary – at birth should be avoided.
• Positions other than "on-back" at birth should be supported.
• After the birth mother and baby should be kept together, it is best for the mother, baby and breastfeeding (Walker et al., 2009; Lamaze International 2019).

Natural birth, respiration and relaxation techniques, communication skills, comfort and evidence-based applications are the bases of the "Lamaze Childbirth Education". Pregnant women are encouraged to participate in education at the beginning of the third trimester. The trainings consist of 12-hour sessions and can be held once a week or in weekend intensive formats. Classes are limited to 12 pregnant women and the person who support them (spouses). All learning and experimental learning methods are applied in the trainings. Cultural values and beliefs of the participants are taken into consideration (Walker et al., 2009; Onat Bayram and Şahin, 2010; Lamaze International 2019).

Lamaze International offers the internationally recognized Lamaze Certified Childbirth Educator (LCCE) program approved by the National Commission for Certifying Agencies (Lamaze International, 2019).

## 5 Bradley Method (Husband-Coached Childbirth)

Method Gynecologist was developed in 1947 by Robert Bradley. In this method, which is designed to prepare pairs in normal and natural form without unnecessary medical interventions or medications, fathers are birth coaches (Walker et al., 2009; Varner, 2015).

Bradley believed that certain conditions (darkness, loneliness, silence, physical comfort, relaxation, controlled breathing and eyes closed and sleep) were necessary for women at birth (Walker et al., 2009; Varner, 2015).

Certified Bradley Method trainers are experts in the field of childbirth education. They have passed a comprehensive training program with the "American Academy of Husband-Coached Childbirth" and must complete their continuing education requirements, and renew them each year (Bradley Method, 2019).

In Bradley Method classes:

- Natural birth is an important goal and it is possible to teach families how to do natural births. The techniques are simple and effective; it is based on knowledge about how the human body works at birth. Couples are taught how to work with their bodies to reduce pain and make birth more efficient.
- A 130-page workbook including the course program, study guides, words used, pregnancy, birth, postpartum, coach/doula training, attachment at birth, staying healthy and being at low risk, nutrition, protein counter, general assignments, birth plans, relaxation exercises, birth rehearsal, certificate of participation, pictures and more are provided for each couple. The workbook provides standardization in trainings.
- Provides excellent coach/doula training. Coaches learn the relaxation techniques and effective birth positions. The training is designed to train, motivate and make them a valuable part of the birth experience.
- Comprehensive training is offered: nutrition, exercise, comfort in pregnancy, the role of coaches, information about birth, advanced techniques for delivery, complications, caesarean section, postnatal care, breastfeeding and care of the newborn baby.
- Average 3–6 or 6–8 couples are preferred in classes.
- Trainings are only provided by Certified Bradley Method ™ trainers (specialists and professionals in childbirth education).
- Courses are given in a period of 12 weeks. The reason why the lessons are 12 weeks is because it is believed that there is a difference between obtaining information and physically preparing the body (Bradley Method, 2019).

# 6 Active Birth

The founder of the Active Birth Movement is Janet Balaskas. Janet started a revolution when she set up the Active Birth Movement in the early 80s. When Janet gave birth to her first child Nina in 1973 at the age of 24, she first encountered traditional obstetric attitudes:

"During her first prenatal visit to London, she found her natal clinic very cold and clinical. She changes her plans and goes to South Africa, where her aunt has had three successful natural births in the past. There she thinks that she has more chance of getting what she wants. When birth begins, she spends most of her time at her aunt's house. When she goes to the hospital, she gets an enema, the hair of the perineum is shaved and she is told to lie on the bed. Everything goes well, but in the end, an unnecessary episiotomy is performed, although it was promised not to. Even though the experience was generally good for her, she decides to give birth at home after an episiotomy, to educate women to resist unnecessary interventions and to lead them to give birth in natural ways (Active Birth Center, 2019).

Janet attends the "National Childbirth Trust" (NCT) and is trained as a childbirth educator. She does yoga-based exercises to help the pelvic area to expand, soften and prepare the body for birth. This was a start in pregnancy yoga throughout the world - the purpose of Janet's pregnancy yoga is not only to relax in pregnancy, but to prepare for an active birth (Active Birth Center, 2019).

Janet realizes the importance of upright (squatting) positions at the birth of her second daughter, Kim, and physically prepares her body before her third childbirth. The third birth takes place in the "four feet" position, comfortably at home, in the desired positions. Inspired by her birth experiences, Janet begins teaching women how to prepare for "Active Birth" and publishes her first book "New Life". Soon after, Janet's methods are heard by the public. They were shown on British television after the work of Michel Odent, a French obstetrician who gained remarkable results using similar approaches in her clinic in Pithiviers (Active Birth Center, 2019).

In April 1982, Janet set up the Active Birth Movement, which published the "Active Birth Manifesto", which revealed important research results in order to remain active at birth. On 4 April, Janet, collaborating with colleagues, Sheila Kitzinger and birth organizations, AIMS (Association for Improvements in Maternity Services), NCT (National Childbirth Trust) and Radical Midwives, organize the "Birthrights Rally" in Hampstead Heath. More than 5,000 people who support active births take part in this event, which is handled by journalists Anna Ford, Sheila Kitzinger and Michel Odent (Active Birth Center, 2019).

In October 1982, Janet organizes the first International Conference on "Active Birth" at the Wembley Conference Center. The speakers include the world-renowned psychiatrist R.D. Laing, Michel Odent, Yehudi Gordon and Sheila Kitzinger alongside Janet. Her second book, "Active Birth", published in 1983, states all the ideas and evidence that are essential for active birth today. In 1986, the Active Birth Center opened and is still one of the most preferred methods in the UK. Birth Centers in the UK are designed to enable active births, like the hospitals (Active Birth Center, 2019)".

Active birth is a natural, spontaneous birth where the mother uses her body as she likes. Unlike other birth philosophies, the position of the woman at birth, the hormones secreted at birth and their effect on the birth and pregnancy and the importance of yoga at birth are emphasized. In addition, during the trainings, massages to be applied at birth, methods for the spouse to support during the positions of the woman at birth and breastfeeding and exercises for the postpartum period are also mentioned (Serçekuş and İşbir, 2012).

Janet Balaskas is still in the world (Australia, New Zealand, Estonia, Finland, Ireland, Turkey, Israel, Brazil, India) is continuing her training.

Janet Balaskas still continues her seminars worldwide (Australia, New Zealand, Estonia, Finland, Ireland, Turkey, Israel, Brazil, India) to this day. Janet Balaskas has provided training in Turkey for the first time in 2010 during an "Active Birth" seminar. The seminars were repeated in 2012 and 2013 (Serçekuş and Yenal, 2015). In 2013, 40 persons received an "Active Childbirth Trainer" certificate.

# 7 Mindfulness-Based Childbirth and Parenting

Mindfulness-Based Childbirth and Parenting (MBCP) program, 1979, is an official adaptation of the Mindfulness-Based Stress Reduction (MBSR) program provided by Kabat-Zinn et al. (Walker et al., 2009; Onat Bayram and Şahin, 2010; Mindfulness-Based Professional Training Institute, 2019).

The MBCP Program was established by Nancy Bardacke, a certified nurse-midwife and mindfulness educator (Bardacke, 2017; http://www.mindfulbirthing.org). In 1994, Bardacke attended a training course attended by Kabat-Zinn and health professionals, and in 1998, she has begun training people in MBCP (Walker et al., 2009; Bardacke, 2017). Nancy has taught the MBCP method to more than 1400 parents in 70 courses in the last 15 years (Mindfulness-Based Professional Training Institute, 2019).

The Mindfulness-Based Childbirth and Parenting program offers a practical and systematic way to engage in a broad relationship with one's own and own experiences, taking its foundation from consciousness and awareness. Awareness-Focused Birth and Parenting program is a childbirth education class for expectant parents, which is built on "awareness", a skill learned by living (Bardacke, 2017).

The MBCP program consists of nine weeks, three hours per week (Walker et al., 2009; Onat Bayram and Şahin, 2010; Mindfulness-Based Professional Training Institute, 2019). After completing this program, participants would learn:

- The relationship between body and mind at birth,
- How the ability to stay in the moment is critical in supporting the normal physiological process of childbirth, and to directly experience ways to train the mind to work at birth,
- How critical the ability to "stay in the moment" is in supporting the normal physiological process of birth,
- How to directly experience the methods to train the mind to work efficiently during the birth,
- How awareness can be used to reduce the fear of birth,
- The importance of the participation and support of the spouse in the birth,
- How a practice of awareness can positively affect the couple's relationship,
- The role of awareness in healthy parent-infant bonding.

The training involves the period of daily meditation, yoga/mindfulness movement and silence by combining didactic, experiential and small group learning (Mindfulness-Based Professional Training Institute, 2019).

## 8  England-Birthing from Within

The method developed by Pam England adopts a holistic approach to birth and postpartum. Pam developed this method after focusing on other women's previous birth experiences, knowledge, fears, needs and desires after their birth experience (Walker et al. 2009; Onat Bayram and Şahin, 2010; Elmas et al., 2017).

Instinctive Birth is a holistic approach that examines birth as an act of deep transition and a self-discovery rather than a medical act. Unlike other methods, it focuses on helping health professionals and parents better understand their own motivations and fears, as well as helping them return to their inner resources to explore their power to guide them (Birthing from Within, 2019).

Pam has also written the book *Birthing from Within: An Extra-Ordinary Guide to Childbirth Education* with Rob Horowitz (Walker et al., 2009; Onat Bayram and Şahin, 2010).

The method encourages couples to pursue freedom and creativity during their education. Inner, experiential self-discovery processes are presented together with practical information. Basic points taught in the method are:

- Natural birth
- An instinctive and holistic approach
- Ability to express yourself
- To deal with difficulties (Walker et al., 2009; Onat Bayram and Şahin, 2010).

# 9 Conclusion

It is argued that birth is a healthy, natural action on the basis of methods used in childbirth education. Although the methods or philosophies used in the trainings may be different, the main goal is to prepare the mother for the birth, and to help her live it as a healthy and beautiful experience for the baby and her spouse.

Studies conducted in Turkey suggest that pregnant women receiving prenatal training have a lower rate of c-section (Çopur et al. 2013; Mete et al. 2017), prepare for birth more consciously (Mete et al. 2017), have fewer birth-related fears and negative thoughts (Subaşı et al., 2013), are able to manage the act of labor and participate in it actively and thus, have higher levels of satisfaction and self-confidence (Coşar and Demirci, 2012; İşbir et al., 2015), are more confident about self-care and infant care and have higher levels of preparedness for discharge (Altıntuğ and Ege, 2013; Burucu and Akın, 2017), perceive their babies positively (Şeker and Sevil, 2015), and have higher rates of feeding only breastmilk within the first six months and higher durations of breastfeeding (Mete et al., 2010; Serçekuş and Mete, 2010). In Turkey, childbirth educations are given both in private institutions, as well as in institutions linked to the state. Nurses should support the couples to prepare for birth by participating in these trainings. In addition, nurses should take an active role in planning and conducting trainings.

# References

Active Birth Centre. (2019). What is Active Birth. http://www.activebirthcentre.com (accessed on 14.02.2019).

Altıntuğ, K. & Ege, E. (2013). Sağlık Eğitiminin Annelerin Taburculuğa Hazır Oluş, Doğum Sonu Güçlük Yaşama Ve Yaşam Kalitesine Etkisi, *Hemşirelikte Araştırma Geliştirme Dergisi*, 15(2), 45–56.

Bardacke, N. (2017). *Farkındalıkla Doğum-Doğum Mucizedir Tadını Çıkar* (Çeviren: Özge Onan). Doğan Egmont Yayıncılık ve Yapımcılık. 1. Baskı.

Buran, G. (2015). Doğum Öncesi Hazırlık Kursu Örneği: Deneyimler ve Sonuçları: 2013–2015, *Journal of Obstetric Women's Health and Diseases Nursing*, 1(1), 25–32.

Burucu, R. & Akın, B. (2017). Gebeliğin Üçüncü Trimesterinde Gebelere Verilen Eğitimin Doğum Sonu Taburculuğa Hazır Oluşluk Düzeyine Etkisi, *Hacettepe Üniversitesi Hemşirelik Fakültesi Dergisi*, 4(2), 25–35.

Coker, H., Karabekir, N. & Varlık, S. (2015). Keşkesiz Doğum Modeli ve Ekibi, *Turkiye Klinikleri Obstetric-Women's Health and Diseases Nursing- Special Topics*, 1(3), 27–37.

Coşar, F. & Demirci, N. (2012). Lamaze Felsefesine Dayalı Doğuma Hazırlık Eğitiminin Doğum Algısı ve Doğuma Uyum Sürecine Etkisi. *Süleyman Demirel Üniversitesi Sağlık Bilimleri Enstitüsü Dergisi*, 3(1), 18–30.

Çopur, A. Kayacık, F., Özkan, T. & Özen, B. (2013). Doğuma Hazırlık Kursuna Katılan Gebelerin Doğum Korkusu Yaşama Durumlarının Belirlenmesi, *Acıbadem Hemşirelik e- Dergi*. http://www.acibademhemsirelik.com/e-dergi/79/docs/bilimsel-calisma-2.pdf (accessed on 22.02.2019).

Discover Birthing from Within. (2019). www.birthingfromwithin.com (accessed on 22.02.2019).

Elmas, S., Yeyğel, Ç. & Saruhan, A. (2017). Doğum Öncesi Eğitim Modelleri Eşliğinde Doğal Doğum, *Anadolu Hem ve Sağ Bil Derg*, 20(4), 299–303.

HypnoBirthing®Institute. (2019). What is HypnoBirthing? www.hypnobirthing.com (accessed on 11.02.2019).

İstanbul Doğum Akademisi (İDA) Doğuma Hazırlık Eğitmeni ve Doula Eğitim Programı Yönetmeliği (DHEDE). http://dogumakademisi.com/tr (accessed on 11.02.2019).

İşbir, G.G., Serçekuş, P. & Çoker, H. (2015). Doğuma Hazırlık Eğitiminin Doğum Deneyimi ve Doğumdan Memnuniyet Üzerine Etkisinin İncelenmesi, *Turkiye Klinikleri Journal of Nursing Sciences (Journal of Obstetric Women's Health and Diseases Nursing-Special Topics)*, 1(1), 10–15.

Keşkesiz Doğum Merkezleri. (2019). http://www.keskesizdogummerkezi.com/ (accessed on 19.02.2019).

Lamaze International. (2019). Healthy Birth Practices. www.lamaze.org (accessed on 14.02.2019).

Mete, S., Yenal, K. & Okumuş, H. (2010). An Investigation into Breastfeeding Characteristics of Mothers Attending Childbirth Education Classes, *Asian Nursing Research*, 4(4), 216–226.

Mete, S., Çiçek, Ö., Tokat, A.M., Çamlıbel, M. & Uludağ, E. (2017). Doğuma Hazırlık Sınıflarının Doğum Korkusu, Doğum Tercihi ve Doğuma Hazır Oluşluğa Etkisi, *Turkiye Klinikleri Journal of Nursing Sciences*, 9(3), 201–206.

Mindfulness-Based Professional Training Institute. (2019). MBCP: Mindfulness-Based Childbirth and Parenting. http://mbpti.org/programs/mbcp/mbcp-mindfulness-based-childbirth-and-parenting/ (accessed on 15.02.2019).

Mindfull Birthing-Training the Mind, Body and Heart for Childbirth and Beyond. http://www.mindfulbirthing.org/ (accessed on 15.02.2019).

Mongan, M.F. (2016). Hypnobirthing Mongan Yöntemi (Ed. Çoker H.), 3. Baskı, İstanbul: Gün Yayıncılık.

Onat Bayram, G. & Şahin, N.H. (2010). Doğuma Hazırlık Eğitimi Modelleri ve Güncel Yaklaşımlar, *Hemşirelikte Eğitim ve Araştırma Dergisi*, 7(3), 36–42.

Serçekuş, P. & İşbir, G.G. (2012). Aktif Doğum Yaklaşımının Kanıta Dayalı Uygulamalar ile İncelenmesi, *TAF Preventive Medicine Bulletin*, 11(1), 97–102.

Serçekuş, P. & Yenal, K. (2015). Doğuma Hazırlık Sınıflarının Türkiyedeki Gelişimi, *Turkiye Klinikleri Journal of Nursing Sciences (Journal of Obstetric Women's Health and Diseases Nursing- Special Topics)*, 1(1), 33–35.

Serçekuş, P. & Mete, S. (2010). Effects of Antenatal Education on Maternal Prenatal and Postpartum Adaptatıon. *Journal of Advanced Nursing*, 66(5), 999–1010.

Subaşı, B., Özcan, H., Pekçetin, S., Göker, B., Tunç, S. & Budak, B. (2013). Doğum Eğitiminin Doğum Kaygısı ve Korkusu Üzerine Etkisi, *Selçuk Tıp Derg*, 29(4), 165–167.

Şeker, S. & Sevil, Ü. (2015). Doğuma Hazırlık Sınıflarının Annenin Doğum Sonu Fonksiyonel Durumuna ve Bebeğini Algılamasına Etkisi, *Turkiye Klinikleri Journal of Obstetric Women's Health and Disease Nursing-Special Topics*, 1(1), 1–9.

The Bradley Method® of Husband Coached Natural Childbirth. (2019). Why Take Classes in the Bradley Method® of Natural Childbirth? http://www. bradleybirth.com (accessed on 12.02.2019).

Varner, C.A. (2015). Comparison of the Bradley Method and HypnoBirthing Childbirth Education Classes, *The Journal of Perinatal Education*, 24(2), 128–136.

Walker, D.S., Visger, J.M. & Rossie, D. (2009). Contemporary Childbirth Education Models, *Journal of Midwifery & Women's Health*, 54(6), 469–476.

Müge Seval and Münevver Sönmez

# 8: Current Approaches in Pain Management for Children and Adults: Integrative Pain Management

## 1 Introduction

Integrative medicine is an integrative medicine practice and includes practices and methods for integrating alternative, complementary and scientific data-based medical practices into each other. In Turkey, the Ministry of Health within the Directorate General of Health Services in legislative decree No. 2014 663 (SCC) pursuant to the "Traditional and Complementary Medicine Practice Department" was established. In the regulation prepared by the Department of Traditional and Complementary Medicine Practices, the initiatives to be carried out at the units and application centers are discussed in 15 sub-headings. These topics include acupuncture, apitherapy, phytotherapy, hypnosis, leech, homeopathy, chiropractic, cup application, larval application, mesotherapy, prolotherapy, osteopathic ozone application, reflexology and music therapy. One of the most frequently used areas of integrative health is pain. Pain affects the individual's body, soul and mental processes. The use of complementary methods in pain management enables the patient to participate more effectively. The main purpose of integrative medicine applications is to increase self-management power by supporting the participation of the individual in the treatment process. Thus, the individual can remain their health management even if their connection with the health team is cut. Integrative health applications form the door-control mechanism in pain, activating the nociceptive afferent system by increasing the release of endogenous opioids. In addition, it strengthens the immune system to facilitate homeostatic balance. In this part of the book, it is aimed to give information about the basic principles of complementary/supportive healing methods that can be integrated with non-pharmacological, non-invasive, patient-centered and modern medical therapies, which can be used in pain management in children and adult patients, and the stages of using in nursing and nursing applications.

## 2 Traditional, Complementary and Integrative Health Practices

The terms "Complementary treatment" and "Alternative treatment" are often used interchangeably but they have different dimensions. The methods applied together with medical treatments in order to support the medical treatment are called "Complementary treatment", while the methods which are applied in place of medical methods (and whose effect has not been scientifically proven) are considered as "alternative treatment" (Peksoy et al., 2018). The name of the National Center for Complementary and Alternative Medicine (NCCAM) of the United States Department of Health (NIH) has been renamed as National Center for Complementary and Integrative Health (NCCIH), "Alternative Medicine" being removed from the name.

National Center for Complementary and Alternative Medicine (NCCIH) defined "Alternative Applications" as methods which are used instead of traditional medicine, and has instead given place to the "Integrative Health" concept (Cırık and Efe, 2017). "Integrative medicine" or "integrative health concept"; covers the methods and practices that are considered as integrative/holistic medicine as a holistic assessment of traditional and complementary medicine, and evidence-based medicine practices (Peksoy et al., 2018).

Turkey's application related to the expansion of the use of traditional and complementary medicine made it necessary to adopt regulations about which occupations would do the applications, their education levels and practice indications. In Turkey, the first arrangements made in this area are in 1991-issued "Regulation of Acupuncture Treatment". In this regulation, acupuncture application methods are defined and occupational fields which have the authority would apply treatment (Uysal, 2016). In October 2014, the "Regulation on Traditional and Complementary Medical Practices" published by the Ministry of Health, the diseases to be applied, the trainings to be taken on the subject, the practitioners who are authorized to implement and the characteristics of the health institutions are clearly stated. In this regulation, 14 applications such as apitherapy, phytotherapy, hypnosis, leech, homeopathy, chiropractic, cup application, larval application, mesotherapy, prolotherapy, osteopathy, ozone application, reflexology and music therapy are included in the scope of more traditional and complementary medicine practice (Uysal, 2016).

## 3 Definition and Types of Pain

Subjective pain makes it difficult to identify (Aslan et al., 2009). For this reason, many opinions have been raised to "describe" pain. According to the definition given in many literature, pain is an "unpleasant biochemical and emotional condition or behavior that is caused by a certain area of the body, caused by tissue damage and/or does not occur, affected by the previous experiences of the person, and is to remove an unwanted situation (IASP, 1986). For the

The Classification of Pain diagram contains the following categories:

| Source | Sensation Type | Etiology | Start Time | Mechanism |
|---|---|---|---|---|
| Somatic | Sudden, Sharp, Sinking | Mechanical | Acute | Nociceptive |
| Visceral | | Inflammatory | Chronic | Neuropathic |
| Sympatetic | Slowly Increasing | | Repetitive | Deafferantation |
| Peripheral | Blunt, Sometimes Flammable | | | Reactive/ Reagent |
| | | | | Psychosomatic |

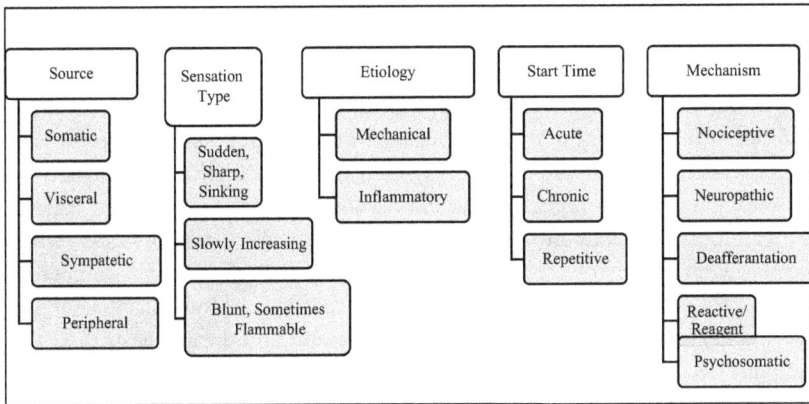

**Fig. 8.1:** The Classification of Pain (Aslan and Uslu, 2016).

pain, McCaffery's definition that "If the patient claims that he/she has pain, it exists, we need to believe in it" is defined as the gold standard (Törüner and Büyükgönenç, 2012; Büyükgönenç and Törüner, 2013). Pain is a subjective and difficult to understand concept, which is subject to individual characteristics and negative health conditions experienced by the individual. In recent years, non-pharmacological methods are used more frequently, in order to increase the effect of pharmacological methods or where situations where pharmacological methods are contraindicated (Akın Korkan and Uyar, 2014; Özveren et al., 2016). The classification of pain is made according to different factors (Fig. 8.1):

## 4 Integrative Health Application Methods Used in Pain Management

The recent current approach to the continuation and reconstruction of physiological, emotional and spiritual well-being is the use of non-pharmacological and integrative treatment methods, one of which is pain. The use of integrative methods in pain management enables the patient to participate more effectively. Individual participatory integrative approaches increase treatment options, reduce symptoms and improve self-management power. Integrative healthcare practices are effective through the release of endogenous opioids by the formation of a door-control mechanism in pain management. Integrative health practices supporting pain management in the Health Regulation on "Traditional and Complementary Medicine Practices" are summarized below:

## 4.1 Acupuncture

Acupuncture is the approach of traditional Chinese medicine with the highest degree of evidence in integrative applications. Acupuncture is a method that facilitates the treatment of many diseases by injecting acupuncture needles into the pressure points in the body (Ovayolu and Ovayolu, 2017). Acupuncture provides pain management by stimulating endorphin release. It is an effective method used especially in the treatment of head, waist, neck, shoulder, elbow, toothache and many diseases (Özveren, 2011). In recent years, it has been reported that acupuncture application can be used as a non-pharmacological method because it decreases the sensory symptoms and the analgesic dose they use, and decreases the frequency of headache in migraine attacks in patients with chemotherapy-related peripheral neuropathic pain management (İzgü, 2017).

## 4.2 Hypnosis

Hypnosis is a state of deep relaxation where cognitive alertness decreases and patient's ability to take the suggestions improve. Hypnosis hampers the emotional relationship between the sensory cortex and the amygdala-limbic system, which is experienced as pain (Yıldız et al., 2013). When hypnosis is applied, it is ensured that the individual is in a comfortable position, breathing deeply and slowly. The patient is advised to reduce his/her interest in the environment, to focus on a positive idea, to dream of the object, to relax and to control the pain and anxiety and to be calm (Özcan, 2018). Especially in the treatment of birth pain, the use of hypnosis gives positive results.

## 4.3 Cup Application

Cup application is one of the fifteen applications adopted in the "Regulation on Traditional and Complementary Medicine" by the Ministry of Health. It is based on the technique of creating negative pressure with millimetric scratches on the skin and apparatus made of various materials. Cup application is applied in two different ways – wet and dry cup application. Vacuuming mugs is placed on the skin on a certain line. Blood circulation is increased in the region of application bythe vasodilatation effect in the blood vessels, while redness on the skin occurs (Sert et al., 2015). According to the door-control theory, painless stimuli in the treatment of cups close the doors that cause painful stimuli (Yıldız et al., 2013). Various studies have shown the efficacy of cup application in painful conditions (headache, myofascial pain and fibromyalgia) (Sert et al., 2015).

## 4.4 Leech

Although leeches have more than 15,000 species, the most commonly used genus in medical applications is Hirudo Medicinalis. Medical leeches do not provide treatment "because they absorb dirty blood", as they are believed. The therapeutic properties are not due to the removal of blood, but because of the *substances* released when blood is absorbed (local anesthetic, histamine-like vasodilators, anticoagulants, spreading factors, etc.). There are many bioactive substances that show anti-inflammatory and anticoagulant effect in leech saliva (Sert et al., 2015). Leeches constitute an important part of conventional pain treatment, since they were used in the treatment of many diseases since ancient times (Yıldız et al., 2015). Studies have shown that leech therapy causes a significant decrease in pain without causing complications in resistant knee pain due to osteoarthritis, and leech application is considered to be a safe option in the treatment of knee osteoarthritis (Michalsen et al., 2003; Andereya et al., 2008; Stange et al., 2012).

## 4.5 Prolotherapy

Prolotherapy is a treatment where an irritant solution is injected into the adjacent joint space instead of small volumes of painful ligaments and/or tendon adhesions. Prolotherapy has been applied since the 1950s as an integrative method to solve the problems of the musculature such as tendinopathy, gonarthrosis, osteoarthritis and low back pain (Özcan and Sert, 2016; Yaman and Vural, 2016).

The aim of prolotherapy is to reduce the trauma caused by pain and accelerate tissue repair. The procedure stimulates the body's natural healing mechanisms, strengthening ligaments and connective tissues, thereby reducing pain by improving joint stabilization and function. (Özcan and Sert, 2016).

## 4.6 Reflexology

There are certain points in the body that are reflected in the hands, feet and ears. Technically, these points are given pressure in reflexology and these warnings are improved by the reactions of the organs. Reflexology practice in pain control is based on door-control theory. Reflexology provides touch stimuli carried by beta-sensory fibers, type A, which can weaken the transmission of pain signals, creating local and lateral inhibition through the dorsal horn of the spinal cord. In addition, the applications to the reflex points stimulate the release of various chemicals, including the release of endorphins in the body, as a result of which it helps to control the pain (Stephenson et al., 2000; Uysal and Kutluturkani, 2016).

When the researches about reflexology are examined; It has been reported that reflexology significantly alleviates pain in fibromyalgia, relieves low back pain, decreases pain in patients with rheumatoid arthritis and also provides improvement in muscle strength and tone in patients with multiple sclerosis, and decreases sensory and urinary symptoms (Quinn et al., 2008; Gunnarsdottir and Peden-McAlpine, 2010).

## 4.7 Music Therapy

It is known that treatment with music is related to and used in many fields in medical science. The use of music as an adjunctive treatment tool in the treatment of diseases encountered in the branches of science such as oncology, cardiology, neurology, psychiatry and pediatrics has a positive effect on the treatment process of diseases (Gençel, 2006). Music therapy is used in patient care as a complementary method in the management of non-pharmacological pain. Music is an effective, inexpensive and easy to use method to control pain (Arslan, 2007; Updike, 2010).

Music therapy affects the neuroendocrine system and the autonomic nervous system. The music played on the low pitch and at a low tempo affects the limbic system of the brain, which is the center of emotion and excitement, reducing the ability of neural transmission to regulate disturbing emotions. It causes physiological and psychological changes in the body by acting on neuroendocrine system and autonomic nervous system. By activating the parasympathetic nervous system, it causes a decrease in physiological findings such as blood pressure, pulse and respiration (Arslan, 2007; Updike, 2010). Music therapy application enhances endorphin release by stimulating the pituitary gland. As a result of the release of endorphins, the body's natural painkiller and mental status regulator, pain and anxiety are reduced and have a positive effect on detection. The music distracts the patient from the pain and reduces the feelings that aggravate the pain, such as anxiety and fear. It provides sedation by affecting the mood of the people. Music reduces the response to stress (Arslan, 2007). In the pain management as a non-pharmacological practice, the use of music therapy has been shown to be effective in reducing the pain in post-operative, painful invasive procedures (Port catheter insertion, blood drawing) and dressing changes, especially in burn dressing (Ovayolu, 2006; Yaşar, 2010; Yiğit, 2017).

## 4.8 Massage

Some aromatherapy oils used in massage are effective in reducing pain in patients. These oils spread rapidly to the painful area, increasing circulation and tissue oxygenation. In addition, by reducing the frequency of using painkillers, both the patient's body and the economic loss is prevented and the use of safe medication is supported. The oils used for this purpose are called volatile oils. The application of essential oils in the treatment of pain by mixing with fixed oils provides an effective support treatment. With the use of essential oils, the dose of pain relief can be reduced and more effective pain control can be achieved. Research suggests that many essential oils are natural analgesics. Essential oils act as a supportive treatment for pain treatment. Massage with these oils reduces anxiety and stress and helps the patient relax and feel less pain. Aromatic oils commonly used in the treatment of pain are as follows:

- **Mint oil:** Cooler, pain relieving, calming
- **Clove oil:** Arthritis and rheumatism pains
- **Sandalwood oil:** Abdominal pain, sedative
- **Rose oil:** Menstrual pain
- **Lavender oil:** Headache, calming
- **Bergamot oil:** Neuropathic pain, chronic pain, sedation
- **Green apple oil:** Migraine pain (http://www.naturenurture.com.tr/blog-detay/aromaterapi-ve-agri-tedavisi/)

In a study, it was observed that lavender with inhalation method was effective in migraine headaches and decreased the severity of migraine pain (Sasannejad, 2012). In another study, it was observed that the application of lavender oil through massage was effective in pain and inflammation as well as prescription products (Silva, 2015).

In another study, it was found that lavender and sage oil were applied to the lower abdomen by massaging and decreasing the duration and intensity of menstrual pain (Ou et al., 2012). In another study conducted in 2013, Cinnamon, clove, rose and lavender oils were mixed with sweet almond oil and started to be applied once a day before the menstruation. It has been shown that the mixture decreases tension, stress and pain due to menstruation (Marzouk, 2013).

# 5 Integrative Health Practices Used in Pain Management for Adults and Nursing Care Principles

Although the use of complementary therapies in the health field has increased in recent years, it is seen that nurses have insufficient knowledge level about nonpharmacological methods and do not use them very often in pain management (Gök, 2015; Özveren et al., 2016; Özcan, 2018).

In recent years, "integrative nursing" concept moves under the roof of "holistic nursing" philosophy. In particular, it is important to use integrative guidelines in order to make sure that integrative treatment approaches are used correctly in clinical applications.

Evidence-based guidelines should facilitate the assessment of the effectiveness of the practices. The effects of the interventions applied with these guidelines on the effectiveness, quality and patient satisfaction of the given care should be evaluated. It is important that the nurses and all the team members who contribute to the application are informed about the effects, side effects and reliability of the methods in order to make the evaluation error-free. Therefore, it is important to continuously update nurses' knowledge about integrative treatment methods, to provide evidence-based care and to plan patient education (Cırık and Efe, 2017).

In the study of Güngörmüş et al. (2012), information about integrative treatment applications in the treatment of pain, patients were informed via mostly (48.8 %) from their spouse/relative/family members, followed by (23.1 %) the media, and (1.9 %) from the nurses only (Güngörmüş and Kıyak, 2012). In a similar study in Malaysia, this was found to be 13.3 % (Thorne et al., 2002). This situation presents the risk of misinformation and application about the content and application of integrative therapies.

To reduce this risk, members of the healthcare team, especially nurses, need to be sensitive about informing patients. Researches conducted in different countries show that nurses and patients informed by them often use alternative treatment methods. A study by Shorofi et al. (2010) in Australia found out that nurses frequently use pain therapy, massage therapy, music therapy, meditation/relaxation techniques and aromatherapy (Shorofi and Arbon, 2010). In Taiwan, a study conducted by Chu et al. (2007) states that nurses use relaxation therapy (74.7 %), massage (69.9 %), music therapy (45.9 %), therapeutic touch (44.7 %) and aromatherapy (27.7 %) in practice of treating patients' pain and bodily discomfort (Chu and Wallis, 2007). In a study conducted by Hassan et al. (2014) with oncology nurses in Qatar, they found that the use of integrative treatment methods – in painful cases – were effective in regulating physical and mental health of patients, improving quality of life and alleviating disease symptoms (Hassan et al., 2014).

In Turkey, Tercan's (2015) in his research with nurses, has determined that nurses do not have enough knowledge about the use of non-pharmacological methods in pain management and therefore prefer not to use it. It is concluded that it is important that nurses are given in-service training programs, seminars and courses related to the current use of non-pharmacological treatment methods, pain assessment is done with internationally valid scales and via legal regulations related to the subject, and they are given the authority to apply these practices.

## 6 Integrative Health Practices Used in Pain Management for Children and Principles of Nursing Care

It is noteworthy that pharmacological methods are objectively preferred by nurses when pain management in children is considered. However, integrative health practices, which include all nonpharmacological, alternative and complementary methods, are easy to use, cheap, without side effects and evidence-based applications to assess and manage children's pain (Landier and Tse, 2010). The main philosophies of pediatric nursing are atraumatic and family centered care. In this context, if there are no medical contraindications, it is important that integrative health practices take place in child care and treatment. Integral health practices should be used to provide children with atraumatic care, especially as bad experiences associated with children's pain may adversely affect subsequent hospital and pain experiences (Birnie et al., 2014; Herrington and Chiodo, 2014).

Acupuncture is one of the applications we can evaluate within the scope of integrative health practices used in pain management in children. In a study of 56 children who underwent tonsillectomy between the ages of 2 and 17, acupuncture was found to be effective on the pain of children in the postoperative period (Ochi, 2013). Since the needle was scary and caused children to refuse acupuncture, a second study was performed and Ochi (2015) applied the Korean Needle Therapy, a needleless acupuncture method, to 29 children aged 1–14 years who had undergone tonsillectomy. As a result, it was reported that this therapy was easy to accept by children and effective on postoperative pain in them (Ochi, 2015).

Integrative health practices have a positive effect on pain because of decreasing fear, anxiety and stress in children (Birnie et al., 2014). For example, anxiety and the amount of pain felt by the children can be reduced by helping him/her loosen by hypnosis (Landier and Tse, 2010; Birnie et al., 2014; Özcan, 2018).

Reiki, acupuncture and music therapy are used to reduce the pain experienced during physical theraphy in children with cerebral palsy (www.ribem.com.tr).

Again, in a study of 832 children with chronic neurological disease, 25 % of mothers applied massage to their children for the pain in the back and waist region (due to long-term hospitalization) and resorted to listening to music when their children could not sleep at night (Çarman et al., 2018).

In infants with infantile colic (also known as gas pains), the 5S method is used: [S]waddling, [S]winging the baby (with tiny jiggly movements), the pacifier ([S]ucking), laying the infant on his/her [S]tomach and the whispering lullabies or the [S]sh sound to the baby's ear. The 5S principles are in synergy with reflexology, massage and music therapy. This is an indication of the use of integrative treatment methods in the neonatal period (Şimsek Orhon, 2016). Uğurlu, Kalkim and Sağkal (2014) in their study with children 0–1 years determined that 77.6 % of the mothers calmed the baby by using massage methods for abdominal pain and shaking on lap. When it is considered that reiki is some kind of massage and lullaby is music therapy, it is seen that integrative methods are used in babies (Uğurlu et al., 2014).

Integrative treatment methods and therapies are used in addition to medical treatment in child-age pediatric patients who have entered the terminal period due to cancer or other chronic disease and who have been taking palliative care. Acupuncture, reiki/reflexology and hypnosis are the methods used to reduce pain related to the complications of cancer and treatment in children (Konuk Şener and Üstüner Top, 2018).

In the study of Soltani et al. (2013), it was observed that the daily dose of paracetamol was decreased in children who had been cured with lavender oil after tonsillectomy.

One of the most comprehensive studies in this area is the evidence-based systematic review of Cura et al. (2018). In this study, 15 Turkish and English articles, which include complementary and alternative medicine applications used in pain relief in the pediatric age group, were examined. Music therapy, as well as mechanical vibration, manual pressure and massage application methods were found to be effective in reducing pain in children.

## 7 Conclusion

It is important that nurses keep their knowledge up-to-date so that they prefer non-pharmacological methods for pain control more frequently in both children and adults. New legal arrangements and special education programs are needed for nurses to use integrative treatment methods in patient care. In addition, it is very important to use data collection forms where nurses can easily apply integrative methods in clinical setting, to ensure their application in all clinics and to be supported by institutions.

## References

Akın Korkan, E. & Uyar, M. (2014). Ağrı Kontrolünde Kanıt Temelli Yaklaşım: Refleksoloji, *Acıbadem Üniversitesi Sağlık Bilimleri Dergisi*, 1, 9–14.

Andereya, S., Stanzel, S., Maus, U., Mueller-Rath, R., Mumme, T., Siebert, C.H., Stock, F. & Schneider, U. (2008). Assessment of Leech Therapy for Knee Osteoarthritis: A Randomized Study, *Acta Orthopaedica*, 79(2), 235–243.

Arslan, S. (2007). *Dokunma, Müzik Terapi ve Aromaterapinin Yoğun Bakım Hastalarının Fizyolojik Durumlarına Etkisi.* Yayınlanmamış Doktora Tezi, Atatürk Üniversitesi, Erzurum.

Aslan, F.E. & Uslu, Y. (2016). Ağrının Sınıflandırılması. (Ed. Aslan F. E.) *Cerrahi Bakım Vaka Analizleri ile Birlikte*, 1. Baskı, Akademisyen Tıp Kitapevi, Ankara.

Aslan, F.E., Badir, A., Arli, S.K. & Cakmakci, H. (2009). Patients' Experience of Pain after Cardiac Surgery, *Contemporary Nurse*, 34, 57–67.

Birnie, K.A., Ons, B.A.H, Noel, M., Parker, J.A., Chambers, C.T., Uman, L.S. & Mcgrath, P.J. (2014). Systematic Review and Meta-analysis of Distraction and Hypnosis for Needle-Related Pain and Distress in Children and Adolescents, *Journal of Pediatric Psychology*, 39(8), 783–808.

Büyükgönenç, L. & Törüner, E.K. (2013). Çocukluk Yaşlarında Ağrı ve Hemşirelik Yönetimi, (Eds. Conk Z., Başbakkal Z., Bal Yılmaz H., Bolışık B.), *Pediatri Hemşireliği*, Akademisyen Tıp Kitabevi, Ankara.

Çarman, K.B., Laçinel Gürlevik, S., Kaplan, E., Dinleyici, M., Yarar, Ç. & Aslantaş, D. (2018). Kronik Nörolojik Hastalığı Olan Çocuklarda Tedavisinde Tamamlayıcı ve Alternatif Tıp Uygulamalarının Kullanılma Durumunun Belirlenmesi, *Haydarpaşa Numune Medical Journal*, 58(3), 117–121.

Chen, Y.F. & Chang, J.S. (2003). Complementary and Alternative Medicine Use among Patients Attending a Hospital Dermatology Clinic in Taiwan, *International Journal of Dermatology*, 42(8), 616–621.

Chu, F.Y. & Wallis, M. (2007). Taiwanese Nurses' Attitudes Towards and Use of Complementary and Alternative Medicine in Nursing Practice: Across-Sectional Survey, *International Journal of Nursing Studies*, 44(8), 1371–1378.

Cırık, V. & Efe, E. (2017). Pediatri Hemşireliğinde Tamamlayıcı Sağlık Yaklaşımlarının Önemi, *Hemşirelikte Eğitim ve Araştırma Dergisi*, 14(2), 144–149.

Cura, Ş., Oğul, T. & Kurt, F. (2018). Pediatrik Yaş Gruplarında Akut Ağrının Giderilmesinde Kullanılan Tamamlayıcı ve Alternatif Tıp Uygulamaları, *Zeynep Kamil Tıp Bülteni*, 49(1), 126–129.

Gençel, Ö. (2006). Müzikle Tedavi, *Kastamonu Eğitim Dergisi*, 14(2), 697–706.

Gök, M. (2015). *Romatoid Artritli Hastalarda Aromaterapi Masajı ve Refleksoloji Uygulamalarının Ağrı Ve Yorgunluğa Etkileri*, Yayınlanmamış Doktora Tezi, Hacettepe Üniversitesi, Ankara.

Güngörmüş, Z. & Kıyak, E. (2012). Ağrı Yaşayan Bireylerin Tamamlayıcı ve
Alternatif Tedaviye İlişkin Bilgi, Tutum ve Davranışlarının Değerlendirilmesi,
*Ağrı Dergisi*, 24(3), 123–129.

Gunnarsdottir, T.J. & Peden-McAlpine, C. (2010). Effects of Reflexology on
Fibromyalgia Symptoms: A Multiple Case Study, *Complementary Therapies İn
Clinical Practice*, 16(3), 167–172.

Hassan, A., Allam, A., Al Kindi, S., Abu Zeinah, G., Eziada, S. & Bashir, A.
(2014). Knowledge, Attitudes and Practices of Oncology Nurses towards
Complementary and Alternative Medicine for Cancer Care in Qatar, *Journal
of Anesthesia and Clinical Research*, 5, 12.

Herrington, C.J. & Chiodo, L.M. (2014). Human Touch Effectively and Safely
Reduces Pain in the Newborn Intensive Care Unit. *Pain Management
Nursing*, 15(1), 107–115.

http://www.naturenurture.com.tr/blog-detay/aromaterapi-ve-agri-tedavisi/
(accessed on 10.01.2019).

IASP. (1986). Classification of Chronic Pain. Descriptions of Chronic Pain
Syndromes and Definitions of Pain Terms, *Pain*, 3, 1–226.

İzgü, N. (2017). *El ve Ayağa Uygulanan Aromaterapi Masajının Kemoterapi
İlişkili PeriferalNöropatik Ağrı ve Yorgunluk Üzerine Etkisi.* Yayınlanmamış
Doktora Tezi, Hacettepe Üniversitesi, Ankara.

Konuk Şener, D. & Üstüner Top, F. (2018). Terminal Dönemdeki Çocuklarda
Ağrı Yönetimi (Ed. Cimete G.) Çocuklarda Palyatif Bakım; *Terminal
Dönemdeki Çocuk ve Aileye Yaklaşım*, 1. Baskı, Türkiye Klinikleri, Ankara.

Landier, W. & Tse, A.M. (2010). Use of Complementary and Alternative Medical
Interventions for Management of Procedure-Related Pain, Anxiety and
Distress in Pediatric Oncology: An Integrative Review, *Journal of Pediatric
Nursing*, 25(6), 566–579.

Marzouk, T.M., El-Nemer, A.M. & Baraka, H.N. (2013). The Effect of
Aromatherapy Abdominal Massage on Alleviating Menstrual Pain in Nursing
Students: A Prospective Randomized Cross-Over Study, *Evidence-Based
Complementary and Alternative Medicine*, 10, 1–6.

Michalsen, A., Klotz, S., Lüdtke, R., Moebus, S., Spahn, G. & Dobos, G.J. (2003).
Effectiveness of Leechtherapy in Osteoarthritis of Theknee: A Randomized,
Controlledtrial, *Annals of Internal Medicine*, 139(9), 724–730.

Ochi, J.W. (2013). Acupuncture instead of Codeine for Tonsillectomy Pain in
Children, *International Journal of Pediatric Otorhinolaryngology*, 77(12),
2058–2062.

Ochi, J.W. (2015). Korean Hand Therapy for Tonsillectomy Pain in Children,
*International Journal of Pediatric Otorhinolaryngology*, 79(8), 1263–1267.

Ou, M.C., Hsu, T.F., Lai, A.C., Lin, Y.T. & Lin, C.C. (2012). Pain Relief Assessment by Aromatic Essential Oil Massage On Outpatients with Primary Dysmenorrhea: A Randomized, Double-Blind Clinical Trial, *Journal of Obstetrics and Gynaecology Research*, 38(5), 817–822.

Ovayolu, N. (2006). Listening to Turkish Classical Music Decreases Patients' Anxiety, Pain, Dissatisfaction and the Dose of Sedative and Analgesic Drugs During Colonoscopy: A Prospective Randomized Controlledtrial, *World Journal of Gastroenterology*, 12(46), 7532–7536.

Ovayolu, Ö. & Ovayolu, N. (2017). Palyatif Bakım Alan Kanser Hastalarının Ağrı Yönetiminde Integratif Yaklaşımlar, *Hacettepe Üniversitesi Hemşirelik Fakültesi Dergisi*, 4(3), 54–64.

Özcan, N. (2018). *Göğüs Tüpü Çıkarma İşlemi Öncesi Uygulanan Progresif Kas Gevşeme Egzersizi, Soğuk Uygulama Ve Lokal Anestezinin Hastanın Ağrı, Konfor Düzeyi Ve Yaşam Bulguları Üzerine Etkisi*, Yayınlanmamış Yüksek Lisans Tezi, Cumhuriyet Üniversitesi, Sivas.

Özcan, G. & Sert, A.T. (2016). Kas İskelet Ağrısı Tedavisinde Proloterapinin Kanıta Dayalı Kullanımı, *Turkish Journal of Physical Medicine and Rehabilitation*, 62(2), 192–198.

Özveren, H. (2011). Ağrı Kontrolünde Farmakolojik Olmayan Yöntemler, *Hacettepe Üniversitesi Sağlık Bilimleri Fakültesi Hemşirelik Dergisi*, 18(1), 83–92.

Özveren, H., Faydalı, S. & Özdemir, S. (2016). Hemşirelerin Ağrının Farmakolojik Olmayan Yöntemlerle Kontrolüne İlişkin Bilgi ve Uygulamaları, *Turkish Journal of Clinics and Laboratory Care*, 7(4), 99–105.

Peksoy, S., Demirhan, İ., Kaplan, S., Şahin, S. & Arıöz Düzgün, A. (2018). Tamamlayıcı ve Alternatif Tedavinin Jinekolojik Kanserlerde Kullanımı, *Türkiye Sağlık Bilimleri ve Araştırmaları Dergisi*, 1(1), 36–47.

Quinn, F., Hughes, C. M. & Baxter, G. (2008). Reflexology in the Management of Low Back Pain: A Pilot Randomised Controlled Trial, *Complementary Therapies in Medicine*, 16 (1), 3–8.

Sasannejad, P., Saeedi, M., Shoeibi, A., Gorji, A., Abbasi, M. & Foroughipour, M. (2012). Lavender Essential Oil in the Treatment of Migraine Headache: A Placebo-Controlled Clinical Trial, *European Neurology*, 67(5), 288–291.

Sert, E., Sakarya, A.A., Yüksel, Ş.B., Sert, A. & Tüfekçi, S. (2015). Tıbbi Sülükler ve Tıbbi Sülük Salyasının Özellikleri, *Integratif Tıp Dergisi*, 3(2), 12–18.

Shorofi, S.A. & Arbon, P. (2010). Nurses Knowledge, Attitudes, and Professional Use of Complementary and Alternative Medicine (Cam): A Survey at Five Metropolitan Hospitals in Adelaide, *Complementary Therapies in Clinical Practice*, 16(4), 229–234.

Silva, G.L., Luft, C., Lunardelli, A., Amaral, R.H., Melo, D.A., Donadio, M.V. & Oliveria, J.R. (2015). Antioxidant, Analgesic and Anti-inflammatory Effects of Lavender Essential Oil, *Anais da Academia Brasileira de Ciências*, 87(2), 1397–1408.

Şimsek Orhon, F. (2016). İnfantil Kolik Tanı ve Tedavisinde Güncel Yaklaşımlar, Ankara *Üniversitesi Tıp Fakültesi Mecmuası*, 69(3), 159–166.

Soltani, R., Soheilipour, S., Hajhashemi, V., Asghari, G., Bagheri, M. & Molavi, M. (2013). Evaluation of the Effect of Aromatherapy with Lavender Essential Oil on Post-Tonsillectomy Pain in Pediatric Patients: A Randomized Controlled Trial, *International Journal of Pediatric Otorhinolaryngology*, 77(9), 1579–1581.

Stange, R., Moser, C., Hopfenmueller. W., Mansmann, U., Buehring, M. & Uehleke, B. (2012). Randomised Controlled Trial with Medical Leeches for Osteoarthritis of Theknee, *Complementary Therapies in Medicine*, 20(1–2), 1–7.

Stephenson, N.L.N., Weinrich, S.P. & Tavakoli, A.S. (2000). The Effects of Foot Patients with Breast and Lung Cancer Reflexology on Anxiety and Pain, *Oncology Nursing Forum*, 27, 67–72.

Tercan, B. (2015). *Hemşirelerin Ağrı Yönetiminde İlaç Dışı Yöntemleri Bilme ve Uygulama Durumları*, İnönü Üniversitesi Sağlık Bilimleri Enstitüsü Hemşirelik Yüksek Lisans Tezi.

Thorne, S., Paterson, B., Russell, C. & Schultz, A. (2002). Complementary/ Alternative Medicine in Chronic Illness as Informed Self-Care Decision Making, *International Journal of Nursing Studies*, 39(7), 671–683.

Törüner, K.E. & Büyükgönenç, L. (2012). *Çocuk Sağlığı Temel Hemşirelik Yaklaşımları*. Göktuğ Yayıncılık. Ankara.

Uğurlu, E., Kalkım, A. & Sağkal, T. (2014). 0–1 Yaş Arası Bebeklerde Sık Karşılaşılan Ağrı Durumları ve Ailelerin Yaklaşımları, *Fırat Tıp Dergisi*, 19(1), 25–30.

Updike, P. (2010). Music Therapy Results for ICU Patients, *Dimensions of Critical Care Nursing*, 9(1), 39–45.

Uysal, H. (2016). Kardiyovasküler Hastalıklarda Tamamlayıcı ve Alternatif Tıp Konusunda Güncel Yaklaşımlar, *Journal of Cardiovascular Nursing*, 7, 69–83.

Uysal, N. & Kutlutürkani, S. (2016) Kanserli Bireylerde Semptom Kontrolünde Refleksoloji Uygulaması, *Bakırköy Tıp Dergisi*, 12(3), 103–109.

Yaman, H. & Vural, R. (2016). Proloterapi: Kronik Ağrı Yönetiminde Etkili Bir Yöntem. *Ankara Medical Journal*, 16(2), 220–224.

Yaşar, E. (2010). *Genel Anestezi Altındaki Hastalarda Müziğin Intraoperatif ve Postoperatif Etkileri*. Uzmanlık Tezi, Aydın Menderes Üniversitesi, Aydın.

Yiğit, Ü. (2017). *Spinal Anestezide Ameliyat Sırasında Dinletilen Müziğin Hastaların Ameliyat Sırası Yaşam Bulguları ile Ameliyat Sonrası Ağrı ve Anksiyetesi Üzerine Etkisi*, Abant İzzet Baysal Üniversitesi Sağlık Bilimleri Enstitüsü Yayınlanmamış Yüksek Lisans Tezi.

Yıldız, Ü.G., Yıldız, S., Kurt, B.B., Ürper, S., Kurt, Y. & Güzel. S. (2013). Doğum Ağrısı ve Hipnoz, *Integratif Tıp Dergisi*, 1(1), 22–27.

# SECTION 2: New Approaches in Medicine

Güliz Dirimen Arıkan, Ebru Em Öztürk and Meliha Güleryüz

# 9: New Approaches in Medicine

## 1 Introduction

Rapid developments in information technologies in modern societies, the use of social media and the rapid dissemination of information continuously change living conditions. This change is manifested itself in health as in many areas of life. Medicine may be one of the disciplines which is most open to innovation and most needed. In medicine, it is necessary to evaluate innovations with regards to service providers and service receivers.

With the development of technology, production patterns, time management, employee profiles and way of working also change. Considering the ratio of technology usage outside of office, a global research from 6,600 workers across 9 countries indicated that 70 % of employees have access to the files also out of office, 57 % of them can attend same conferences and have same messaging tools. According to the same data, 43 % of employees request better health and well-being, while 37 % of them request to be interested in their family responsibilities (http://www.fuze.com/files/documents/Fuze-WorkforceFutures.pdf). The fulfillment of these expectations is possible by the use of technology and the formation of non-office working environments. Otherwise, work-private life balance cannot be achieved; this situation mentally overburdens individuals. Cognitive disorders are important problems of our age in this challenging and mental burden–increasing environment and cause dependence and disability. Cognitive disorders are also associated with a significant increase in health expenditures.

According to World Health Organization (WHO), 47 million people have severe cognitive impairment worldwide; this number has been estimated to reach 75 million in 2030 (Wallin et al., 2018). New approaches using high technologies are needed to overcome these problems. Lean thinking is one of the new approaches that are inspired by engineering and adapted to health services. The principles of lean thinking can be used in many services, such as emergency, oncology and radiology services. For example, these principles have led to the development of solutions ranging from the use of high-precision troponin-T tests in emergency services to shorten patient wait time for a hospital bed (Wallin et al., 2018).

In this section, innovative approaches that are prominent in some areas of medicine will be discussed.

## 2 Innovation in Medicine

Nowadays, due to intense work pressure, time management problems and increased costs, it has become more difficult for individuals to share their health problems or to have physical check-up going to hospitals. For example, the programs such as HealthTap, Teladoc helps people to communicate with medical doctors via phone and web video and to ask medical questions directly to physicians through a secure, private web platform (https://www. christenseninstitute.org/blog/can-telemedicine-make-the-leap/).

Preventive medicine is one of the most important field of medicine. By means of innovative approaches using technology, diseases can be prevented before they occur and reduction in treatment costs can be provided. The best example of preventive medicine is vaccination; there have been very promising recent developments in this field. The latest vaccines have been developed against diseases as Human Immunodeficiency Virus (HIV) and breast cancer and worked on to put them into practice (Emens, 2018). Another preventive service is the early diagnosis of cancer. Recently, Swiss researchers tried to achieve the early diagnosis of cancer by making visible increase of calcium levels on the skin by an implant in human cells by biotechnological methods (Smart Tattoo) (Tastanova et al., 2018). Genetic analyzes, which are used for early diagnosis, especially in individuals having family members with cancer, have become increasingly popular. They are currently not widely used due to high costs, but it is foreseen that its use will increase in the future with cost reduction.

Whole exome sequencing (WES) is one of the most important test panels developed by using genetic technology. With this test, changes in functional regions of the genome called exon can be determined. Exome is all of the DNA sequences of genes that provide the production of proteins necessary for the function of our body. Many of the mutations that cause diseases were detected in the exon regions of DNA. While most of the genetic tests screened few genes that were thought to be related to the disease, WES tests can screen thousands of genes simultaneously. In families with genetic diseases, the definitive diagnosis of diseases by mutation detection is important for keeping the family name alive. In addition, genetic analysis in in vitro fertilization allows the prevention of diseases (Demirci, 2016).

Colon cancer is among the cancers causing the highest number of deaths, especially in men. Colonoscopy has been started to implement by family physicians in colorectal cancer screening. In a review article of McClellan et al., 1155 colonoscopy applications of family physicians between 2011 and 2014 were evaluated under the supervision of four board certified family physicians. Colonoscopy tests revealed that 38.15 % of the men and 25.96 % of women over 50 years of age had adenoma. The results of the studies have emphasized the positive results of colonoscopies performed by the family physicians for screening; this situation is also stated by various organizations such as American Gastrointestinal Endoscopy Association (ASGIE) (McClellan et al., 2015).

For the treatment of cancer, a biomaterial was produced to deliver drugs to tumor cells without damaging healthy cells (Ruskowitz et al., 2018). Recently, stem cell therapies have been increasingly applied in many different fields of medicine. Organoids produced from the stem cell in cell culture go to the damaged organs and help repairing them (Dye et al., 2015).

The aging of societies and the increase of health expenditures increased the demand for preventive care and primary health care. New application models have been brought to agenda in order to meet this demand (Auerbach et al., 2013a). The patient-centered treatment house model and health centers managed by nurses are among these innovative and integrated healthcare models. These models are expected to improve the quality of the provision of primary healthcare services in particular. The two important functions of treatment houses are teamwork based care and the adaptation of technology into care. In this team, doctors, advanced practice nurses and nurses in other fields, doctors' assistants, pharmacists, nutritionists, social workers, educators and care coordinators are included. The innovations of this model being carried into practice are electronic health record systems and coordination of care. Comprehensive primary care and some specialty services are provided by nurses-managed health centers (known as nurse centers). Today, these centers are typically affiliated to the academic health centers. It is foreseen that the need in primary care will be greatly reduced when these centers become widespread (Auerbach et al., 2013a). Possible obstacles to the implementation of these models are the presence of care process requiring physicians in law and the perceptions of physicians and nurses. Another innovation of the study was that offered an online tool which can modify future predictions by changing the number of health personnel. When these innovative care models are combined with technology and self-management of patients, they will be able to change the way of providing health care significantly (Auerbach et al., 2013b).

According to the World Health Organization (WHO), the most important cause of death in the world is cardiovascular diseases (World Health Organization, 2018). In order to prevent the development of cardiovascular disease, numerous campaigns and educational seminars are organized as a product of innovative thinking, which will lead people for being physically more active, quit smoking and having healthier diet.

Ultrasonography has an important role in the diagnosis of cardiovascular diseases as much as EKG. In a study of Bornemann et al. (2015), the use of pocket-sized USG as a screening tool for left ventricular hypertrophy was investigated; it was shown that left ventricular hypertrophy, which was important for the comorbidities of hypertensive patients, could be evaluated by using technological opportunities in the first line of the treatment.

In the treatment of cardiovascular diseases, third generation biomaterials provide both organ function as well as the stents used in the heart vessels and take part in the treatment by releasing a drug into circulation. Some synthetic peptides are released into circulation as pieces, and they find damaged tissues and repair them (Royal Academy of Engineering, 2014).

One of the most important diseases causing cardiovascular complications is diabetes. The survival and life quality is directly related to patient compliance in patients with diabetes which is known to occur due to a decrease in insulin sensitivity of the surrounding tissues and/or inadequate insulin release from the pancreas (International Diabetes Federation, 2009). One of the programs developed with the use of technology to facilitate patient compliance is the Diabetes Conversation Map (http://www.journeyforcontrol.com/diabetes-educator/about-conversation-map/). This program consists of four different game-like educational tools. Through this tool, the systolic blood pressure levels of the individuals in the case group decreased of 5.4 mmHg in comparison with initial levels (p= 0.014). This study showed that the computer-aided program of the Diabetes Conversation Map improves diabetes performance measurements compared to classical lectures (Crawford and Wiltz, 2015). In another recent study, patients were given education with home visits for 6 weeks about monitoring blood glucose, actions to be taken in possible complications, coordinating of the treatment, body care and help people who need to be reached when necessary; this program was awarded (Codner et al., 2018).

Capillary blood glucose monitoring is very important for diabetes; however, constant finger pricking is a disturbing method and complicates patient compliance with treatment. In order to solve this problem, nanotechnological methods have been developed which less bother patients (Washington State University, 2018; Siwach et al., 2019). Bio prostheses apply to the skin with these methods provide blood glucose monitoring as desired time and frequency without disturbing patients. GlucoModicum Ltd.'s new glucose monitoring technique with the IFUS system developed at the University of Helsinki measures glucose from interstitial fluid without needle puncture (Lautala, 2018).

For the treatment of diabetes, new products that provide ease of use to patients bring out such as buccal and inhaler insulin and patch pump insulin (Easa et al.,

2018). There is no definitive treatment of diabetes yet, but pancreatic islet cell transplantation and stem cell studies are promising (Hart and Powers, 2019).

One of the most important diseases of our age is multiple sclerosis (MS). MS is a chronic, inflammatory and neurodegenerative disease with demyelination and axonal damage of the central nervous system (CNS). The disease can cause progressive and irreversible physical and cognitive disability (Ziliotto, 2018). In young adults, being the second reason after the trauma as a cause of disability increases the importance of MS (Cree, 2008). The invention and becoming widespread of magnetic resonance imaging (MRI) is an important step in the diagnosis and follow-up of MS. In conventional MRI, white matter lesions are seen as hyperintense on T2 sequences, whereas gray matter lesions are not seen because they retain normal proton concentrations (Poloni et al., 2011). Diffusion Tensor Imaging (DTI), Magnetisation Transfer Imaging (MTI) and H-Magnetic Resonance Spectroscopy (MRS) are advanced imaging techniques, which are found to be more sensitive to demonstrate gray matter abnormalities and to monitor the change of these lesions over time (Geurts et al., 2009; Flippi and Rocca, 2011).

In the 1990s, there was no specific treatment for MS and almost only MS attacks could be treated. The studies on the treatment of MS gained momentum over the last 10 years. In recent years, molecularly targeted monoclonal antibody therapies have been introduced in addition to the current prophylactic classical therapies in MS. The clinical trials on many novel molecules also continue. In MS, treatment targets head towards preventing irreversible damage beyond preventing attacks. Monoclonal antibodies are promising for patients who do not respond to current treatments (Gündüz et al., 2018). It has been possible to pass the blood brain barrier and make determinations at the molecular level with nanotechnology. It is expected that nanotechnology, which is a potential area for the diagnosis of MS and development of new treatment models, will increase the quality of life of patients in the future (Ojha and Kumar, 2018). The studies on walking and balance with the help of exoskeletons and robots are promising in MS patients with severe disability (Kozlowski et al., 2017; Straudi et al., 2017).

With increasing life expectancy, today Alzheimer's disease (AD) is an important health problem. Dementia is the loss of one or more of the brain functions in a way that disrupts daily life due to various reasons (Kulaksızoglu, 2018). AD, a type of dementia, was firstly identified in 1906 by Alois Alzheimer (Toodayan, 2016; Kulaksızoğlu, 2018). In this disease, the etiology is not precisely determined, the lack of adequate success in the treatment increases the importance of patient care. The purpose of patient care is to maintain patients' mental functions at the highest level and to make their life quality better. Nowadays, electronic devices are increasingly used to help patients to remember their daily activities. The methods have been developed for reminding their daily schedules to individuals through messages for recording personal information, medical history and medicines, making a shopping list. A safer environment can be provided to patients through assistive technologies such as gas alarms, fire alarms and detectors that report falling (Imbeault et al., 2014). Conducting individual-centered studies with ergo therapy, patients are provided to use assistant tools and adaptations; it is aimed to improve the daily activities of patients using assistive technology and education (Tarakçı, 2018). In recent years through nanotechnology based drug delivery systems in, the active substances enable to pass the blood brain barrier and to be released in brain at the desired concentration, at a constant rate for the desired time. Therefore, it is thought that nanotechnology-based drug delivery systems will improve the clinical response and improve the quality of life in the treatment of AD (Dereli et al., 2016; Aliev et al., 2018).

Acupuncture is a treatment method that has been increasingly used in more fields of medicine and of which origin is based on ancient times. The battlefield acupuncture is an application that was first used for acute injuries of the soldiers and was named after it. In this relatively easy-to-learn technique, family physicians place the needle on the outer ear; the complication rates of the technique are quite low. In addition to the widespread use of acupuncture, Moss and Crowford reported that family physicians used this method in acute sore throat (Moss and Crawford, 2015).

The use of robotic diagnosis and treatment methods in medicine can be life-saving for patients having hard to access higher-level healthcare facilities. An example of this is the prenatal evaluation of a pregnant woman living in northern Canada. USG was applied by remote assistance of a robot for a pregnant woman who was living in Saskatchewan in Canada and had acute problems in her baby. In addition, the nurse taking care of the patient was able to perform intravenous administration with the same guidance (World Economic Forum, 2018).

It would be appropriate to summarize some important examples of new approaches in medicine, each may be a separate book subject, as follows (Raconteur, Wearable Healthcare Tech, 2018):

One of the new technological products, 3D *(three dimensional) virtual glasses* are used in psychiatry. The therapy has been provided by allowing patients to face their phobias in 3-D environment and providing relaxation techniques, which can help patients to overcome this situation.

With an application called *MUSE* and its earphones, the waves are sent to individuals to correct stress, depression and anxiety and focusing problem by determining their moods. Changing challenging living conditions lead to many psychological problems in humans.

UV radiation has an important role in skin cancer. By help of innovation, it is possible to determine the duration of exposure to the sun by means of *UV-sensing sunglasses*. Another recent interesting product is *digestible micro robots*, which go to target body areas or blocked veins, mechanically clear them and provide treatment by secreting drugs when necessary.

*Smart watches*, which are inspired by watches being used in our daily life and have been widely used in recent years, allow the detection of cardiac arrhythmias and transmission of these information to patients' physicians when necessary.

By help of *smart lenses*, blood glucose monitoring will be possible in the near future without using needles. Researchers work on smart contact lenses to measure glucose levels by using tears.

*Virtual consultations* have started to gain momentum, particularly since 2017. Numerous applications have been introduced that allow direct communication of surgeons and primary care physicians without being in the same physical environment.

*Wearable ECG* with the original name of QardioCore is a wireless electrocardiogram developed for the purpose of detecting and monitoring cardiac diseases to minimally disrupt daily life. It is placed on the chest with a light band and has no cables and adhesive tapes as in conventional ECG.

*Smart insulin bands* are wearable microfluidic bands which follow blood glucose levels and automatically administer insulin directly to blood. At the same time, these bands can also be used to administer the drugs that stimulate the pancreas to secrete more insulin.

*The ingestible sensors* provide a new understanding of the health-related patterns of patients and the effectiveness of drug treatments. A microscopic sensor offered by the digital company of Proteus is activated when contacting with the stomach. This sensor is connected with a wearable band that monitors the action of the drug.

*Smart tattoos* are health sensors developed by the researchers at Harvard University and the Massachusetts Institute of Technology (MIT) and embedded in human skin. These sensors use smart tattoo inks that change color according to biochemical materials in the body's interstitial fluid. Meanwhile, the researchers at the University of Illinois study on flat, flexible sensors to apply to temporary tattoos for monitoring the electrical signals generated by heart, brain and muscles.

## 3 Conclusion

As in all areas of life, the main goal of innovation in medicine is to increase the quality and length of life. Registered and accessible public health information is important for both patients and healthcare providers. One of the most important reflections of information technologies in our country are e-government/e-pulse applications, which allow that patients can see their medical histories and share them with their physicians when necessary.

Education is the basis of innovation; it is even claimed that education also has a relationship with life span. In a study, the life expectancy of women with low education level was found to be low (Renard et al., 2019). In today's education systems, such as in the Continuing Medical Education Commission of Istanbul University – Cerrahpaşa Faculty of Medicine, it is tried to gain an understanding being in tune with the time by including educative staff as well as patients and students receiving medical education into medical education programs with the new regulations (Cerrahpaşa Tıp Fakültesi, 2019).

One of the most important recent topics of debate in medicine is whether health-related practices are cost-effective because economy plays an important role in the development of societies. The most outstanding examples of innovative applications are organ transplantations (e.g. face transplantation, hair transplantation, limb transplants) (Berglund et al., 2019; Joshi et al., 2019; Özer and Çolak, 2019). Organ transplants are the implementations that significantly increases patient's quality of life and are successfully performed in Turkey. With the contribution of such practices, the authorities stated that health tourism also creates a remarkable economy in Turkey (Sağlık Bakanlığı, 2019). In our country, there are many innovations in the surgical interventions that may cause increase in health tourism. Perhaps the most important of these innovations is robotic surgery (Esen et al. 2019). With the help of these applications, it is aimed to increase success rate and to decrease complication rates by remotely controlled surgical operations.

In the near future, especially in the field of health, with the use of many technological products and applications that are probably the subjects of science fiction movies previously, times, which important part of intractable diseases will be treated and patient's quality of life will increase, have been waiting for us (Akalın, 2016).

## References

Akalın, E. (2016). Sağlık Politikaları Üzerine, Tıpta İnovasyon ve Ezber Bozan "Disruptive" Teknolojiler, http://saglikpolitikalari.omegacro.com/tipta-inovasyon-ve-ezber-bozan-disruptive-teknolojiler, (accessed on: 30.01.2019).

Aliev, G., Ashraf, G.M., Tarasov, V.V. & et al. (2018). Alzheimer Disease-Future Therapy Based on Dendrimers, *Current Neuropharmacology*, 17(3), 288–294.

Auerbach, D.I., Chen, P.G., Friedberg, M.W. & et al. (2013a). *New Approaches for Delivering Primary Care Could Reduce Predicted Physician Shortage*, RAND Corporation, Research Highlight, http://www.rand.org/pubs/research_briefs/RB9752.html, (accessed on: 21.01.2019).

Auerbach, D.I., Chen, P.G., Friedberg, M.W. & et al. (2013b). Nurse-Managed Health Centers and Patient-Centered Medical Homes Could Mitigate Expected Primary Care Physician Shortage, *Health Affairs*, 32(11), 1933–1941.

Berglund, E., Andersen Ljungdahl, M., Bogdanović, D., Berglund, D., Wadström, J., Kowalski, J. & et al. (2019). Clinical Significance of Alloantibodies in Hand Transplantation – A Multicenter Study, *Transplantation*, 30, 163.

Bornemann, P., Johnson, J., Tiglao, S. & et al. (2015). Assessment of Primary Care Physicians' Use of a Pocket Ultrasound Device™ to Measure Left Ventricular Mass in Patients with Hypertension, *Journal of the American Board of Family Medicine*, 28, 706–712.

Cerrahpaşa Tıp Fakültesi. (2019). Sürekli Tıp Eğitimi Etkinlikleri, http://www.ctf.edu.tr/stek/stek.htm, (accessed on: 11.03.2019).

Codner, E., Acerini, C.L., Craig, M.E., Hofer, S.E. & Maahs, D.M. (2018). International Society for Pediatric and Adolescent Diabetes. ISPAD Clinical Practice Consensus Guidelines. (2018). International Society for Pediatric and Adolescent Diabetes. http://www.ispad.org/page/ISPADGuidelines2018, (accessed on: 30.01.2019).

Crawford, P. & Wiltz, S. (2015). Participation in the Journey to Life Conversation Map Improves Control of Hypertension, Diabetes, and Hypercholesterolemia, *Journal of the American Board of Family Medicine*, 28, 767–771.

Cree, B.A.C. (2008). Multiple Sclerosis and Demyelinating Diseases. (Ed. Brust, J.C.M.). Current Diagnosis and Treatment. McGraw-Hill, New York.

Demirci, H. (2016). Genome Analysis Techniques, TÜBİTAK İleri Genom ve Biyoenformatik Araştırma Merkezi (İGBAM), *Türkiye Klinikleri J Med Genet-Special Topics*, 1(2), 8–12.

Dereli, N., Gün, Ö. & Hasçiçek, C. (2016). Nano-Sized Drug Delivery Systems for Alzheimer Disease Treatment, *Journal of Faculty of Pharmacy of Ankara*, 40(1), 54–73.

Dye, B.R., Hill, D.R., Ferguson, M.AH. & et al. (2015). In Vitro Generation of Human Pluripotent Stem Cell Derived Lung Organoids, *Elife*, 4, e05098.

Easa, N., Alany, R.G., Carew, M. & Vangala, A. (2018). A Review of Non-invasive Insulin Delivery Systems for Diabetes Therapy in Clinical Trials over the Past Decade, *Drug Discovery Today*, 24(2), 440–451.

Emens, L. (2018). Treatment of Aggressive Breast Cancer Improved by Immunotherapy-Chemotherapy Combination, EurekAlert! *Science News*, http://eurekalert.org/pub_releases/2018-10/uops-toa102018.php, (accessed on: 30.01.2019).

Esen, E., Aytac, E., Ozben, V., Bas, M., Bilgin, I.A., Aghayeva, A. & et al. (2019). Adoption of Robotic Technology in Turkey: A Nationwide Analysis on Caseload and Platform Used, *International Journal of Medical Robotics*, 15(1), e1962.

Flippi, M. & Rocca, M.A. (2011). MR Imaging of Multiple Sclerosis, *Radiology*, 259, 659–681.

Geurts, J.J., Stys, P.K., Minagar, A., Amor, S. & Zivadinov, R. (2009). Gray Matter Pathology in (Chronic) MS: Modern Views on an Early Observation, *Journal of Neurological Science*, 282, 12–20.

Gündüz, T., Yüksel, B., Tamam, Yusuf., İrkeç, C. & Karabudak, R. (2018). Multiple Sklerozda Monoklonal Antikorlar. (eds. Efendi, H., Yandım Kuşçu, D.), *Multiple Skleroz Tanı ve Tedavi Klavuzu 2018*. İstanbul: Galenos.

Hart, N.J. & Powers, A.C. (2019). Use of Human Islets to Understand Islet Biology and Diabetes: Progress, Challenges and Suggestions, *Diabetologia*, 62(2), 212–222.

http://www.fuze.com/files/documents/Fuze-WorkforceFutures.pdf, (accessed on: 30.01.2019).

http://www.journeyforcontrol.com/diabetes-educator/about-conversation-map/, (accessed on: 27.01.2019).

https://www.christenseninstitute.org/blog/can-telemedicine-make-the-leap/, (accessed on: 30.01.2019).

Imbeault, H., Bier, N., Pigot, H., Gagnon, L., Marcotte, N., Fulop, T. & Giroux, S. (2014). Electronic Organiser and Alzheimer's Disease: Factor Fiction?, *Neuropsychological Rehabilitation*, 24(1), 71–100.

International Diabetes Federation. (2009). IDF Diabetes Atlas, Fourth Edition, http://idf.org/e-library/epidemiology-research/diabetes-atlas/21-atlas-4th-edition.html, (accessed on: 30.01.2019).

Joshi, R., Shokri, T., Baker,A., Kohlert, S., Sokoya, M., Kadakia, S. & et al. (2019). Alopecia and Techniques in Hair Restoration: An Overview for the Cosmetic Surgeon, *Oral & Maxillofacial Surgery*, 23(2), 123–131.

Kozlowski, A.J., Fabian, M., Lad, D. & Delgado, A.D. (2017). Feasibility and Safety of a Powered Exoskeleton for Assisted Walking for Persons with Multiple Sclerosis: A Single-Group Preliminary Study, *Archives of Physical Medicine and Rehabilitation*, 98(7), 1300–1307.

Kulaksızoğlu, IB. (2018). Demans Tanımı ve Alzheimer Hastalığı. (ed. Ünal, M.), *Alzheimer'a Dair Her Şey (Alzheimer Hastası Olmak, Alzheimer'lı Hasta ile Yaşamak)*, İstanbul: İstanbul Tıp Kitabevi.

Lautala, E. (2018). GlucoModicum: Needle-Free and Painless Health Monitoring, University of Helsinki, http://helsinki.fi/en/news/health-news/glucomodicum-needle-free-and-painless-health-monitoring, (accessed on: 30.01.2019).

McClellan, D.A, Ojinnaka, C.O., Pope, R. & et al. (2015). Expanding Access to Colorectal Cancer Screening: Benchmarking Quality Indicators in a Primary Care Colonoscopy Program, *Journal of the American Board of Family Medicine*, 28, 713–721.

Moss, D.A. & Crawford, P. (2015). Ear Acupuncture for Acute Sore Throat: A Randomized Controlled Trial, *American Board of Family Medicine*, 28, 697–705.

Ojha, S. & Kumar, B. (2018). A Review on Nanotechnology Based Innovations in Diagnosis and Treatment of Multiplesclerosis, *Journal of Cellular Immunotherapy*, 4(2), 56–64.

Özer, K. & Çolak, O. (2019). Micro-Autologous Fat Transplantation Combined with Platelet-Rich Plasma for Facial Filling and Regeneration: A Clinical Perspective in the Shadow of Evidence-Based Medicine, *Journal of Craniofacial Surgery*, 30(3), 672–677.

Poloni, G., Minagar, A., Haacke, E.M. & Zivadinov, R. (2011). Recent Developments in Imaging of Multiple Sclerosis, *Neurologist*, 17, 185–204.

Raconteur, Wearable Healthcare Tech. (2018). http://res.cloudinary.com/yumyoshojin/image/upload/v1/pdf/future-healthcare-2018.pdf, (accessed on: 30.01.2019)

Renard, F., Devleesschauwer, B., Van Oyen, H., Gadeyne, S. & Deboosere, P. (2019). Evolution of Educational Inequalities in Life and Health Expectancies at 25 Years in Belgium between 2001 and 2011: A Census-Based Study, *Archives of Public Health*, 77(6), 1–10.

Royal Academy of Engineering. (2014). Innovation in Materials, http://raeng.org.uk/publications/reports/innovation-in-materials, (accessed on: 30.01.2019).

Ruskowitz, E.R., Comerford, M.P., Badeau, B.A. & DeForest, C.A. (2018). Logical Stimuli-Triggered Delivery of Small Molecules from Hydrogel Biomaterials. *Biomaterials Science*, 7, 542–546.

Sağlık Bakanlığı, Sağlık Hizmetleri Genel Müdürlüğü, Sağlık Turizmi Daire Başkanlığı. (2019). https://saglikturizmi.saglik.gov.tr/TR,175/saglik-turizmi-hakkinda.html, (accessed on: 11.03.2019).

Siwach, R., Pandey, P., Chawla, V. & et al. (2019). Role of Nanotechnology in Diabetic Management, *Recent Patents on Nanotechnology*, 13(1), 28–37.

Straudi, S., Manfredini, F., Lamberti, N. & et al. (2017). The Effectiveness of Robot-Assisted Gait Training versus Conventional Therapy on Mobility in Severely Disabled Progressive Multiple Sclerosis Patients (RAGTIME): Study Protocol for a Randomized Controlled Trial. *Trials*, 18(1), 88.

Tarakçı, E. (2018). Alzheimer Hastalığında Ergoterapi. (ed. Ünal, M.), *Alzheimer'a Dair Her Şey (Alzheimer Hastası Olmak, Alzheimer'lı Hasta ile Yaşamak)*, İstanbul: İstanbul Tıp Kitabevi.

Tastanova, A., Folcher, M., Müller, M. & et al. (2018). Synthetic Biology-Based Cellular Biomedical Tattoo for Detection of Hypercalcemia Associated with Cancer, *Science Translational Medicine*, 10(437), eaap8562.

Toodayan, N. (2016). Alois Alzheimer (1864–1915): Lest We Forget, *J Clin Neurosci*, 31, 47–55.

Wallin, A., Kettunen, P., Johansson, P.M. & et al. (2018). Cognitive Medicine – A New Approach in Health Care Science, *BMC Psychiatry*, 18(1), 42.

Washington State University. (2018). 3D-Printed Glucose Biosensors, *ScienceDaily*. www.sciencedaily.com/releases/2018/12/181207112658.htm, (accessed on: 30.01.2019).

World Economic Forum. (2018). How Robots Are Helping Doctors Save Lives in the Canadian North. http://weforum.org/agenda/2018/12/how-robots-are-helping-doctors-save-lives-in-the-canadian-north/?utm_source=Facebook%20Videos&utm_medium=Facebook%20Videos&utm_campaign=Facebook%20Video%20Blogs,

World Health Organization. (2018). The Top 10 Causes of Death. http://who.int/news-room/fact-sheets/detail/the-top-10-causes-of-death, (accessed on: 30.01.2019).

Ziliotto, N., Bernardi, F., Jakimovski, D. & et al. (2018). Hemostasis Biomarkers in Multiple Sclerosis, *Neurology*, 25, 1169–1176.

Mümtaz Taner Torun

# 10: Robotic Surgery from Past to Future and Its Applications in Otorhinolaryngologic Surgery

## 1 Introduction

Technological developments cause major changes in health care in recent years. With the integration of industrial robots in the medical field, many risky and challenging surgeries become easier. Robotic surgical techniques started to be used in the late 1980s. In the 2000s da Vinci robot has become widespread after the approval of the Food and Drug Administration (FDA) (Pugin et al., 2011). There were 1.745 million robotic surgeries performed in the USA between the years of 2000 and 2013 and it increases every year (Usluoğulları et al., 2017). At first, robots were used for biopsy by the neuro-surgical department. After the developments in robotic surgery, advanced robots have started to be used in various medical fields such as cardiovascular surgery, orthopedics, urology, otorhinolaryngologic diseases and general surgery.

In the future, robots may be able to perform surgical interventions by their own special techniques. It can be predicted that they will be able to suture and perform various operations autonomously.

## 2 The History of Robotic Surgery

Al-Jazari, who lived in the 12th century, was accepted the father of robotic science with his invention of the first robot. In 1917, Czechoslovakian Josef Ćapek mentioned about automatons in his short story "Opilec" and his brother Karel Ćapek first used the word of robot in his book "Rossum's Universal Robots" in 1920 and then this word had been used worldwide (Ćapek, 1920; Ćapek, 1925). Robotics deals with the design, construction, operation and use of robots, as well as computer systems for their control, sensory feedback and information processing. These technologies are used to develop machines that can substitute for humans and replicate human actions.

Industrial robots are used in various surgical techniques. Robotic surgery is a type of surgical procedure that is done using robotic systems completely or partially. The introduction of robots in medicine began in the 1980s with the robotic surgery studies of the engineers of AMES Research Center (work for the National Aeronautics and Space Administration [NASA] in the USA) and Stanford Research Institute (Lanfranco et al., 2004). PUMA 560, the first robot used in surgery, was used in computed tomography (CT) assisted brain tissue sampling in 1985. Three years later, PROBOT was developed by Imperial College London and started to be used in transurethral prostatic surgeries (Harris et al., 1997).

In 1992, ROBODOC was developed by Integrated Surgical Systems and International Business Machines Corporation and it was approved by the FDA and was used in femoral head replacement (Hockstein, 2007). In 1993, a voice controlled robotic system was developed and was approved with the name of AESOP 1000 (Automated Endoscopic System for Optimal Positioning, Computer Motion, Inc., Goleta, CA) by the FDA, in 1994. In the following years, AESOP 2000, AESOP 3000 and AESOP HR models have been introduced with the new functions of sound control such as operation table position and illumination of the operation room. (Lanfranco et al., 2004). Key features in these models are having a robotic arm holding the endoscope and the presence of a special sound control system for the surgeon.

In 1997, a new robotic surgical system (RSS) called MONA was developed and used in robotic-assisted laparoscopic cholecystectomy for the first time in Belgium (Shah, 2014). This system with power-feedback and three dimensional (3D) display would have been the prototype of modern da Vinci robots (Intuitive Surgical, Sunnyvale, CA). As technological advances continue, the AESOP systems have not been abandoned and the ZEUS (Computer Motion, Inc., Goleta, CA), where all systems are placed into a telemanipulator (a device remotely controlled by a live operator), is produced. This model has received FDA approval for a limited number of surgeries in 2001. Similar to the AESOP model, the arm that holds the endoscope is sound controlled and the other two arms are designed in a structure that can be controlled by the surgeon with joystics and use various instruments. The use of ZEUS by Reicherspurner has also been widely used in various areas such as tubal ligation, pelvic lymph node dissection and cholecystectomy following the first robotic aortocoronary bypass application (Reichenspurner, 1999; Guillonneau, 2001).

In 2001, a transatlantic operation was performed by Professor Jacques Marescaux and his assistants for the first time with the help of the SOCRATES system (Computer Motion, Inc., Santa Barbara, CA) (Marescaux, 2001). A laparoscopic cholecystectomy was performed on a 68-year-old female patient in Paris with a delay of approximately 150 msec from Strasbourg.

ZEUS and da Vinci RSS were developed in the same years. Da Vinci has received FDA approval for general laparoscopic surgeries in RSS 2000 and its new models were developed in 2002, 2006 and 2009. This system is used in cardiac, colorectal, gynecological, head and neck, thoracic and urological surgeries.

The various Rsss such as HERMES (it is a voice controlled robotic system and robotic arms are not used), Orthopilot (it is used in large joint replacements and is FDA approved), Artemis (it is used in minimally invasive abdominal surgeries), Raven 1 and 2 (they are tele-operative systems and are available in different disciplines, such as engineering and computer science except for surgery), Sofie (it is the first robotic system that provides force feedback), Amadeus (it is developed in Canada and it is used for laparoscopic surgeries), Endo Stitch Suturing (it is developed for automatic suturing) and Cyber Knife (it is an image-guided robotic tecnology for non-invasive radiation procedures, and is FDA approved) are also used (Dwivedi and Mahgoub, 2012).

In this area, which is dominated by the da Vinci RSS, among other systems with FDA approval, there are also RSSs like the Sensei X robotic catheter system (it is designed for cardiac catheterization by Hansen Medical Inc, Mountain View, CA, and it received FDA approval in 2007), FreeHand v1.2 (it was developed by FreeHand 2010 Ltd, Cardiff, UK, it is a robotic camera carrier system in minimally invasive surgery and it received FDA approval in 2009), Invendoscopy E200 system (it was developed by Invendo Medical GmbH, Germany, it has handheld and processing unit for colonoscopy and it received FDA approval in 2016), the Flex robotic system (it designed for transoral surgeries in otorhinolaryngology, designed by Medrobotics Corp, Raynham, MA and it received FDA approval in 2009), Senhance (it is a console type robotic platform, produced by TransEnterix, Morrisville, NC and received FDA approval in 2017), Auris robotic endoscopic system (it was designed for visualization of the respiratory system during bronchoscopy by Auris Surgical Robotics, Silicon Valley, CA, USA and it received FDA approval in 2016) and NeoGuide Endoscopy System (it is used in colonoscopy, designed by NeoGuide Endoscopy System Inc, Los Gatos, CA and it received FDA approval in 2009) (Peters et al., 2018). However, there are various RSSs which have not received FDA approval yet, such as MiroSurge (it is a system for better haptic return to the surgeon and created by RMC, DLR, German Aerospace Center, Oberpfaffenhofen-Weßling), ViaCath system (Biotronik, Berlin, Germany), SPORT surgical system (Titan Medical Inc, Toronto, Ontario), The SurgiBot (TransEnterix, Morrisville, NC), Versius Robotic System (Cambridge Medical Robotics Ltd, Cambridge, UK), master and slave transluminal endoscopic robot (Nanyang Technological University and National University Health System), Verb Surgical (Verb Surgical Inc, J&J/Alphabet, Mountain View, CA, USA), Miniature in vivo robot (Virtual Incision, CAST, University of Nebraska Medical Center, Omaha, Nebraska, USA) and the Einstein surgical robot (Medtronic, Minneapolis, MN) (Peters et al., 2018).

## 3 Robotic Surgery Equipments

The da Vinci RSS has the most use in its field and consists of 4 basic elements:

**Surgical Console:** It is the part where the surgeon will be able to sit comfortably and control robotic instruments by watching a 3D image of the operation area.

**Robot and Carrier Platform:** This part consists of robotic arms and the platform on which the patient is placed. There are three or four arms under the command of a surgeon who will perform the operation. One of these arms, which has the ability to rotate in its pivot points, holds the 3D camera while the other three hold surgical instruments to be used during the operation.

**Surgical Instruments:** It consists of the instruments with 7 degrees of free movement and 2 degrees of axial rotation which can rotate 540 degrees around their axis.

**Imaging Systems:** It contains the system which is the same as 3D image that the human eye perceives in real life. Two high-resolution optical fiber camera systems are used for this purpose. Each camera transmits its image to one of the surgeon's eyes via the optical device. A 3D image is created by producing an image by the right camera for the right eye and an image by the left camera for the left eye of the surgeon.

## 4 Advantages and Disadvantages of Robotic Surgery

Robotic systems, which are defined as master-slave, are used by the surgeon sitting on the console and directing the robot remotely nowadays. RSS prevents surgeons not only stand up for a long time but also fatigue. So they can complete surgeries in a healthier way. In addition, although the tremor of hands of the surgeon operating in the console, a software measure this tremor and the effect of it is reduced to zero. RSS instruments can mimic the human wrist reflexes such as holding and cutting in smaller areas, even with a much higher degree of curve and sensitivity.

In laparoscopic surgeries, the images are 2-dimensional (2D) as they are produced with a single camera. Da Vinci can produce 3D images in its robotic camera, instead of 2D images. Thus, surgeons have the chance to perform their operations in a much more sensitive way. RSSs can also provide remote operation, such as tele-surgery, even transoceanic surgeries.

In recent systems, haptic vibrations have been transmitted to surgeons and this is no longer the disadvantage of RSS.

Robotic Simultaneous Image Joining System is the combination of robot and imaging methods such as x-ray, CT, magnetic resonance imaging (MRI) and ultrasonography (Curiel et al., 2007). In this way, a simultaneous step-by-step images can be taken during surgery.

Hard accessibility and high costs are the most important disadvantages of robotic surgeries. Today, da Vinci RSS costs approximately 1.55 million pounds, the annual service fee 125000 pounds and its instruments are around 2000 pounds (Ashrafian et al., 2017). In many studies, the researchers have found out that the RSS operations have been more expensive than laparoscopic and open surgeries (Yu et al., 2012; Yang et al., 2014). However, when funding is not limited, robotic surgery can be used to provide surgical care to patients without direct access to the surgeon.

The long preparation time of the system, heaviness and largeness are the other disadvantages. These problems are expected to be overcome in following years.

## 5 Usage Fields of Robotic Surgery Systems

**Urological Surgery:** The robotic surgery has the most common usage in urology. It is used extensively in the pelvis where mobility is difficult and the movement is restricted. RSS is used in operations such as radical and partial nephrectomy, pyeloplasty, radical prostatectomy, radical cystectomy, adrenalectomy, pelvic lymph node dissection and sacrocolpopexy. In addition, it is used in pediatric ureteropelvic junction strictness surgeries. In a study, it has been reported that robotic-asisted cystroprostatectomies have shorter postoperative catheterization period and less bleeding. The erectile function returns faster, too (Menon et al., 2003). Similar results have been reported in different studies, but it has been emphasized that its cost was higher than laparoscopic and open surgeries (Ficarra et al., 2013).

**Cardiothoracic Surgery:** The most important usage of robotic surgery is coronary artery bypass operations. Instead of median sternotomy, the lower morbidity, shorter postoperative recovery period and less incisions are the main advantages of the robotic surgery. Mitral valve repair, pericardiectomy, retromediastinal tumors and atrial septal defect repair are other usage areas of RSSs.

**Gynecologic Surgery:** The first animal studies with RSSs were reported in uterine horn and tubal anastomosis operations, in 1998 (Margossian et al., 1998a, 1998b). Hysterectomy, salpingooferectomy, myomectomy and endometriosis surgeries on humans have been reported since 2000 (Degueldre et al., 2000; Falcone et al., 2000).

**Gastroeneterologic Surgery:** Nowadays capsule endoscopy is used clinically. These capsules move forward with peristaltic movements and take images from the gastrointestinal tract (Ashrafian et al., 2017). In addition, it is used in a wide range of operations such as antireflux operations, Heller myotomy, gastric bypass, gastrojejunostomy, esophogectomy, gastrectomy, gastric band operations, colectomy, splenectomy and pancreatic resection.

**Other Surgeries:** RSSs are used in many other fields such as orthopedic surgeries (hip prosthesis, total knee arthroplasty, fracture repositioning etc.), pediatric surgeries (congenital heart diseases, ureteropelvic stenosis procedures etc.) and transplantation and brain surgery operations (brain tumor resection, microsurgery).

## 6 Robotic Surgery and Its Applications in Otorhinolaryngologic Diseases and Head and Neck Surgery

The use of robotic surgery in head and neck surgery began in 2003 by neck dissection and submandibular gland excision on pigs (Hauys et al., 2003). After the studies have demonstrated the feasibility of robotic surgery in canine and human cadaver models with transoral robotic surgery (TORS) techniques in 2005, TORS has been used widespread in otorhinolaryngologic diseases (Hockstein et al., 2005; Weinstein et al., 2005). In 2009, the FDA approved da Vinci RSS in T1 and T2 oropharynx, larynx and hypopharynx tumor operations. Multiple arms have difficulty in maneuvering and reaching to the operational area in the oral cavity so it is possible to use only two arms (one of them is to catch and hold the tissue and the other one is to dissect). The single port is a system with 3-joint instrument and a flexible 3D camera that can be used with a 25 mm cannula (Remacle et al., 2005).

Nowadays, RSSs are safely used in the benign and malignant diseases of the pharynx (including tongue, tongue base and tonsils) as well as in the pathologies of the larynx (supraglottis, glottis), hypopharynx, parapharynx, and nasopharynx. After Vicini et al. has reported the first RSS usage in tongue base procedures in 2010, it has been used widespread in sleep apnea operations (Vicini et al., 2012). In transoral procedures recovery is faster, postoperative pain is less and the operation time is shorter than the other procedures (Vicini et al., 2010).

Weinstein et al. developed and performed the robotic supraglottic laryngectomy technique for the first time (Weinstein et al., 2007).

The most important advantages of TORS are less bleeding and short recovery period. Also, there is no incision scar and no need to tracheotomy. In 2013, Lawson et al. developed robotic total laryngectomy technique by combining transoral supraglottic laryngectomy and hypopharyngectomy procedures (Lawson et al., 2013). Maximum mucosal protection, minimal pharyngotomy defect and direct vision of neofarenx are the main advantages of the transoral total laryngectomy technique.

It was started to be used in thyroidectomy with hemithyroidectomy operations in 2005 (Tae et al., 2019a). Cosmetic results are excellent with RSSs when the transoral (access to the thyroid area is achieved by blunt dissection after 3 incisions from the inner side of the lower lip), postauricular facelift (access to the thyroid area is achieved by the dissection throughout the sternocleidomastoid muscle after a retroauricular incision) and transaxillary (access to the thyroid area is achieved by dissection over the pectoralis major muscle with an axillar incision) approaches are applied in thyroid surgeries (Tae et al., 2019b).

Although postauricular incisions have often been preferred for the neck dissection (radical, modified radical and functional), transoral (it has been preferred for retropharyngeal lymph node dissection) and transaxillary (it is hard to access to I and IIb regions of the neck) approaches have also been used. The neck dissection procedures were performed via the transaxillary approach and it was reported as case series in the literature (Lörincz et al., 2013; Yu et al., 2018).

Chan et al. reported that TORS can also be used in head and neck reconstructions. They presented a patient with hypopharyngeal cancer who underwent transoral resection and transoral reconstruction with a jejunum flap (Chan et al., 2017).

There has not been enough information for robotic paranasal sinus surgery in the literature, yet. In 2007, Hanna et al. described transnasal access to the anterior skull base by performing superior vestibular incisions from the canine fossa on four cadavers, followed by osteotomies and inserting the endoscope through the nostril (Hanna et al., 2007). At the same year, Strauss et al. developed an endoscope holder for endonasal etmoidectomy procedures and tested it in 49 total ethmoidectomy operations (Strauss et al., 2007).

It is aimed that robotic anterior and middle skull base procedures (especially for infratemporal fossa, nasopharynx, pituitary and dura approaches) should be performed without transfacial incision and bone excisions. There are several cadaver studies in the literature (Schuler et al., 2015; Friedrich et al., 2017a). Robotic sinus surgery and skull base procedures are currently under investigation and there is no routine system available.

RSSs has also started to be used in ear surgeries. After the promising cadaveric studies on mastoidectomy and cochlear implantation surgeries, the first clinical trial (robotic cochlear implantation) was presented by Caversaccio et al. in 2017 (Caversaccio et al., 2017).

The use of rigid and linear scopes in da Vinci RSS may be inadequate in access to curved areas such as tongue base and pharynx. To use rigid and linear

**Tab. 10.1:** The Development Process of RSSs in Otorhinolaryngology and Head and Neck Surgery (Ashrafian et al., 2017).

| Year | Development |
| --- | --- |
| 2000 | FDA approval of da Vinci System for laparoscopy. |
| 2003 | Application of the first head and surgical procedure by using da Vinci System. |
| 2005 | First head and neck surgery on a human by using da Vinci System. |
| 2009 | FDA approval of da Vinci System for transoral robotic surgery. |
| 2012 | Use of FLEX Robotic System on a cadaver. |
| 2014 | The first use of FLEX Robotic System on a human with CE approval. |
| 2015 | FDA approval of FLEX Robotic Sytem for transoral robotic surgery. |

scopes in da Vinci RSS may be inadequate to access curved areas such as tongue base and pharynx. The Flex Robotic System (Medrobotics, Raynham, MA) was designed for head and neck surgery procedures. This system increases the field of view with its flexible endoscopic instrument and it has 2 consoles. The consoles contain carrier robotic scope, monitor and joystick. Various semi-flexible devices can also be added to lengthen the robotic arm. Remacle et al. conducted the first study on this system that received European CE approval in 2014 (Remacle et al., 2015).

In 2015, the Flex Robotic System was approved by FDA for oropharynx, hypopharynx, and larynx surgery in patients older than 22 years. Animal model and cadaver studies have demonstrated its feasibility in laryngectomy, Zenker diverticulum excision, thyroid lobectomy, neck dissection, submandibular gland excision, skull base and nasopharyngeal procedures (Schuler et al., 2015; Friedrich et al., 2017b). In addition, Lerner et al. found similar results with other methods in terms of oropharynx and hypopharynx abrasion and blunt trauma (Lerner et al., 2017). Table 10.1 summarizes the development of the RSSs in otolaryngology and head and neck surgery.

# 7 Conclusion

There have been important developments in the robotic surgery since 2000. Simple-function devices turned into the sophisticated and capable robots and they become widespread. Although it was first used in the cardiac surgery, it was started to be used in all surgical fields. The most common usage field of RSSs is urological surgeries.

It's possible to integrate the navigation systems, CT and MRI to RSS in the future. With such technological advancement, it may be easier to control the operations by performing simultaneous imaging in the surgery. If elastography, spectroscopy, histopathological screening and nanoparticle technology combine with RSSs, surgical margin control and pathological tissue typing can be simultaneously performed in the surgery. Thus, postoperative pathological examination may not be needed.

Studies are currently in progress to identify macroscopically invisible nerves during surgery. The development of such a system and its integration into RSS can greatly increase the success in nerve-sparing surgery.

Scientists are working on a technology to prevent the loss of image due to fog, bleeding and debris accumulation during the operation. It is aimed to overcome this problem by creating a carbon dioxide barrier on the lens and cleaning the lens automatically and quickly. Although there is intense bleeding, intervention and suturing may be performed within the bloody area instead of open surgery in the future.

NASA is exploring the use of surgical robots for emergency surgery on astronauts in a submarine to simulate conditions in space in a project called NEEMO 7. The Pentagon is investing $12 million in a project to develop a "trauma pod" surgical robot to operate on soldiers wounded away from home (Poon et al., 2018).

In the future, the plan is to implement the Trauma Pod in combat areas via telesurgery and telecommunications while protecting the actual surgeons in a remote location.

In a four step process, the first step involves loading the wounded soldier into the pod via a fully automated machine. The second step involves complete initial scan and administration of oxygen, fluid or blood infusion, as well as processing and prep work for triage and treatment. The third step involves the remote surgeon teleoperating the instruments to stabilize the patient. The final step is airlifting the injured via evacuation helicopters to the nearest field hospital (Yu et al., 2012).

It is possible that robots will be able to perform surgical interventions with their own special techniques. It's also possible that they will be able to move, cut and suture autonomously during a surgery. The autonomous movements of robots will be synchronized with surgeons for various standard operation procedures in the future, too. Different simulation programs can help the researchers to find the informations that they need about different types of surgeries. For instance, when the datas of the approximate size of a kidney cancer and its distance to other organs uploaded to the robot, it can be possible to predict the complications then the surgeons can solve the problem easily.

We have seen that a robot can get into a human organ through small holes. We do not mention about a treatment with scalpel and knife. In future, robots should eliminate the problems and eradicate the diseases completely by delivering drugs to relevant areas. Moreover, various capsules should be able to diagnose and cure the diseases.

In the future, robotic surgery may be as in the novel of "Fantastic Voyage" by Isaac Asimov. Magnetic manipulation of robotic capsules in human veins may facilitate the treatment of these capsules by reaching the most difficult parts of our circulatory system. Why not?

## References

Ashrafian, H., Clancy, O., Grover, V. & Darzi, A. (2017). The Evolution of Robotic Surgery: Surgical and Anaesthetic Aspects, *Br J Anaesth*, 119(1), 72–84.

Čapek, J. (1925). Opilec, *Aventinum*, Prague: Lelio A Pro DelWna.

Čapek, K. (1920). *Rossum's Universal Robots*, (Eds. P Selver, N Playfair, Trans), Mineola, Dover Pub. Inc.

Caversaccio, M., Gavaghan, K., Wimmer, W., Williamson, T., Ansò, J., Mantokoudis, G. & et al. (2017). Robotic Cochlear Implantation: Surgical Procedure and First Clinical Experience, *Acta Oto-Laryngol*, 137(4), 447–454.

Chan, J.Y.W., Chan, R.C.L., Chow, V.L.Y., Tsang, R.K.Y., Wong, S.T.S. & Wei, W.I. (2017). Transoral Robotic Total Laryngopharyngectomy and Free Jejunal Flap Reconstruction for Hypopharyngeal Cancer, *Oral Oncol*, 72, 194–196.

Curiel, L., Chopra, R. & Hynynen, K. (2007). Progress in Multimodality Imaging: Truly Simultaneous Ultrasound and Magnetic Resonance Imaging, *IEEE Trans Med Imaging*, 26(12), 1740–1746.

Degueldre, M., Vandromme, J., Huong, P.T. & Cadière, G.B. (2000). Robotically Assisted Laparoscopic Microsurgical Tubal Reanastomosis: A Feasibility Study, *Fertil Steril*, 74(5), 1020–1023.

Dwivedi, J. & Mahgoub, I. (2012). *Robotic surgery – A Review on Recent Advances in Surgical Robotic Systems*, Florida Conference on Recent Advances In Robotics, Boca Raton, Florida, May 10–11.

Falcone, T., Goldberg, J.M., Margossian, H. & Stevens, L. (2000). Robotic-Assisted Laparoscopic Microsurgical Tubal Anastomosis: A Human Pilot Study, *Fertil Steril*, 73(5), 1040–1042.

Ficarra, V., Wiklund, P.N., Rochat, C.H., Dasgupta, P., Challacombe, B.J., Sooriakumaran, P. & et al. (2013). The European Association of Urology

Robotic Urology Section (ERUS) Survey of Robot-Assisted Radical Prostatectomy (RARP), *BJU Int*, 111(4), 596–603.

Friedrich, D.T., Scheithauer, M.O., Greve, J., Rotter, N., Doescher, J., Hoffmann, T.K. & Schuler, P.J. (2017a). Application of a Computer-Assisted Flexible Endoscope System for Transoral Surgery of the Hypopharynx and Upper Esophagus, *Eur Arch Otorhinolaryngol*, 274(5), 2287–2293.

Friedrich, D.T., Sommer, F., Scheithauer, M.O., Greve, J., Hoffmann, T.K. & Schuler, P.J. (2017b). An Innovate Robotic Endoscope Guidance System for Transnasal Sinus and Skull Base Surgery: Proof of Concept, *J Neurol Surg B Skull Base*, 78(6), 466–472.

Funk, E., Goldenberg, D. & Goyal, N. (2017). Demonstration of Transoral Robotic Supraglottic Laryngectomy and Total Laryngectomy in Cadaveric Specimens Using the Medrobotics Flex System, *Head Neck*, 39(6), 1218–1225.

Guillonneau, B., Cappele, O., Martinez, J.B., Navarra, S. & Vallancien, G. (2001). Robotic Assisted, Laparoscopic Pelvic Lymph Node Dissection in Humans, *J Urol*, 165(4), 1078–1081.

Hanna, E.Y., Holsinger, C., DeMonte, F. & Kupferman, M. (2007). Robotic Endoscopic Surgery of the Skull Base: A Novel Surgical Approach, *Arch Otolaryngol Head Neck Surg*, 133(12), 1209–1214.

Harris, S.J., Arambula-Cosio, F., Mei, Q., Hibberd, R.D., Davies, B.L., Wickham, J.E., Nathan, M.S. & Kundu, B. (1997). The Probot – An Active Robot for Prostate Resection, *Proc Inst Mech Eng H*, 211(4), 317–325.

Haus, B.M., Kambham, N., Le, D., Moll, F.M., Gourin, C. & Terris, D.J. (2003). Surgical Robotic Applications in Otolaryngology, *Laryngoscope*, 113(7), 1139–1144.

Hockstein, N.G., Gourin, C.G., Faust, R.A. & Terris, D.J. (2007). A History of Robots: From Science Fiction to Surgical Robotics, *J Robot Surg*, 1(2), 113–118.

Hockstein, N.G., Nolan, P., O'Malley, J. & Woo, Y.J. (2005). Robot-Assisted Microlaryngeal Surgery: Results of Robotic Cadaver Dissections, *Laryngoscope*, 115(6), 1003–1008.

Lanfranco, A. R., Castellanos, A. E., Desai, J.P. & Meyers, W. C. (2004). Robotic Surgery: A Current Perspective, *Ann Surg*, 239(1), 14–21.

Lawson, G., Mendelsohn, A.H., Van Der Vorst, S., Bachy, V. & Remacle, M. (2013). Transoral Robotic Surgery Total Laryngectomy, *Laryngoscope*, 123(1), 193–196.

Lerner, M.Z., Tricoli, M. & Strome, M. (2017). Abrasion and Blunt Tissue Trauma Study of a Novel Flexible Robotic System in the Porcine Model, *Am J Otolaryngol*, 38(4), 447–451.

Lörincz, B.B. & Knecht, R. (2013). Transoral Robotic Total Laryngectomy and Neck Dissection: The Concept of Robotic Combo Surgery, *Laryngorhinootologie*, 92(9), 585–588.

Marescaux, J., Leroy, J., Gagner, M., Rubino, F., Mutter, D., Vix, M., Butner, S.E. & Smith, M.K. (2001). Transatlantic Robot-Assisted Telesurgery, *Nature*, 413(6854), 379–380.

Margossian, H., Garcia-Ruiz, A., Falcone, T., Goldberg, J.M., Attaran, M. & Gagner, M. (1998a). Robotically Assisted Laparoscopic Microsurgical Uterine Horn Anastomosis, *Fertil Steril*, 70(3), 530–534.

Margossian, H., Garcia-Ruiz, A., Falcone, T., Goldberg, J.M., Attaran, M., Miller, J.H. & Gagner, M. (1998b). Robotically Assisted Laparoscopic Tubal Anastomosis in a Porcine Model: A Pilot Study, *J Laparoendosc Adv Surg Tech A*, 8(2), 69–73.

Menon, M., Hemal, A.K., Tewari, A., Shrivastava, A., Shoma, A.M., El-Tabey, N.A., Shaaban, A., Abol-Enein, H. & Ghoneim, M.A. (2003). Nerve-Sparing Robot-Assisted Radical Cystoprostatectomy and Urinary Diversion, *BJU Int*, 92(3), 232–236.

Peters, B.S., Armijo, P.R., Krause, C., Choudhury, S.A. & Oleynikov, D. (2018). Review of Emerging Surgical Robotic Technology, *Surg Endosc*, 32(4), 1636–1655.

Poon, H., Li, C., Gao, W., Ren, H. & Lim, C.M. (2018). Evolution of Robotic Systems for Transoral Head and Neck Surgery, *Oral Oncol*, 87, 82–88.

Pugin, F., Bucher, P. & Morel, P. (2011). History of Robotic Surgery: From Aesop® and Zeus® to da Vinci, *J Visc Surg*, 148(5), 3–8.

Reichenspurner, H., Damiano, R.J., Mack, M., Boehm, D.H., Gulbins, H., Detter, C., Meiser, B., Ellgass, R. & Reichart, B. (1999). Use of the Voice-Controlled and Computer-Assisted Surgical System Zeus for Endoscopic Coronary Artery Bypass Grafting, *J Thorac Cardiovasc Surg*, 118(1), 11–16.

Remacle, M., Prasad, V.M.N., Lawson, G., Plisson, L., Bachy, V. & Van der Vorst, S. (2015) Transoral Robotic Surgery (Tors) with the Medrobotics Flex™ System: First Surgical Application on Humans, *Eur Arch Otorhinolaryngol*, 272(6), 1451–1455.

Schuler, P.J., Scheithauer, M., Rotter, N., Veit, J., Duvvuri, U. & Hoffmann, T.K. (2015). A Single-Port Operator-Controlled Flexible Endoscope System for Endoscopic Skull Base Surgery, *HNO*, 63(3), 189–194.

Shah, J., Vyas, A. & Vyas, D. (2014). The History of Robotics in Surgical Specialties, *Am J Robot Surg*, 1(1), 12–20.

Strauss, G., Hofer, M., Kehrt, S., Grunert, R., Korb, W., Trantakis, C., Winkler, D., Meixensberger, J., Bootz, F., Dietz, A. & Wahrburg, J. (2007). Manipulator

Assisted Endo-Scope Guidance in Functional Endoscopic Sinus Surgery: Proof of Concept, *HNO*, 55(3), 177–184.

Tae, K., Ji, Y.B., Song, C.M. & Ryu, J. (2019a). Robotic and Endoscopic Thyroid Surgery: Evolution and Advances, *Clin Exp Otorhinolaryngol*, 12(1), 1–11.

Tae, K., Lee, D.W., Song, C.M., Ji, Y.B., Park, J.H., Kim, D.S. & Tufano, R.P. (2019b). Early Experience of Transoral Thyroidectomy: Comparison of Robotic and Endoscopic Procedures, *Head Neck*, 41(3), 730–738.

Usluoğulları, F.H., Tıplamaz, S. & Yaycı, N. (2017). Robotic Surgery and Malpractice, *Turk J Urol*, 43(4), 425–428.

Vicini, C., Dallan, I., Canzi, P., Frassineti, S., Nacci, A., Seccia, V., Panicucci, E., Grazia La Pietra, M., Montevecchi, F. & Tschabitscher, M. (2012). Transoral Robotic Surgery of the Tongue Base in Obstructive Sleep Apnea-Hypopnea Syndrome: Anatomic Considerations and Clinical Experience, *Head Neck*, 34(1), 15–22.

Vicini, C., Dallan, I., Frassinet, S., La Pietra, M.G. & Montevecci. F. (2010). Transoral Robotic Tongue Base Resection in Obstructive Sleep Apnoea-Hypopnoea Syndrome: A Preliminary Report, *ORL J Otolaryngol Relat Spec*, 72(1), 22–27.

Weinstein, G.S., O'Malley, B.W. & Hockstein, N.G. (2005). Transoral Robotic Surgery: Supraglottic Laryngectomy in a Canine Model, *Laryngoscope*, 1115(7), 1315–1319.

Weinstein, G.S., O'Malley, B.W. Jr, Snyder, W. & Hockstein, N.G. (2007). Transoral Robotic Surgery: Supraglottic Partial Laryngectomy, *Ann Otol Rhinol Laryngol*, 116(1), 19–23.

Yang, D.Y., Monn, M.F., Bahler, C.D. & Sundaram, C.P. (2014). Does Robotic Assistance Confer an Economic Benefit During Laparoscopic Radical Nephrectomy? *J Urol*, 192(3), 671–676.

Yu, H.W., Chai, Y.J., Kim, S.J., Choi, J.Y. & Lee, K.E. (2018). Robotic-Assisted Modified Radical Neck Dissection Using a Bilateral Axillo-Breast Approach (Robotic Baba Mrnd) for Papillary Thyroid Carcinoma with Lateral Lymph Node Metastasis, *Surg Endosc*, 32(5), 2322–2327.

Yu, H.Y., Hevelone, N.D., Lipsitz, S.R., Kowalczyk, K.J. & Hu, J.C. (2012). Use, Costs and Comparative Effectiveness of Robotic Assisted, Laparoscopic and Open Urological Surgery, *J Urol*, 187(4), 1392–1398.

Yılmaz Güzel and Yılda Arzu Aba

# 11: A New Reagent in Determining Ovarian Reserve: Antimullerian Hormone (AMH)

## 1 Introduction

The number of women who are in the tendency to postpone pregnancy plans to advanced ages has increased day by day. Following reasons can be aligned for this postponement: will to start to domesticity, being increasingly gained economic freedom by women, expectancy to raise their children better in better environmental conditions in advanced ages. Especially the tending to marry and have children late makes aging of ovaries that is the essential organ of reproduction skill quite important. Diminishing ovarian reserve is called as ovarian aging. Ovarian reserve is a concept that reflects the quality and number of oocyte and defines the functional potential of ovarium. Much as there can be thought treatment approaches toward problems arising from aging ovarium, there has not been found an approach that stops or regress this process as of yet. However, there are various applications to determine ovarian reserve in the early stage. A large number of tests and reagents have described to evaluate ovarian reserve in literature. However, recent studies show that Antimullerian Hormone (AMH) is a remarkable reagent in women. Changes in AMH levels of women lifetime are detailedly analyzed and argued. It is especially clear that the AMH test is the vital hormonal test before treatment in infertility patients. Moreover, AMH concentration measurement is a similar indicator in terms of estimating ovarian reserve when it is compared with follicular stimulant hormone concentration and age factor.

## 2 Tests on Determining Ovarian Reserve

Studies that survey aging and its clinical results make us think that ovarian reserve measurement is necessary for patients who want to become pregnant in the later reproductive age that defines size and quality of ovarian follicle pool in the last 15 years. It is aimed in all of the methods of several techniques to foresee possible fecundabilities and success of treatment in infertile women.

The question called 'Should ovarian reserve tests be applied in all the women?' comes to mind. An international screening program can be implemented for all women as well as it is suggested to apply ovarian reserve tests in women based on characteristics below (Nikolaou and Templeton, 2003):

- 35 years and older,
- Having early menopause history in the family,
- Having a single ovary or ovary surgery (cystectomy, drilling),
- Having chemotherapy or pelvic radiation therapy story,
- Being in an unexplained infertile patient group independent from age,
- Smoke,
- Weakly react to gonadotropins,
- Planning treatment by assisted reproductive techniques (ART),

A large number of tests and reagents to evaluate ovarian reserve in literature until today. A good ovarian reserve test needs to have the characteristics below:
- Cheap and easily applicable,
- Having the ability to specify conception possibility with treatment or without treatment,
- Having the ability to the chance of live birth,
- Having the ability to estimate how long this measured activity continues at the same level before ovarian aging,
- Being an instructive in determining the optimal dose and foreseeing personal prognosis in ovarian stimulation protocol planned (Maheshwari et al., 2006).

Ovarian reserve tests are grouped as statics, ultrasonographic and dynamic tests. There are age, serum basal follicle stimulating hormone (FSH), estradiol (E2), inhibin B, anti-mullerian hormone (AMH) level, ultrasonographic ovary volume, number of the basal antral follicle, ovarian stromal stream measurements and ovarian biopsy among statics tests. There is clomiphene citrate test (CCCT), GnRH agonist stimulation test (GAST) and exogen FSH ovarian reserve test (EFORT) (İnceboz, 2005) among the dynamic tests. There is not a certain standardization in specifying ovarian reserve all over the world. Discussions and opponent studies can be seen about what the securest parameter is.

**Age:** Chronological age of a woman is the simplest way to get information about ovarian reserve in terms of both quantitatively and qualitatively. There is shown a specific correlation between serum FSH levels, average ovarian volume, and AFS along with age variable (Ng et al., 2003). Fertility capacity differs between women in similar ages in spite of the number and quality of oocyte decreases after the age increases.

**Basal Serum FSH:** This is the simplest and most common test that is utilized to determine basal FSH ovarian reserve in the second and fourth days of the menstrual cycle. Values start to increase by age. The high value of FSH (10–20 mIU/mL) is associated with a weak response to ovarian stimulation and decreasing the chance of pregnancy formation (Zapantis and Santoro, 2002).

**Basal Serum Estradiol:** Since basal E2 level can be a predictor of ovary response that is measured in the third day of the cycle, it is assumed that it is an indirect indicator of ovarian reserve (Bükülmez and Arici, 2004).

**Basal Serum Inhibin B:** Inhibins are the hormones in glycoprotein structure which belongs to the family of Transforming Growth Factor-β (TGF-β). Inhibin B that is secreted by granulosa and theca cells inhibits FSH secretion at the pituitary level. Serum basal inhibin B level pg/ml and values under it are accepted as abnormal (Ramalho de Carvalho et al., 2012).

**Clomiphene Citrate Challenge Test (CCCT):** This is a more sensitive provocative test than basal FSH. Serum FSH level is measured in the third day of a cycle; Clomiphene citrate (100 mg/per day) is given between 5th and 9th days; serum FSH value is remeasured in the 10th day. The value that is higher than 14.9 IU/L is accepted as abnormal (Ramalho de Carvalho et al., 2012).

**GnRH Agonist Stimulation Test (GAST):** This is a test that is applied in the 2nd day of a cycle before applying GnRH agonist; it shows estradiol change in the 3rd day of the cycle. It is evaluated as decreasing <180 pg/ml ovarian reserve for estradiol change (İnceboz, 2005).

**Exogen FSH Ovarian Reserve Test (EFORT):** It is based on determining the increase of E2 and inhibin B after giving 300 IU recombinant as recombinant subcutaneous in the third day of the cycle. Being related value 30 pg/ml or less is evaluated in favor of diminished ovarian reserve (İnceboz, 2005).

**Ultrasonographic Ovarian Volume:** The fact that both of the ovarian volumes were under 3 cm$^3$ was a good indicator of the diminished ovarian reserve and the ovarian response skill (Vanden et al., 2013).

**A number of Antral Ultrasonographic Follicle:** It is defined as the number of follicles that have a volume less than 10 mm that is found by AFS early follicular phase transvaginal ultrasonography. It is confirmed that AFS is as valuable as AMH in evaluating ovarian reserve and ovarian response skill (Muttukrishna et al., 2005).

**Ovarian Stromal Blood Stream:** There is seen a negative correlation between preovulatory perifollicular bloodstream and age that are analyzed in stimulant cycle (Costello et.al, 2006). Since there is used a different stream parameter in a meta-analysis that scrutinizes ovarian bloodstream, there are no certain deductions about clinical values as an ovarian reserve (Gibreel et al., 2009).

**Ovarian Biopsy:** This application that is an invasive method shows the follicle intensity and a number of the follicle in the ovarian cortex in unit volume. With reference to an idea, it could be used for showing the ovarian reserve of follicle intensity by conducting a biopsy from the ovary. However, it is not beneficial to confirm the ovarian reserve (Lambalk et al., 2004).

## 3  AMH Changes in Reproduction Physiology

AMH that is also called as MIS (Mullerian Inhibiting Substance) is synthesized by granulosa cells in primer, preantral and antral follicles whose size is up to 6 mm in women ovarian. Hormone that is in glycoprotein structure is accepted as a member of the TGF-β family (Aboulghar, 2014; Grynnerup et al., 2012).

AMH is defined by its significant role in sex differentiation as a gonadal factor in men. First of all, French anatomist Dr. Alfred Jost crystalized to the process in men 70 years before. Experiments of Professor Jost confirmed testosterone is insufficient for duty without a helper (Jost, 1947). Sertoli cells that are a resource of MIS/AMH in men were defined after more than twenty years (Josso, 1973). AMH is secreted by Sertoli cells of testicles in boys; it remains high during the childhood period. However, it regresses in pubertal and adulthood. While it provides a normal male reproductive system and Mullerian channels to regress in the improvement of a male fetus; it also ensures lack of AMH and uterine tubes, improvement of the uterus and upper part of the vagina (Kim et al., 2014).

AMH in women is produced by theca granulosa cells of ovarian follicles in early stages of follicle improvement. After the increase till early adulthood, AMH concentrations become gradually indeterminable when the reserve of primordial follicles deplete almost 5 years before menopause. A number of critical oocyte number that determines the menopause is almost 1000. Personal AMH serum concentration reflects the size of the antral follicle pool that shows the amount of the remained primordial follicle (Broer et al., 2014). It is the criterion of the amount of oocyte rather than the quality of oocyte; it shows the reproductive potential of a woman (Andersona et al., 2012).

It is pointed out that AMH has an essential role in decreasing primordial follicle pool and organizing the transition speed of follicles from the primordial stage to the growth phase. Moreover, AMH plays a protective role by decelerating the consumption rate of the primordial follicle pool. It also organizes the growth rate of follicles by inhibiting follicle growth based on FSH in the early antral period. The extra primordial follicle is stimulated by follicle FSH as the result of the lack of AMH. Thus, more follicles enter the growth phase (Sarıyıldız and Akdağ, 2013).

As is known, ovarian reserve decreases by age, and the quality of oocyst is impaired after 35 years. Typical morphological changes are seen in oocytes that are obtained by assisted reproductive techniques in advanced ages. Mechanism of reserve decrease cannot be perfectly known. However, oxidative damage and hormonal balance bring follicle to atresia by environmental effects. Age-specific serum AMH values of 17120 women who appeal to a fertility center in the USA, both medium and average AMH values decrease so as to be associated with advanced age (Seifer et al., 2011).

## 4  Antimullerian Hormone in Evaluating Ovarian Response

AMH is utilized in clinical use for purposes such as evaluating fertility potential; estimating the starting period of menopause and evaluating the possibility of polycystic ovary syndrome. For literature, the AMH test is mostly used in women over 35 years and who have early menopause story in family, single ovarium, received ovarian surgery, chemotherapy and pelvic radiation therapy, unexplained infertility facts, given diminished react gonadotropin warning, planned assisted reproductive techniques (Artini et al., 2013; Mutlu and Erdem, 2012). The general run of studies in literature mostly center on infertile women; AMH values are analyzed in women who have chronic diseases and were applied ovarian surgery (Grynnerup e al., 2012).

Accordingly, AMH has emerged as an indicator of ovarian reserve recently (Oktem and Oktay, 2008). It is utilized for evaluating fertility potential in women; estimating the starting period of menopause and interpreting the possibility of polycystic ovary syndrome.

AMH measurement at one sitting gradually becomes widespread to show the available amount of oocyte, namely the ovarian reserve; it starts to be accepted as well. Main benefits of AMH measurement and knowing ovarian reserve are as follows; informing patient about pregnancy ratio; being directed to life fertility plan by the patient; determining the cost in treatment; oocyte donation or adoption (Şahmay, 2015). Moreover, the level of AMH may be a decision-maker in ovarian tissue and oocyte freeze before possible chemotherapy and radiotherapy applications within the frame of fertility preserver approach.

One of the most significant advantages of AMH is remaining stable when it is evaluated in different periods such as hormonal contraception, GnRH agonist use, menstruation and pregnancy. This is because evaluation can be carried out on any day of the menstrual cycle.

There is no internationally accepted reference method for AMH serum level as of yet as well as AMH results can be analyzed under five different groups based on ovarian reserve (Tsepelidis et al., 2007).

$\leq 0.38$ ng/ml terrible ovarian reserve
$>0.39-\leq2.19$ ng/ml low ovarian reserve
$>2.20-\leq4$ ng/ml normal ovarian reserve
$>4.1-\leq6.79$ ng/ml increased ovarian reserve
$\geq6.8$ ng/ml polycystic ovary syndrome

Barad et al. conducted a study that reveals the relationship between age and AMH concentration and emphasized the importance of the use of serum AMH concentration among current screening tests as ovarian reserve test in young women in terms of fertility preservative approaches (Barad et al., 2011). In a similar manner, with reference to the study results of Letterie et al., there is a need for counseling services by determining AMH levels and reproductive potential of young women in the early period (Letterie et al., 2015).

Fanchin et al. (2005) used AMH, basal FSH, inhibin-B, E2 concentrations and basal AFC in three following menstrual cycle to determine ovarian reserve in 47 norma-ovulatory infertile patient in 25–40 age group. For research results, the best and most cost-effective reagent is AMH besides being the reagent that least differs between cycles within hormonal parameters. The reason for this is while AMH secretion is independent of gonadotropins, concentrations of other hormonal parameters are interrelated.

# 5 Conclusion

Ovarian-aging is an unstoppable process today. This circumstance is based on some changes in ovarian functions that emerge by age. AMH is a reagent that has a high potential in evaluating ovarian pathophysiology in sexual health. Its level at the follicular phase is not affected by GnRH. This is because it can be tested on any day of the spontaneous cycle (3,5 ng/mL). A single test is enough because of high intercycle correlation. Analyzing AFS is as important as AMH to foresee the bad ovarian response.

# References

Aboulghar, M. (2014). Anti-Mullerian Hormone in the Management of Infertility, *Middle East Fertil Soc J*, 19, 1–7.

Andersona, R.A., Nelsonb, R.M. & Wallace, W.H. (2012). Measuring Anti-Müllerian Hormone for the Assessment of Ovarian Reserve: When and for Whom Is It Indicated?, *Maturitas*, 71, 28–33.

Artini, PG., Ruggiero, M., Uccelli, A., Obino, M.E. & Cela, V. (2013). Fertility Management of Patients with Reduced Ovarian Reserve. Reproductive System & Sexual Disorders. http://omicsonline.org/fertility-management-of-patients-with-reduced-ovarian-reserve-2161-038X.S5-006.pdf (accessed on 04.06.2015).

Barad, D.H., Weghofer, A. & Gleicher, N. (2011). Utility of Age-Specific Serum Anti-Mullerian Hormone Concentrations, *Reprod Bio Med*, 22, 284–291.

Broer, S.L., Broekmans, F.J., Laven, J.S. & Fauser, B.C. (2014). Anti-Müllerian Hormone: Ovarian Reserve Testing and Its Potential Clinical Implications, *Hum Reprod Update*, 20(5), 688–701.

Bükülmez, O. & Arici, A. (2004). Assessment of Ovarian Reserve, *Curr Opin Obstet Gynecol*, 16, 231–237.

Costello, M.F., Shrestha, S.M., Sjoblom, P., Mcnally, G., Bennett, M., Steigrad, S.J. & Hughes, G.J. (2006). Power Doppler Ultrasound Assessment of The Relationship between Age and Ovarian Perifollicular Blood Flow in Women Undergoing in Vitro Fertilization, *J Assist Reprod Genet*, 23, 359–65.

Fanchin, R., Taieb, J., Lozano, D.H., Ducot, B., Frydman, R. & Bouyer, J. (2005). High Reproducibility of Serum Anti-Mullerian Hormone Measurement Suggests a Multi-Staged Follicular Secretion and Strengthen Sits Role in the Assessment of Ovarian Follicular Status, *Hum Reprod*, 20, 923–7.

Gibreel, A., Maheshwari, A., Bhattacharya, S. & Johnson, N.P. (2009). Ultrasound Tests of Ovarian Reserve; A Systematic Review of Accuracy in Predicting Fertility Outcomes, *Hum Fertil (Camb)*, 12, 95–106.

Grynnerup, A.G., Lindhard, A. & Sørensen, S. (2012). The Role of Anti-Mullerian Hormone in Female Fertility and Infertility – An Overview, *Acta Obstet Gynecol Scand*, 91, 1252–1260.

İnceboz, Ü. (2005). Klinik Praktikte Yaşlanan Over, *TJOD-Uzmanlık Sonrası Eğitim ve Güncel Gelişmeler*, 2, 15–20.

Josso, N. (1973). In Vitro Synthesis of Mullerian-Inhibiting Hormone by Seminiferous Tubules Isolated from the Calf Fetal Testis, *Endocrinology*, 93, 829–34.

Jost, A. (1947). Recherches sur la Differenciation Sexuelle de l'embryon de Lapin, *Arch Anat Microsc Morphol Exp*, 36, 271–315.

Kim, J.H., MacLaughlin, D.T. & Donahoe, P.K. (2014). Müllerian Inhibiting Substance/Anti-Müllerian Hormone: A Novel Treatment for Gynecologic Tumors, *Obstet Gynecol Sci*, 57(5), 343–357.

Lambalk, C.B, de Koning, C.H, Flett, A., Van Kasteren, Y., Gosden, R. & Homburg, R. (2004). Assessment of Ovarian Reserve, Ovarian Biopsy Is Not a Valid Method for the Prediction of Ovarian Reserve, *Hum Reprod*, 19, 1055–1059.

Letterie, G., Klein, N. & Criniti, N. (2015). Predictive Value of Anti-Mullerian Hormone Levels (AMH) in a Young Non Infertile Donor Population, *Fertil Steril*, 103(2), 28.

Maheshwari, A., Fowler, P. & Bhattacharya, S. (2006). Assessment of Ovarian Reserve – Should We Perform Tests of Ovarian Reserve Routinely, *Hum Reprod*, 21(11), 2729–2735.

Mutlu, M.F. & Erdem, A. (2012). Evaluation of Ovarian Reserve in Infertile Patients, *J Turkish-German Gynecol Assoc*, 13, 196–203.

Muttukrishna, S., McGarrigle, H., Wakim, R., Khadum, I., Ranieri, D.M. & Serhal, P. (2005). Antral Follicle Count, Anti-Müllerian Hormone and Inhibin B: Predictors of Ovarian Response in Assisted Reproductive Technology, *BJOG*, 112, 1384–1390.

Ng, E.H., Yeung, W.S., Fong, D.Y. & Ho, P.C. (2003). Effects of Age on Hormonal and Ultrasound Markers of Ovarian Reserve in Chinese Women with Proven Fertility, *Hum Reprod*, 18, 2169–2174.

Nikolaou, D. & Templeton, A. (2003). Early Ovarian Aging: A Hypothesis: Detection and Clinical Relevance, *Hum Reprod*, 18, 1137.

Oktem, O. & Oktay, K. (2008). The Ovary: Anatomy and Function Throughout Human Life, *Ann NY Acad Sci*, 1127, 1–9.

Ramalho de Carvalho, B., Gomes Sobrinho, D.B., Vieira, A.D., Resende, M.P., Barbosa, A.C, Silva, A.A. & Nakagava, H.M. (2012). Ovarian Reserve Assessment for Infertility Investigation, *ISRN Obstet Gynecol*, 57, 6385.

Şahmay, S. (2015). *Anti-Müllerian Hormon (Amh) Ölçümünün Klinik Uygulamaları*, Üreme Tıbbı ve Cerrahisi Derneği. https://docplayer.biz. tr/11886346-Anti-mullerian-hormon-amh-olcumunun-klinik-uygulamalari. html (accessed on 27.05.2015).

Sarıyıldız, L. & Akdag, S.A. (2013). New Predictor AMH (Anti-Mullerian Hormone) to Determining Ovarian Reserve and Menopausal Aging in the Women, *J Clin Anal Med*, 4(3), 241–244.

Seifer, D.B., Baker, V.L. & Leader, B. (2011). Age-Specific Serum Anti-Mullerian Hormone Values for 17120 Women Presenting to Fertility Centers within the United States, *Fertil Steril*, 5, 747–750.

Tsepelidis, S., Devreker, F., Demeestere, I., Flahaut, A., Gervy, C.H. & Englert, Y. (2007). Stable Serum Levels of Anti Mullerian Hormone during the Menstrual Cycle: A Prospective Study in Normo Ovulatory Women, *Hum Reprod*, 22(7), 1837–1840.

Vanden Brink, H., Chizen, D., Hale, G. & Baerwald, A. (2013). Age-Related Changes in Major Ovarian Follicular Wave Dynamics during the Human Menstrual Cycle, *J North Am Menopause Soc*, 20(12), 1–12.

Zapantis, G. & Santoro, N. (2002). Ovarian Aging and the Menopausal Transition, *Best Prac Res Clin Obstet Gynaecol*, 16(3), 263–276.

Derya Kanza Gül

# 12: New Approaches in Fetal Aneuploidy Scan

## 1 Introduction

Aneuploidy is a chromosomal disease arising from numerical excess or shortage of our euploidic genetic structure with 46 chromosomes. Different clinical pictures vary between abortus, inutero fetal loss, motor-mental retardation and infertility in the early period (Chaveeva et al., 2016). Literature shows that fetal aneuploidy is seen for once every 150 birth. Autosomal trisomies are the most frequent type of fetal aneuploidy (Dashe, 2016). Trisomy 21 (down syndrome) is seen for once every 800 birth; trisomy 18 (Edward syndrome) is seen for once every 6500 birth; and trisomy 13 (Patau syndrome) is seen for once every 12500 birth (Spencer, 2007). Turner syndrome (45, X0) and Klinefelter syndrome (47, XXY) are the most frequent sex chromosomal abnormalities. Almost 30 % of the fetus with trisomy 21, and also 80 % of trisomy 18 and 13 lose their lives in the early intrauterine period (Snijders et al., 1999).

Fetal aneuploidy diagnosis is made by invasive methods such as chorionic villus sampling, amniocenteses, and cordocentesis. Since there is a possibility to face with fetal abortion for once every 500 pregnancies, the preference to take action should be up to the parents (American College of Obstetricians and Gynecologists ACOG, 2016; the international society of ultrasound in obstetrics and gynecology ISUOG, 2016). It is suggested to be applied non-invasive scanning methods before invasive diagnostic tests. The goal is to specify the high-risk group for chromosome anomaly of the fetus. Fetal aneuploidy screen tests are risk identification tests, not diagnostic tests. This does not mean that fetuses in high-risk groups have chromosome anomaly or the low-risk groups have no chromosome anomaly. All the pregnant women should be informed on chromosomal screen tests; the tests need to be applied in the ones who demand them (ACOG, 2007; Benn et al., 2013; ACOG, 2016).

## 2 Ultrasonography Screening

### 2.1 Nuchal Translucency (NT)

NT distance is defined as the anechogenic (black) area between cervical spine behind head-neck of the fetus and the skin covers the spine (Nicolaides et al., 1992). NT measurement is carried out between 11th and 14th weeks and also between 38–45 mm and 84 mm of crown-to-rump length. The image should be

**Tab. 12.1:** NT Measurement Gestational Week and CRL Measurements (Created by the Author)

| Gestational Week | CRL | NT Median(mm) | 90th | 95th | 99th |
|---|---|---|---|---|---|
| 11.3–11.7 | 45–50 | 1.2 | 1.7 | 1.9 | 2.5 |
| 11.8–12 | 51–54 | 1.3 | 1.7 | 1.9 | 2.5 |
| 12.1–12.3 | 55–58 | 1.4 | 1.8 | 2.0 | 2.5 |
| 12.4–12.7 | 59–63 | 1.5 | 2.0 | 2.2 | 2.6 |
| 12.8–13 | 64–67 | 1.6 | 2.1 | 2.4 | 2.8 |
| 13.1–13.4 | 68–72 | 1.7 | 2.2 | 2.5 | 2.9 |
| 13.5–14.2 | 73–84 | 1.8 | 2.4 | 2.5–2.7 | 2.9–3.3 |

at the size so as to cover the head, neck, and upper part of thorax within the full screen of ultrasound. The fetus needs to be at midsagital plan (there is seen nasal bone, palate, and anechogenic diencephalon). Length of fetus needs to be at a neutral position; amnion membrane needs to separately be seen. Measurement ought to be carried out as vertical to the fetal axis in the largest area. Measurement signals should be inwardly put as "+". NT measurement varies by gestational weeks and CRL measurements (Jelliffe-Pawlowski et al., 2015). (Tab. 12.1).

Being NT measurement over 99th (3.5 mm) percentile based on the gestational week is defined as increased NT thickness (Bakker et al., 2014). NT measurements of the risk of fetal chromosomal anomaly are relatively expressed approximately as 7 %, 20 %, 50 % and 75 % for 3.5 mm (99th percentile), 3.5–4.4mm, 5.5–6.4 mm and ≥8.5 mm (Kagan et al., 2006). The mechanisms like circulatory disorder, lymphatic drainage disorder, increase in the amount of skin collagen and hyaluronan and intrathoracic pressure increase are thought in NT increase (Bakker et al., 2014). It is also accepted that being suggested diagnostic invasive tests instead of biochemical tests will be in better taste if NT is 3.5 mm and above (Chaveeva et al., 2016).

NT increase upgrades the possibility of fetal structural abnormalities and genetic syndromes besides chromosomal abnormalities. The major congenital cardiac defect is seen almost in 4–5 % of euploid fetuses with NT increase. Cardiac defect prevalences in fetuses whose NT is 3.5 and 8.5 mm are relatively mentioned as 2.5 % and 64 % (Bakker et al., 2014). It is also pointed out that the ratio of orafacial abnormalities increases with NT increase besides heart anomalies (Timmerman et al., 2010). Structural abnormalities in euploid fetuses with NT increase need to be exhaustively evaluated by detailed ultrasonography and fetal echocardiography. The relationship between the genetic syndrome and NT increase is determined in a large number of adverse conditions such as Noonan syndrome, Smith-Lemli-Opitz syndrome, spinal muscular atrophy and other musculoskeletal disorders (Bakker et al., 2014).

## 2.2 Ultrasonographic Markers of the First Trimester

The absence of nasal bone, reverse a-wave in ductus venosus and tricuspid insufficiency is relatively seen in 60 %, 66 % and 55 % of fetuses with trisomy 21; 2.5 %, 3 % and 1 % of euploid fetuses. Determination possibility of adding these ultrasonographic markers in the combined test is 93–96 % for fetuses with down syndrome even though there is 3 % of a false positive ratio (Chaveeva et al., 2016).

## 2.3 Major Structural Abnormalities Accompanying Fetal Aneuploidy

AV canal defects, cardiac anomalies, duodenal atresia, ventriculomegaly, cystic hygroma, and nonimmun hydrops fetalis are mostly observed in trisomy 21. Cardiac abnormalities, central nervous system anomalies, micrognathia, omophalocele, radial aplasia, overlapping fingers, club foot, cerebellar dysgenesis, and nonimmun hydrops are more frequently seen in trisomy 18. Heart anomalies, SSS anomalies, omophalocele, cleft palate-lip, urinary system abnormalities, Rocker bottom food, diaphragmatic hernia, middle line facial anomalies, and nonimmun hydrops fetalis are the structural anomalies accompanying trisomy 13 (Chaveeva et al., 2016).

## 2.4 Minor Findings Found in the Second Trimester Ultrasonography

Minor ultrasound findings are not anomalies on their own; they are ultrasound indicators that may show chromosomal aberration in the fetus. The ratio between observation frequencies of minor ultrasonography findings in fetuses with trisomy 21 and euploid fetuses shows positive likelihood ratio (+ LHR) for the related indicator. Approximately 1/3 of fetuses with down syndrome has a major or minor ultrasonographic indicator (Rink and Norton, 2016). Tab. 12.2 shows the effects of ultrasonographic minor indicator on chromosomal aberration (Agathokleous et al., 2013). Choroid plexus cyst, intracardiac hypoechogenic focus, light pyelectasis, short femur, and short humerus as isolated indicators have no significant effect on Down syndrome (Agathokleous et al., 2013; Norton, 2013; Sonek and Croom, 2014). Risk of trisomy 21 increases in case of determining more than one soft indicators (Tab. 12.2).

Tab. 12.2: Ultrasonographic Soft Indicators (Created by the Author).

| Indicator | Trisomy 21 (%) | Euploid (%) | +LHR | +LHR Isolated Indicator |
|---|---|---|---|---|
| Intracardiac hypoechogenic focus | 24.4 | 3.9 | 5.85 | 0.95 |
| Light hydronephrosis | 13.9 | 1.7 | 7.63 | 1.08 |
| Short humerus | 30.3 | 4.6 | 4.81 | 0.78 |
| Short femur | 27.7 | 6.4 | 3.72 | 0.61 |
| Hyperechogenic bowel | 16.7 | 1.1 | 11.44 | 1.65 |
| Ventriculomegali | 7.5 | 0.2 | 27.52 | 3.81 |
| Nukkalfold>6 mm | 26.2 | 1.2 | 19.18 | 3.12 |
| Aberant right subclavian arter (ARSA) | 30.7 | 1.5 | 21.48 | 3.94 |
| Hypoplasic nasal bone | 59.8 | 2.8 | 23.26 | 6.58 |

## 3 Maternal Serum Biochemical Screening

Maternal biochemical indicators in fetal aneuploidy screen are as follows: pregnancy-associated placental protein A (PAPP-A), free beta human chorionic gonadotrophin (fβHCG), unconjugated estriol (uE3), alfa-fetoprotein (AFP), and inhibin A (Chasen, 2014). Level of placental hormones may vary by gestational week, race, weight, smoking, pregnancy formation by assisted reproduction techniques, diabetes, and features of kits (Spencer, 2007). Median values peculiar to gestational weeks are computed by considering all these characteristics; the level of a hormone that will be analyzed in sample pregnant is accepted as multiple of median (MoM) value and the week variability is removed. For example, if the value in sample pregnant is 400 IU/ml, it is 4 MoM; if the value in sample pregnant is 30 IU/ml, it is 0.3 MoM based on the β-hCG value as 100 IU/ml in the 11th gestational week. Again, for example, if we want to determine the risk of trisomy 21, the likelihood ratio is found by computing the ratio among log10 (MoM) values of pregnants who have fetuses with normal karotype and trisomy 21; maternal-age dependent risk is turned into the risk peculiar to the pregnant (Rink and Norton, 2016). The difference between MoM values in normal fetuses and the fetuses with aneuploidy needs to be more and the gestational week when the related difference is most should be selected. Tab. 12.3 shows the average MoM values of placenta-induced hormones that are used in aneuploidy screen in aneuploid fetuses (Cuckle et al., 2015; Cuckle and Maymon, 2016).

**Tab. 12.3:** MOM Values of Placental Hormones in Fetal Aneuploidic Fetuses (Created by the Author)

|  | Trisomy 21 | Trisomy 18 | Trisomy 13 |
| --- | --- | --- | --- |
| **1st Trimester** |  |  |  |
| s-BhCG | 2.29 | 0.25 | 0.51 |
| PAPP-A | 0.50 | 0.20 | 0.25 |
| **2nd Trimester** |  |  |  |
| BhCG | 1.91 | 0.39 | - |
| s-BhCG | 2.20 | 0.50 | 1.35 |
| İnhibin-A | 2.00 | 0.56 | - |
| AFP | 0.74 | 0.66 | 0.98 |
| uE3 | 0.61 | 0.36 | 0.91 |

PAPP-A, s-βHCG, age, NT is applied in the first-trimester screen; age, AFP, s-BhCG, uE3 (triple test) and age, AFP, s-BhCG, uE3, inhibin A (quad test) are applied in the second-trimester screen (Chaveeva et al., 2016). Alldred et al. (2015) conducted Cochrane meta-analysis with 158,878 pregnant and 1430 fetuses with down syndrome. Related analysis includes 31 investigations and concluded that sensitivity of maternal age, PAPP-A, and s-BhCG in determining fetuses with down syndrome by a 5 % false positive ratio is 68 % (95 % CI 65–71); specificity of maternal age, PAPP-A, and s-BhCG in determining fetuses with down syndrome 95 % (95 % CI 95–95). The related sensitivity is 73 % (95 % CI, 67–79) and the specificity is 93 % (95 % CI, 91–94) when the value is accepted as 1/250. Cochrane meta-analysis of Alldred et al. (2012) found that the sensitivity of maternal age, AFP, s-BhCG, and uE3 (triple test) in determining fetuses with down syndrome is 65.1 % (95 % CI, 46.4–80.1) by 5 % false positive ratio; sensitivity of maternal age, AFP, s-BhCG, uE3, and inhibin A in determining fetuses with down syndrome is 74 % (95 % CI, 58–85) by 5 % false positive ratio.

Although the full integrated test (NT, PAPP-A, AFP, uE3, sBhCG, inh-A) is more effective than a fetal aneuploidy screen, it is more difficult to be applied in practice (Tab. 12.4). The method in which there is no NT measurement is called a serum integrated test. Determining power of the integrated test for fetuses with down syndrome is 96 % by 5 % false positive ratio; determination possibility for fetuses with down syndrome is 1:26–42 per invasive procedure (Benn et al., 2013; Cuckle and Maymon, 2016).

**Tab. 12.4:** Predictive Ratios of Combined Tests (Created by the Author)

| Down Syndrome Screening | DR | FPR | PPV |
|---|---|---|---|
| **1st Trimester Combined test** | | | |
| PAPP-A+sBhCG (10 gh)+NT (12 gh) | 82–87 | 3–5 | 1:29–46 |
| PAPP-A+sBhCG(12 gh)+NT (12 gh) | 80–87 | 3–5 | 1:29–46 |
| **2nd Trimester** | | | |
| Triple test AFP, free β-hCG, uE3 (15–19gh) | 65–70 | 3–5 | 1:59 |
| Quad test AFP, sβ-hCG, uE3, inhibin A (15–19 gh) | 70–75 | 3–5 | 1:36–54 |
| Full Integrated Test 1st trimester Combined + 2nd Trimester quad test | 92–96 | 5 | 1:30–42 |
| Serum integrated 1st trimester PAPP-A + 2nd Trimester quad test | 76–88 | 5 | 1:35–51 |

DR: Detection Rate, Sensitivity, FPR: False Positive Ratio, PBD: Positive Predictive Value

# 4 Extracellular Free DNA in Maternal Blood (cffDNA, NIPT)

Extracellular free DNA in maternal blood is an effective screen test (Society for Maternal-Fetal Medicine SMFM, 2015; American College of Medical Genetics and Genomics ACMG, 2016). Use of cffDNA test in maternal blood in fetal aneuploidy started in 2011. This method is also called a noninvasive prenatal screen test (NIPT). Mackie et al. (2016) conducted a meta-analysis that evaluates 31 investigations and 148,344 tests. With reference to the analysis results, the sensitivity of cffDNA for trisomy 21 diagnosis is 99.4 % (95 % CI, 98.3–99.8); specificity of cffDNA for trisomy 21 diagnosis is 99.9 % (95 % CI, 99.9–100). They expressed the sensitivity for cTrizomi 18 (24 studies, 146,940 tests) is 97.7 % (95 % CI,95.2–98.9); specificity is 99.9 % (955 CI 99.8–100). Besides, they also computed sensitivity for trisomy 13 (16 studies, 134,691 test) is 90.6 % (95 % CI, 82.3–95.8); specificity is 100 % (95 % CI 99.9–100). Sensitivity and specificities for monosomy X, fetal gender and Rh D relatively are 92.9 %, 98.9 %, 99.3 % ve 99.9 %, 99.6 %, 98.4 % (Mackie et al., 2016).

# 5 Conclusion

For the suggestion of American College of Medical Genetics and Genomics (ACMG) (2016), all the pregnant should be informed about aneuploidy screen tests and cffDNA test as the most effective test; preference should be up to the parents. ACOG (2015) also pointed out that all the pregnant ought to be informed about the cffDNA test; pregnants need to know that conventional screen methods are more effective in terms of benefit-cost; cffDNA test can be offered as the second option test for the pregnant in high-risk group for conventional screen test; cffDNA test can be offered as the first option test for pregnants who are in the high-risk group and have kids with trisomy and balanced translocation parents. For SMFM (2015), conventional tests as the first option screen tests for the low-risk group. However, the families should also be informed on the cffDNA test. With reference to the international federation of gynecology and obstetrics (FIGO, 2015), pregnants should be applied the 1st-trimester test; if the risk result is over 1:100, invasive procedure and cffDNA test need to be suggested. cffDNA test can be offered for pregnant whose risk result is 1:101 and 1:2500. There is no need for extra tests who are in low-risk group and whose risk result is less than 1:2500.

# References

Agathokleous, M., Chaveeva, P., Poon, L.C.Y. & et al. (2013). Meta-analysis of Second-Trimester Markers 0, For Trisomy 21, *Ultrasound Obstet Gynecol*, 41, 247–261.

Alldred, S.K., Deeks, J.J., Guo, B. & et al. (2012). Second Trimester Serum Tests for Down's Syndrome Screening, *Cochrane Database Syst Rev*, 6.

Alldred, S.K., Takwoingi, Y., Guo, B. & et al. (2015). First Trimester Serum Tests Fordown's Syndrome Screening. *Cochrane Database Syst Rev*, 11.

American College of Medical Genetics and Genomics. (2016). Noninvasive Prenatal Screening for Fetal Aneuploidy, 2016 Update: A Position Statement of the American College of Medical Genetics and Genomics, *Genet Med*, 18, 1056–1065.

American College of Obstetricians and Gynecologists (ACOG). (2007a). Practice Bulletin No. 77. Screening for Fetal Chromosomal Abnormalities, *Obstet Gynecol*, 109(1), 217–227.

American College of Obstetricians and Gynecologists (ACOG). (2007b). Practice Bulletin No. 88, December 2007, Invasive Prenatal Testing for Aneuploidy, *Obstet Gynecol*, 110, 1459–1467.

American College of Obstetricians and Gynecologists (ACOG). (2015). Committee Opinion No. 640: Cell-Free DNA Screening for Fetal Aneuploidy, *Obstet Gynecol*, 126(3), e31–7.

American College of Obstetricians and Gynecologists (ACOG). (2016). Practice Bulletin, No. 163. Screening for Fetal Aneuploidy, *Obstet Gynecol*, 127 (5), e123-37.

Bakker, M., Pajkrt, E. & Bilardo, C.M. (2014). Increased Nuchal Translucency with Normal Karyotype and Anomaly Scan: What Next?, *Best Pract Res Clin Obstet Gynaecol*, 28, 355–366.

Benn, P., Borell, A., Chiu, R. & et al. (2013a). Position Statement from the Aneuploidy Screening Committee on Behalf of the Board of the International Society for Prenatal Diagnosis, *Prenat Diagn*, 33, 622–629.

Benn, P., Cuckle, H. & Pergament, E. (2013b). Non-invasive Prenatal Testing for Aneuploidy: Current Status and Future Prospects, *Ultrasound Obstet Gynecol*, 42, 15–33.

Chasen, S.T. (2014). Maternal Serum Analyte Screening for Fetal Aneuploidy, *Obstet Gynecol*, 57, 182–188.

Chaveeva, P., Agathokleous, M. & Nicolaides, K.H. (2016). *Fetal Aneuploidies.* Coady, A.M. & Bower, S. (Eds). Twining's Textbook of Fetal Abnormalities, Third Edition, Churchill Livingstone, London.

Cuckle, H. & Maymon, R. (2016). Development of Prenatal Screening – A Historical Overview, *Semin Perinat*, 40(1), 12–22.

Cuckle, H., Benn, P. & Pergament, E. (2015). Cell-free DNA Screening for Fetal Aneuploidy, as a Clinical Service, *Clin Biochem*, 48(15), 932–941.

Dashe, J.S. (2016). Aneuploidy Screening in Pregnancy, *Obstet Gynecol*, 128, 181–194.

FIGO. (2015). Committee Report. Best Practice in Maternal – Fetal Medicine, *Int J Gynecol Obstet*, 128, 80–82.

ISUOG. (2016). Practice Guidelines: Invasive Procedures for Prenatal Diagnosis, *Ultrasound Obstet Gynecol*, 48, 256–268.

Jelliffe-Pawlowski, L.L., Norton, M.E., Sha, G.M. & et al. (2015). Risk of Critical Congenital Heart Defects by Nuchal Translucency Norms, *Am J Obstet Gynecol*, 212, 518–518.

Kagan, K.O., Avgidou, K., Molina, F.S. & et al. (2006). Relation between Increased Fetal Nuchal Translucency Thickness and Chromosomal Defects, *Obstet Gynecol*, 107, 6–10.

Mackie, F.L., Hemming, K., Allen, S. & et al. (2016). The Accuracy of Cell-Free Fetal DNA-Based Non-invasive Prenatal Testing in Singleton Pregnancies: A Systematic Review and Bivariate Meta-analysis, *BJOG*, 1–15.

Nicolaides, K.H., Snijders, R.J., Gosden, C.M. & et al. (1992). Ultrasonographically Detectable Markers of Fetal Chromosomal Abnormalities, *Lancet*, 340, 704–707.

Norton, M.E., Jacobsson, B., Swamy, G.K. & et al. (2015). Cell-free DNA Analysis for Noninvasive Examination of Trisomy, *N Engl J Med*, 372, 1589–1597.

Rink, B.D. (2016). Screening for Fetal an Euploidy, *Seminar Perinat*, 40, 35–43.

Snijders, R.J.M., Sundberg, K., Holzgreve, W. & et al. (1999). Maternal Age and Gestation-Specific Risk for Trisomy 21, *Ultrasound Obstet Gynecol*, 13, 167–170.

Society for Maternal-Fetal Medicine (SMFM). (2015). Committee Opinion No. 640: Cell-Free DNA Screening for Fetal Aneuploidy, *Obstet Gynecol*, 126, 31–37.

Sonek, J.I.R. & Croom, C. (2014). Second Trimester Ultrasound Markers of Fetal Aneuploidy, *Clin Obstet Gynecol*, 57, 159–181.

Spencer, K.(2007). AneuploidyS in the First Trimester, *Am J Med Genet C Semin Med Genet*, 145C(1), 18–32.

Timmerman, E., Pajkrt, E., Maas, S.M. & et al. (2010). Enlarged Nuchal Translucency in Chromosomally Normal Fetuses: Strong Association with Orofacial Clefts, *Ultrasound Obstet Gynecol*, 36, 427–432.

# Section 3: New Approaches in Healthcare Management

Aysu Zekioğlu

# 13: A Consumer Behavior Tendency in Healthcare Services: "Doctor Shopping"

## 1 Introduction

Behaviors of patients who are in the consumer position in healthcare services irrational. The main factor of this circumstance is information asymmetry. The patient who has no knowledge of the content and results of the treatment appoints doctor as an agent during the decision-making process. However, increasing applications toward patient rights in health care and becoming popular of optional healthcare consumption have changed the role and expectations of patients today.

The population that is not in the scope of the health insurance, the high ratio of out of pocket expenses, lack of the number of health facility and medical personnel, physical and technical infrastructure problems obstruct to access healthcare services. Policies have been developed to remove inequalities resulting from the access problem to healthcare services. While these policies cancel the access restrictions to healthcare services in some of the countries, it has caused to become popular doctor shopping (DS) behavior. Health systems enable individuals to appeal to healthcare organizations without being transferred by a doctor and paying an extra fee or patient share. Consulting a doctor to prescribe increases health expenses and triggers negative outputs such as drug resistance and drug-related deaths. Countries struggle with DS behavior via applications like legislative regulations, information technologies, and monitorization problems.

This chapter presents the DS definition, reasons for DS, the prevalence of DS, regulations and studies about DS.

## 2 Concept of Doctor Shopping

DS is defined in different sources in different manners. Much as the scope of definitions are the same, the content varies by criteria like health system structures and the number of application. In the most general sense, DS is the behavior of the patient to continuously change his doctor without a professional transfer in disease period. For Macpherson et al. (2001), DS is being come into contact with three or more than three doctors by the patient. With reference to the definition of Ohira et al. (2012), DS is the behavior of patients who consult two or more than two doctors before consulting a university hospital because of the same complaint; the same patient applies to university hospital without being transferred then. For Rouby et al. (2012), DS means a patient to be prescribed for a few times by more than one doctor; the same patient buys much more medicine more than required. Yeung et al. (2004) defined the concept of DS as the behavior of patients to be performed to eliminate the cost of long waiting lists even though they are pleased with the high service quality ill pay in public hospitals. The related concept has started to be commonly seen in the USA by the consumption increase in healthcare services in the 1970s (Lo et al., 1994).

DS is different from the concept of getting a second option. Patients want to confirm the diagnosis by consulting another doctor with available laboratory and examination results in the concept of getting a second option. In DS behavior, the patient gets medical service once and again by consulting different doctors. This circumstance also results in negative outcomes such as duplicated laboratory and visualization examinations, unnecessary prescriptions, increasing the workload of healthcare providers. Being frequently observed DS behavior in health services also causes increasing the healthcare costs at the same time.

With regard to OECD Health at a Glance report (2017), the average of OECD is found as 6.9 when the rate of applications per person to doctor in 2015 is analyzed. This ratio that was approximately 11.0 in 2000 in Korea where the rate of applications per person to doctor is highest reached 16.0 in 2015. This related ratio that was about 14,5 in 2000 in Japan regressed to 12.7 in 2015; the ratio is still high in spite of regression. While this ratio was almost 2.5 in 2000 in Turkey, it increased to 8.4 in 2015. The countries where the rate of applications per person to the doctor is lowest are Colombia (1.9), South Africa (2.5) and Mexico (2.7). Being low the related ratio in these countries results from the restrictions in access healthcare service, not the conscious attitudes of individuals. OECD's average in 2015 is 2.295. Three countries whose number of appeal to the doctor is highest, respectively, are Korea (7140), Japan (5385) and Turkey (4651). On the other hand, with reference to the report of U.S. Government Accountability Office, 170.000 people who are in scope of Medicare in 2008 to be prescribed by consulting 5 or more than 5 doctors; 65.000 people who are in scope of Medicaid consulted 6 or more than 6 doctors. The average cost of those applications, respectively, is $148 million and $63 million (Worley and Hall, 2012).

There are several different reasons for consulting a doctor and being prescribed. Features of the health system, communication between doctor and patient, costs to be borne, propensity to consume towards healthcare service can be shown as related reasons. There is a need for determining these reasons correctly; solutions need to be developed at the same time.

## 3 Reasons for Doctor Shopping and Prevalence

Reasons that push individuals toward DS behavior stem from both person and the health system. Kasteler et al. (1976) explained the reasons for the related behavior as follows:

- Being dissatisfied by the performance of the doctor consulted and doubting the doctor,
- Being negatively affected by the personal features of the doctor,
- Dissatisfying from the conditions such as location, length of waiting-period and costs,
- Having a high level of Hypochondriasis tendency.

Sansone and Sansone (2012) analyzed DS tendencies of individuals under two key reasons as the doctor-related factor and patient-related factor. Related reasons can be seen below:

- Doctor-related factors: Length of waiting-periods, behavior, and attitudes of doctors, unproper the locations of doctor's office, lack of time for the communication between doctor and patient.
- Patient-related factors: Not to understand the diagnosis or treatment of the previous doctor, progression of the disease, having a chronic disease.

Health systems, socio-cultural structures of countries and personal characteristics and disease state of the patient change the frequency and effect of DS behavior. Literature has several studies on this issue.

There was a study conducted with 1088 patients in Japan; 23 % of participants having a chronic disease displayed DS behavior that, doubting about the diagnosis of the previous doctor, not to understand the explanations of the doctor (Sato et al., 1995). Another study that was performed with 303 patients in Japan concluded that 27,7 % of the patients displayed DS behavior. It was also emphasized that the tendencies of patients who found explanations of doctor insufficient or did not understand related explanations increased (Hagihara, 2005).

A study was conducted in 2000–2001 in Hong Kong where there was a colony of the United Kingdom. Entirely 6459 patients participated in research; 26.4 % of them exhibited DS behavior because of the length of the waiting-periods. Although 74.1 % who exhibited related behavior mentioned that they accept healthcare services as a social right, they buy medical services from the private sector and make HK\$ 100 extra payment to bring forward for 2 weeks (Leung et al., 2006).

Investigators researched by 1079 patients who applied to a first-line health-care organization in France. For research findings, 27.7 % of the participants got medical service for 6 or more than 6 times in the last 6 months. 72 % of those individuals consulted the same General Practitioners (GPs); 10 % of them consulted two GPs; 15 % of them consulted 3 GPs; and 3 % of them consulted 4 or more general practitioners. Following reasons were expressed by the patients about consulting different GPs; length of waiting-periods, being dissatisfied from the previous GPs; the chance to pay by credit card (Norton et al., 2011).

It was found in a study in orthopedics clinic of a hospital in the USA that DS prevalence of 130 patients with orthopedic trauma is 20,8 %. As the educational level decreases, DS tendency increases by 3.2 times at the same time (Morris et al., 2014). There can be seen a cohort study about DS tendency of patients with attention deficit, hyperactivity disorder through U.S. retail prescription database. Patients who consult different doctors more than 5 times within 18 months are called as 'heavy shopper'. It is pointed out in related research which analyzed 4,402,464 data that women are more 'heavy shopper' in comparison with men (Cepeda et al., 2015).

One of the countries where DS tendency is high is Taiwan. Being easily accessible of medical care services is one of the primary reasons that trigger this related behavior. In addition to all these, Ds behavior becomes widespread because of the low patient share and refundment in a national health system that is based on fee-for-service of the global budget (Tseng and Chen, 2015). With reference to the cohort study that was performed by analyzing data of 200.000 people through National Health Insurance Research Database in Taiwan, 17,3 % of patients who applied to hospital in 2002 applied to a different health facility in the same day; 23,5 % of the same patients applied to the same field of specialization in different health facility in 7 days (Chen et al., 2006). It was found in another research in Taiwan in 2013 that 66 of 143 patients with eye floaters displayed DS behavior. Since the symptoms of only 16 of 66 patients lost ground consulted a doctor again, the rest 50 patients are 'true doctor shoppers'. For the research results, factors like failing to satisfy the expectations in consultation affect DS behavior (Tseng and Chen, 2015).

It was found in a study in which DS behaviors of obese individuals and non-obese individuals were compared in the USA that obese or overweight individuals exhibit DS behavior in emergency use when compared with non-obese ones (Gudzune et al., 2013). On the other hand, for results of a study that was conducted in Australia, obese and overweight individuals display DS behaviors less than the people who have a normal body mass index (Feng, 2013).

Another study analyzed applications that were made between the years 2015 and 2017 in a public hospital in Turkey. For the research results, 7,775 of

1,083,553 applications are the re-applications. The ratio of re-applications within three years is 0,72 %. Furthermore, the rate of re-applications of female patients is 20 % more than male patients (Yorulmaz et al., 2017).

It is seen when looking at the results of related studies that differences in cultural norms and health systems affect DS tendency of individuals and also cause differences in behavior frequency. Therefore, countries need to actualize the original application and regulations to avoid DS tendencies.

## 4 Legislative Regulations toward Doctor Shopping

DS embodies consuming healthcare services by consulting a large number of doctors and hospitals besides negativities such as excessive drug consumption. The most remarkable effect of these behaviors that impose a managerial and financial burden in healthcare delivery is on personal health. For example, according to the data of Centers for Disease Control and Prevention (CDCP), more than 70.000 people died because of overdose drug utilization in the USA in 2017. The reason for more than 61.000 of those deaths is overdose drug utilization via unnecessary prescriptions by DS (https://wonder.cdc.gov). Legislative regulations have been performed toward prescriptions to avoid such results of DS tendency in many countries, notably the USA.

Legislative regulations in the USA are performed in two ways as State Law and Federal Law.

**State Law:** The reference point is 'The Uniform Narcotic Drug Act'. Following expression can be seen in this act; "nobody can obtain or try to take a narcotic drug via mispresentation, trick or hiding a material fact". Specific state law examples are as follows (https://healthcare.findlaw.com/patient-rights/doctor-shopping-laws.html; https://www.cdc.gov/phlp/docs/menu-shoppinglaws.pdf; https://definitions.uslegal.com/d/doctor-shopping/):

**Arizona:** Misinformation that is transmitted from patient to doctor to supply a drug (medication) is not kept as a privileged communication.

**Kansas:** Being misinformed by a patient to supply a controlled item (medication) by convincing a practitioner is illegal.

**Montana:** It is forbidden for patients to supply the same or similar medication from another source within 30 days.

**Louisiana:** Patients need to explain the names and number of medications which they bought in the last 30 days.

**Rhode Island:** Government has two acts that forbid such movements; "fraud, trick, mispresentation" and "hiding a material fact".

**California:** Nobody can obtain or try to take a controlled item (medication) via fraud, trick, mispresentation or hiding a material fact.

**Maine:** The person is guilty if he supplies a controlled item (medication) via fraud.

**Kentucky:** Receiving a prescription for a controlled item by mispresentation is the crime.

**Connecticut:** A person who received a controlled item (medication) from a practitioner (physician) cannot ask for a prescription to supply a controlled item (medication) from a practitioner (physician).

**Federal Law:** It defines supplying medication by prescriptions and DS behavior as "having a controlled item (medication) on purpose". Since regulations define this situation as illegally supplying medication, it is accepted as a crime (https://healthcare.findlaw.com/patient-rights/doctor-shopping-laws.html).

While there is emphasized that doctors must look out for patients in basic laws that are determined for DS in Australia, obeying legislative regulations about doctor shoppers is among the primary duties of the doctors (Brand et al., 2013).

Following expression can be seen on the sub-heading of "1.8.1 - Doctor and Dentist Examination Share in Ambulatory Treatment" of "1.8 Patient Share" title of Health Application Notification in Turkey; "(6) Provided that to reserve the general provisions in this article; the first-line health organizations receive patient share by increasing 5 (five) Turkish Lira in applications to different medical service providers in the same medical specialty within 10 days except for chronic diseases and urgent situations that are specified by the institution. 5TL increased is received by income and salaries for people who receive a salary from the institution; it is also received from persons in pharmacies for other people".

There were no special methods to measure DS behaviors in health systems around the world until quite recently. Therefore, a number of prescriptions per patient were used as a criterion. However, refundment databases have been used as a specific indicator in recent years. Related databases determine whether prescriptions are legally used or obtained by DS behavior by reviewing the prescriptions that are written by different doctors for a patient (Pradel et al., 2009).

Uncontrollable increase in drug consumption and mortality rate of doctor shoppers in the USA in recent years have started to create pressure on policymakers (Islam and McRae, 2014). Prescription Drug Monitoring Programs (PDMP) was developed to control the DS habit and follow individuals who have this habit. Related programs are the central databases that are utilized to monitor the payment of prescription drugs. While those programs are used in 49 states, Missouri is the single state which has no authorized program. The issues such as usage of medications that are reported to database; people who inform the data, frequency of reporting (monthly, weekly, transiently); whether the data can be shared with other states and finally, people who have access authorization vary from state to state (Garcia, 2013).

Prescription Monitoring Program was established by General Healthcare Fund in France in 2004. Especially the opioid use has been tried to control by reviewing the written prescriptions via this program (Pradel et al., 2009).

E-prescription application started by Social Security Institution (SSI) in Turkey as from 2013. This application provides authorized doctors to see the medications that are written in the last six months, certificated drugs within the last one year, duration and content of reports, medications within the repayment cover, medication lists with normal-red-orange-purple-green prescription (Akıcı and Altun, 2013). E-prescription application placed a restriction to prescribe unnecessary medications because of DS behavior. Ministry of Health created a form called 'Data Analysis Form of Ratio and Number of Patients who Applied to Emergency Service by the Same Complaint Within 24 Hours' within the scope of quality works in health for emergency services where DS behavior is mostly seen. The goal of this form is to find the number and ratio of patients who apply to emergency service by the same complaint within 24 hours (https://dosyamerkez.saglik.gov.tr/Eklenti/4257,30acilindpdf.pdf?0). Repetitive laboratory and monitoring examinations should also be controlled besides unnecessary prescriptions that are written as a result of DS behavior. In this regard, e-pulse is an important application that is used in Turkey. The doctor can evaluate health records of citizens, and unnecessary examination requests can be avoided via this application which provides individuals and authorized medical personnel to easily access the personal health data. This health database also ensures to increase the quality of diagnosis and treatment process.

## 5  Conclusion

Revealing the reasons for DS, analyzing the type of patients who mostly exhibit this behavior, determining demographic features like gender and age of groups who are in the tendency to display related behavior is essential for health insurance companies, policy makers and service providers.

Healthcare service is demanded in case of occurring a need by nature. Individuals do not ask for healthcare without becoming sick. Individuals do not demand medical service to not face their diseases by displaying an irrational attitude. However, adopting a patient-oriented holistic approach and becoming widespread of programs and sharings relating to health applications via social media and mass communication have caused healthcare services to turn into an optional consumption area, not a need-based area. Thus, a 'health culture' should be constituted in individuals to avoid DS behavior. Having a health culture means comprehending the need for living without a doctor, hospital, medicine-oriented. For example, a person who knows negative effects of radiation during unnecessary and repetitive computarized tomography (CT) will not ask for this from the doctor; or the person will not describe the doctor who does not needlessly apply CT as 'careless doctor'. The health culture that is aimed to bring in the person can be provided by increasing health literacy and popularizing services toward health promotion. The person who is taught health conscious by services toward health promotion takes his own health responsibility.

Generalizing primary care health services and developing transfer chain are vital factors in preventing DS behavior. However, the thing that should be emphasized here is to shorten long waiting periods that can occur because of the transfer chain. Because the studies pointed out that individuals prefer DS behavior to shorten the waiting periods. Therefore, opportunities of the first line health institutions in terms of physical, technological and human resources ought to be improved; a number of population per family doctor needs to be kept in acceptable boundaries.

Organizing people who appeal to emergency services will provide DS behavior to be controlled. The most critical point here is to explain that emergency services are not the areas where ambulatory care services are rendered. Red, yellow and green area application that was established on the purpose of triage in emergency services is a remarkable step. However, there is still a high ratio of green area application; this circumstance shows that there has not been achieved the goal. Rearranging the extra payments of green area and laying a financial burden on the patient may minimize the number of applications to this area. Besides, putting into practice the shift system for family doctors may be beneficial.

Lack of time that is spared for the patient is one of the reasons that trigger DS behavior. Since the number of doctors and allied health personnel is different from the number of daily patient applications to the polyclinic, every hospital should specify the standards by performing a time study by considering own opportunities.

DS behavior is one of the topic titles that is seen and endeavored to be avoided in all the countries. Related behaviors should be controlled to prevent wastage and provide sustainability in healthcare services, protect individual and community health care. Besides determining the reasons for individuals to prefer DS behavior, systemic failures and factors should objectively be revealed and countries need to take original precautions to accomplish related policy and regulations.

# References

Akıcı, A. & Altun, R. (2013). Elektronik (E) Reçete Uygulaması ve Akılcı İlaç Kullanımına Katkısı, *Türkiye Aile Hekimliği Dergisi*, 17(3), 125–133.

Brand, E., Farquharson, I., Hartwig, K. & Loh, K.H. (2013). *Drugs and Doctors: How the Law Responds to Doctor-Shopping in Australia*, Uq Pro Bono Centre – Manning St Project, 1–25.

Cepeda, M.S., Fife, D., Berwaerts, J., Friedman, A., Yuan, Y. & Mastrogiovanni, G. (2015). Doctor Shopping for Medications Used in the Treatment of Attention Deficit Hyperactivity Disorder: Shoppers Often Pay in Cash and Cross State Lines, *The American Journal of Drug and Alcohol Abuse*, 41(3), 226–229.

Chen, T.J., Chou, L.F. & Hwang, S.J. (2006). Patterns of Ambulatory Care Utilization in Taiwan, *BMC Health Services Research*, 6(1), 54–61.

Feng, X. (2013). On The Relationship between Weight Status And Doctor Shopping Behavior-Evidence From Australia, *Obesity*, 21(11), 2225–2230.

Garcia, A.M. (2013). State Laws Regulating Prescribing of Controlled Substances: Balancing the Public Health Problems of Chronic Pain and Prescription Painkiller Abuse and Overdose, The *Journal of Law, Medicine & Ethics*, 41, 42–45.

Gudzune, K.A., Bleich, S.N., Richards, T.M., Weiner, J.P., Hodges, K. & Clark, J.M. (2013). Doctor Shopping by Overweight and Obese Patients Is Associated with Increased Healthcare Utilization, *Obesity*, 21(7), 1328–1334.

Hagihara, A., Tarumi, K., Odamaki, M. & Nobutomo, K. (2005). A Signal Detection Approach to Patient – Doctor Communication and Doctor-Shopping Behaviour among Japanese Patients, *Journal of Evaluation in Clinical Practice*, 11(6), 556–567.

https://definitions.uslegal.com/d/doctor-shopping/ (accessed on 15.01.2019).

https://dosyamerkez.saglik.gov.tr/Eklenti/4257,30acilindpdf.pdf? (accessed on 24.01.2019).

https://healthcare.findlaw.com/patient-rights/doctor-shopping-laws.html (accessed on 15.01.2019).

https://wonder.cdc.gov (accessed on 02.01.2019).

https://www.cdc.gov/phlp/docs/menu-shoppinglaws.pdf (accessed on 10.01.2019).

Islam, M.M. & McRae, I.S. (2014). An Inevitable Wave of Prescription Drug Monitoring Programs in the Context of Prescription Opioids: Pros, Cons and Tensions, *BMC Pharmacology and Toxicology*, 15(1), 46–51.

Kasteler, J., Kane, R. L., Olsen, D. M. & Thetford, C. (1976). Issues Underlying Prevalence of "Doctor-Shopping" Behavior, *Journal of Health and Social Behavior*, 328–339.

Leung, G.M., Yeung, R.Y.T., Wong, I.O.L., Castan-Cameo, S. & Johnston, J.M. (2006). Time Costs of Waiting, Doctor-Shopping and Private–Public Sector Imbalance: Microdata Evidence from Hong Kong, *Health Policy*, 76(1), 1–12.

Lo, A.Y., Hedley, A.J., Pei, G.K., Ong, S.G., Ho, L.M., Fielding, R. & et al. (1994) Doctor-Shopping in Hong Kong: Implications For Quality of Care, *International Journal for Quality in Health Care*, 6(4), 371–381.

Macpherson, A.K., Kramer, M.S., Ducharme, F.M., Yang, H. & Bélanger, F.P. (2001). Doctor Shopping before and after a Visit to a Paediatric Emergency Department, *Pediatrics & Child Health*, 6(6), 341–346.

Morris, B.J., Zumsteg, J.W., Archer, K.R., Cash, B. & Mir, H.R. (2014). Narcotic Use and Postoperative Doctor Shopping in the Orthopaedic Trauma Population, *Journal of Bone and Joint Surgery*, 96(15), 1257–1262.

Norton, J., De Roquefeuil, G., David, M., Boulenger, J. P., Ritchie, K. & Mann, A. (2011). The Mental Health of Doctor-Shoppers: Experience from a Patient-Led Fee-For-Service Primary Care Setting, *Journal of Affective Disorders*, 131(1–3), 428–432.

OECD. (2017). *Health at a Glance 2017: OECD Indicators*, OECD Publishing, Paris.

Ohira, Y., Ikusaka, M., Noda, K., Tsukamoto, T., Takada, T., Miyahara, M. & et al. (2012). Consultation Behaviour of Doctor-Shopping Patients and Factors That Reduce Shopping, *Journal of Evaluation in Clinical Practice*, 18(2), 433–440.

Pradel, V., Frauger, E., Thirion, X., Ronfle, E., Lapierre, V., Masut, A. & et al. (2009). Impact of A Prescription Monitoring Program on Doctor-Shopping For High Dosage Buprenorphine, *Pharmacoepidemiology and Drug Safety*, 18(1), 36–43.

Rouby, F., Pradel, V., Frauger, E., Pauly, V., Natali, F., Reggio, P. & et al. (2012). Assessment of Abuse of Tianeptine From A Reimbursement Database Using 'Doctor-Shopping' as An Indicator, *Fundamental & Clinical Pharmacology*, 26(2), 286–294.

Sansone, R.A. & Sansone, L.A. (2012). Doctor Shopping: A Phenomenon of Many Themes, *Innovations in Clinical Neuroscience*, 9(11–12), 42–46.

Sato, T., Takeichi, M., Shirahama, M., Fukui, T. & Gude, J.K. (1995). Doctor-Shopping Patients and Users of Alternative Medicine among Japanese Primary Care Patients, *General Hospital Psychiatry*, 17(2), 115–125.

Tseng, G.L. & Chen, C.Y. (2015). Doctor-Shopping Behavior among Patients with Eye Floaters, *International Journal of Environmental Research and Public Health*, 12(7), 7949–7958.

Worley, J. & Hall, J. (2012). Doctor Shopping: A Concept Analysis, *Research and Theory for Nursing Practice*, 26(4), 262–278.

Yorulmaz, M., Karaalp, F., Bükecik, N. & Özyılmaz, A.F. (2017). Acil Servise Tekrar Başvuru Oranı Değerlendirmesi, *Selçuk Üniversitesi Sosyal Ve Teknik Araştırmalar Dergisi*, 14, 92–99.

Yeung, R.Y., Leung, G.M., McGhee, S.M. & Johnston, J.M. (2004). Waiting Time and Doctor Shopping in A Mixed Medical Economy, *Health Econ.*, 13(11), 1137–44.

Burcu Aracıoğlu

# 14: Innovation in Health Sector: The Use of IoT and Its Reflections on Efficiency

## 1 Introduction

The technological, socio-cultural and societal developments in the last 20 to 30 years have triggered each other in a cycle and created a change in human life more than that in the previous 100 years. The reflections of this change can be seen in many different areas from as the individual at the micro level to as the social structure at the macro level (social structure) and from information and communication technologies to the forms of trade. These can be considered as a reflection but they are also the triggers of development and change.

Innovation is one of the indispensable concepts for all fields, which was added in the literature by changes. Although the concept of innovation is defined in different ways and there is no consensus on its definition, the common view in these different definitions is that innovation is a new and different phenomenon in terms of product, process, management and marketing approaches.

The concept of innovation has led to significant changes in the health sector as in many other sectors. In this section, the effects of IoT based applications, which are among the innovative approaches that are effective in terms of both product and process in the health sector and recently been very popular, will be evaluated.

Within the scope of this section, firstly the concept of innovation will be defined, and then the application examples in the field of health will be examined. In the following topics, the internet of things in health that constitutes the main point of the study, application examples, and its effects on efficiency, will be investigated.

## 2 Concept of Innovation

Innovation, a word with a Latin origin, is not clearly understood although it has become very important in daily life. The concept of innovation is often confused with some concepts such as invention and discovery.

Gault (2018) has defined innovation by emphasizing two points. According to this definition, innovation is the application for new or having major changes in the product (product or service) or the production, marketing or other managerial units' process. As can be understood from this definition, innovation is not only a product/ service but also a process with continuous development. Farchi and Salge (2017) emphasize this aspect in their study and state that innovation can be considered as an umbrella concept by exemplifying its' ability in order to define as a product, a process or even a business model.

When the studies in the literature are examined, it is seen that there is not a clear definition of how innovation can be interpreted exactly, but the employees, working on innovation, had generally accepted points. The first of them is the definition of innovation within the context of 4 categories such as product, process, organization and marketing, which was made by Schumpeter (1934) (Varis and Littunen, 2010) and accepted and published in 2005 (OECD, 2005; Varis and Littunen, 2010). The other point is the degree of change. The Oslo Manual is an internationally recognized guideline for the identification and measurement of innovation activities. When the definitions of the types of innovation are explained through this guide and considered with current examples (OECD, 2005):

- Product innovation is defined as innovation and significant improvement in products and services. The first generation touch screens can be seen as exemplified. Then these screens have been used in a wide variety of fields, from computers to phones.
- Process innovation is the innovation made in the processes such as production and distribution. An example of process innovation is the fact that banks have started to carry out a banking transaction via mobile phone applications.
- Marketing innovations is the innovation that takes place in different stages from product design to pricing. For example, advertising on social media, which has become widespread with the use of technology in recent years, is a marketing innovation.
- Organizational innovation involves that the change in the structure of an enterprise and/or the way of doing business. Home–Office applications, which have become widespread in recent years and give significant cost advantages to businesses in certain areas, can be cited as an example.

As can be understood from all these definitions and examples, it is not a very correct approach to split innovation types from each other with very clear lines. Innovation types can sometimes complement each other and also sometimes trigger each other.

Another point should be considered is the degree of change. While the word of innovation defines a radical change/novelty which is completely new, there is also the definition of incremental innovation in it, which can be defined as a smaller scale change. As stated by Kahn (2018), the most important point that is missed by individuals and operations is that the changes with incremental structure are not accepted as innovation.

To give an example for this definition, a product, process and approach, that is new for the world, is defined as radical innovation. The appearance of smartphone is an example of radical innovation. However, it is seen that smartphone do not remain as they were first used; they are introduced to the market in a new version day by day. Nowadays, smart phones can be used as a small size computer. In fact, instant monitoring of many data and sharing these data with devices on other platforms can be done via smart phones. This change is an incremental innovation.

When both the basic types of innovation described above and the process of change are discussed in detail, it is not possible to distinguish them with sharp lines as previously mentioned. Nowadays, it is very important that all enterprises in all sectors such as manufacturing, tourism, health and information sectors need to use innovation at the right time and in the right way to have a competitive advantage, decreased costs and increased productivity and quality.

## 3  Innovation in Health with Examples

In today's conditions, it is seen that the enterprises that can make innovation correctly and effectively with the technological and managerial approaches gain a competitive advantage in all sectors. Although the understanding of innovation as just the technology-based creates an idea that innovation can be used by certain sectors, innovation has become an important competitive tool in a wide range of sectors from manufacturing to service sector as mentioned before.

Also, the health sector has many examples of innovation in terms of product, process, managerial/structure. Before examining the concept of innovation in health with examples, it would be more accurate to define the concept of innovation in health. Innovation in health is addressed under the concept of social innovation, aiming to eliminate the problems of poverty, education and health, used as the basis of an assessment of human development measures (Kimble and Massoud, 2017). The World Health Organization has defined health innovation as policies, products, practices and approaches to improve the individuals' quality of life and new and/or improved elements in their ways of delivery (https://www.who.int/topics/innovation/en/). The innovations to be realized can be preventive and curative and auxiliary care services provided in the field of health and the method to be used in the provision of training are related to these products, technologies and/or processes.

In parallel with the developing and changing structures, it is seen that the innovative outputs in the health sector increase as the individuals become more conscious in terms of prolongation of life expectancy and quality of life. The goal of innovation is to reduce costs while increasing the quality and efficiency. Varkey et al. (2008) stated that significant innovations have occurred in medicines (statins, antibiotics, proton pump inhibitors… etc), diagnostic methods (magnetic resonance, mammography, computed tomography… etc.) and applied procedures (balloon angioplasty, cataract extraction etc.) in recent years.

Herzlinger (2006) classified innovation in health care into three groups and stated that service provided with these innovations will be of better quality and cost-effective:

- Nowadays, individuals want to reach health services with diversity, speed, quality and low costs like in other products and services. The first group can be defined as the innovations in the field of health to facilitate purchasing and using of services by patients and patient relatives as consumers. For example, making doctor's appointments via smartphone applications, internet or telephone makes it easier for individuals to access the services with less effort.
- The second group consists of innovations related to the technology used in health service delivery. It is aimed to improve the education, treatment, maintenance and control processes by using computer, sensor and RFID-based tools in health field. In this context, robotic operations or chemotherapy applications can be given as examples of technological-based innovations.
- The third group includes innovations for the business model in healthcare delivery. Herzlinger (2006) addressed business model innovations based on horizontal and vertical structures. The Associations of Public Hospitals in Turkey which were created to benefit from the advantages provided by scale economy can be given as an example of horizontal business models which was defined by Herzlinger and acting of independents structures as whole. With this structure, the materials needed in the provision of health services can be purchased at very low costs. In the vertical structuring, it can be ensured that health service which may require different expertise areas can be combined under one roof and thus all points within the integrated structure can be controlled. This situation is considered as a point that increases the quality of service delivered to patients.

Although the health sector has many innovations in terms of product, process and structure, it is not easy for innovation to become widespread as in other sectors (Omachonu and Einspruch, 2010). Innovation in healthcare service is very different compared to other sectors due to the material, social and, more importantly, ethical risks because health care is about human life. Within the framework of the laws in the field of health, the innovation process can be extended to a longer period and these applications can be abandoned when high potential risk is determined for an innovation (Länsisalmi et al., 2006). For example, the drug development process consists of a total of five stages. These are preclinical studies and clinical studies consisting of 4 phases in accordance with Good Clinical Practice (GCP). This five-stage process lasts 10–15 years on average. The fact that the process is so long which leads to an increase in costs and a longer entry time. Although the process is so long, it is seen that innovative studies are continuing rapidly. One of the most important indicators of this situation is the expenditures of R and D. In the sector report by KPMG, it was stated that the total expenditure on R and D activities until 2015 was over 1.1 trillion dollars. For the 2015–2020 period, R and D expenditure are expected to be 900 billion dollars (KPMG, 2018).

Berwick (2003) emphasized some rules such as the spread of innovation in the health sector, finding and supporting innovation, investing in early adapters and leadership with examples. Berwick also stated that the leaders who understand innovation and how it become widespread, respect the differences in the structure of change and know how to benefit from the stakeholders, are required in order to make significant differences in the health sector in the future.

In health system, there are stakeholders from many different fields such as patients, hospitals, organizations producing medical materials or equipments, pharmaceutical manufacturers and governments. Each of these stakeholders approaches the innovation to be created for the health sector in different ways. The important thing is that the common benefit should be increased for all stakeholders. As a result of the innovation to be successfully applied, the quality level of the service to be acquired by patient increases and thus the satisfaction level increases, institutions will have a chance to optimize their profit.

## 4 Internet of Things in Health and Application Examples

Nowadays, human life is prolonged worldwide; the population, which can be defined as elderly, is on the increase. Increasing elderly population means increasing demand for health services. When we take into consideration the changing socio-cultural structure, it is seen that individuals are much more aware in terms of both preventive and protective and therapeutic applications and improving the quality of life. Individuals' level of awareness about the quality of life increases with their increasing level of compliance to developing technology.

One of the common points of innovations in the field of health is the applications based on internet of things. Nowadays, individuals over 65 years, who may be defined as "elderly", can obtain some health data such as body temperature, blood sugar and electrocardiogram without having to leave their homes and share these data on different platforms with related departments. Thus, necessary interventions can be performed by health professionals (Jimenez and Torres, 2015).

The concept of technology-based innovation, which is at the core of the applications, is the Internet of Things. The Internet of Things (IoT) can be considered as a platform that connects the structures in processes in the simplest term. A more comprehensive definition of IOT includes structures that connect the relevant machinery/equipment/tools directly or via cloud systems and enable the rapid collection, storage and analysis of data when needed (Kulkarni and Sathe, 2014).

IoT is a concept that have become more widespread and complex in parallel with the development of radio frequency identification (RFID), Wi-Fi, Bluetooth which are considered as open wireless technology and sensor-like structures (Gubbi et al., 2013; Vashi et al., 2017). IoT applications, which are based on the use of sensors and data conversion, have become widespread in a short time from production to service delivery; their examples have been seen in the field of health.

In the study conducted by Gope and Hwang (2016), it was emphasized that the elderly population increases rapidly and approximately 80 % of individuals over 65 years would have at least one chronic disease in line with the studies in the field of health; IoT would enable the delivery of quality health services to these individuals without any time and place limitation.

In their study, Tyagi et al. (2016) gave computed tomography and magnetic resonance screenings as examples within the scope of cloud-IoT integrations. By storing the results of these screenings in a cloud system, relevant stakeholder such as health institutions, doctors, etc. have access to patients' medical profiles regardless of their locations. Not only imaging, but also blood groups, allergies, laboratory results of patients can be accessed in this way. These structures are given in Fig. 14.1.

Explaining the ways of using IoT structure in healthcare services by the examples is useful for a clear understanding of both the system and its benefits.

It is very difficult to measure the body temperature of children from infancy to a certain age. In addition, patients' body temperature should be frequently measured in certain situations. The body temperature of individuals can be instantly transferred to mobile device by means of smart thermometers which

E-PRESCRIBING SYSTEM

PATIENTS

Contacting patients for treatment

HOSPITALS

Receiving Health Record

Patient ID

EHR

Writing Prescription

Saving Prescription in the corresponding patient data

Receiving Health record, Lab Reports and all information about patients

DOCTORS

EHR

Saving Health Record

Cloud

Receiving the information about patient history records

PHARMACIST

More detailed information about Medicines Prescribed

Entering the Lab Reports into the Patient Database

LABS

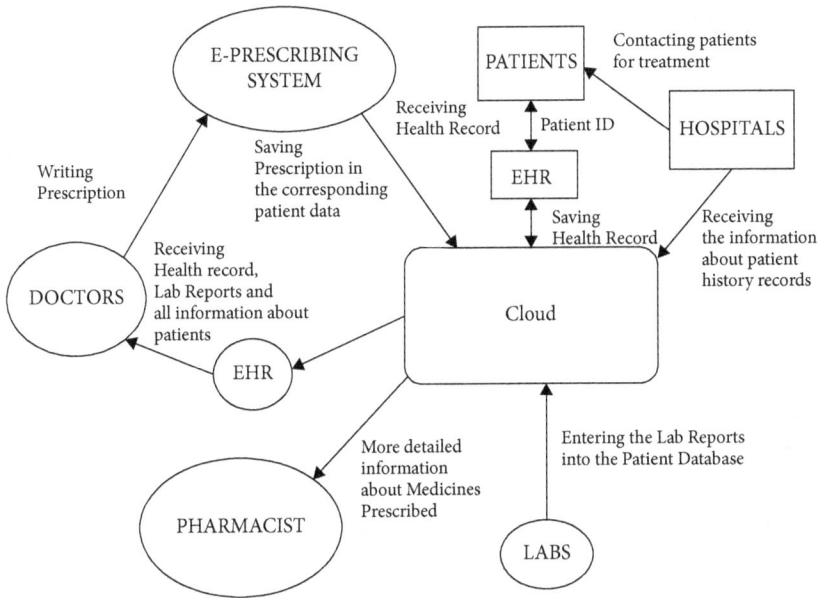

**Fig. 14.1:** Cloud – IoT Based Healthcare Frameworks (Tyagi et al., 2016)

are applied on the skin, have a 24–72 hour lifetime and Bluetooth feature. Since these data are transferred to monitoring devices instantly, the changes in the body temperature of patients at home and in health institutions can be instantly monitored more easily. This structure, which increases the quality of health services, provides an opportunity to health staff to follow up patients more easily, quickly and efficiently. (https://temptraq.healthcare/).

One of the IoT examples brought into use for infants is the "Smart Diapers". Urinary tract infections occur when a bacterium in the intestine passes through the urinary tract to the bladder and causes infection in it by rapid multiplication. These infections can cause significant damage to the kidneys. (http://www.health.vic.gov.au/edfactsheets/downloads/turkish-urinary-tract-infections.pdf). In particular, irregular diapers change during infancy among the causes of such infections. The time of diaper change can be monitored by placing a very thin sensor in diapers which was developed by the researchers at the University of Tokyo. These sensors are also important because they allow parents to perform simple screening for urinary tract infections, dehydration or kidney problems (Yeole and Kalbande, 2016)

Another tool is the Body Sensor Networks. It is in the form of a Body Sensor Network (BSN) and allows monitoring of body functions and the environment through sensors in, on or around the body. While the sensor network in the body provides the connection between the implanted part and the base station, the sensor network on the body provides communication between the devices defined as wearable and the platform to which it is connected (Gope and Hwang, 2016). The medical monitoring provided by the BSN can be of great importance because it provides access to individuals' health records and, more importantly, communication services in emergencies (Darwish and Hassanien, 2011).

Activity trackers follow up patients during cancer treatment. These tools allow patients' activities to be monitored before, during and after the treatment. Although the treatment is same, the effects of drugs may change as the structure of each individual is different. With such tools, the efficacy of the treatment and patient-specific outcomes can be followed up more clearly. Follow up is also important in terms of improving the quality of service. There are also studies conducted for the treatment process of different types of cancer in terms of benefits for both patients and healthcare providers. In the study conducted by Rosenberg et al. (2016), it was stated that the awareness levels of the patients towards physical activities increased with activity trackers devices.

The insulin hormone secreted by the pancreas is needed to use glucose, which is seen as the main nutritional source for all organs. Insulin Dependent Diabetes Mellitus, also known as Type 1 diabetes, means low insulin levels; patients with type 1 DM need to inject insulin into their bodies. (https://www.turkdiab.org/diyabet-hakkinda-hersey.asp?lang=TRandid=47). In the application of the artificial pancreas, the patient's glucose level is continuously measured by the continuous glucose measurement sensor placed under the skin. The data collected via Bluetooth is transferred to devices such as smart phones and computers. The algorithms in these devices analyze the data to determine the time when the patient needs glucose. When a necessity is determined, control platforms provide insulin injection by stimulating the insulin pump through the cannula in the body (Kovatchev, 2018; www.renfrewgroup.com/portfolio/insmart-artificial-pancreas/; http://www.metabolikcerrahi.com/blog/tip-1-diyabet-icin-umut-yapay-pankreas/). Patients do not need tools and equipment for regular measurements or insulin injections. With this system, insulin balance is maintained without affecting the quality of life of individuals.

An application example for the use of IoT in health institutions is patient follow up systems. Patient information is entered through the system and access to information can be provided by means of the device with RFID tag attached to the patient. By making certain definitions on RFID, the patient's exit from the room and his/her path can be followed. One of the most important areas of use is baby monitoring. A small bracelet attached to the baby after the delivery sends alerts directly to the relevant platforms when the baby moves away from the mother.

E-pulse system which was initiated in Turkey provides support for the solution of the problems related to instant access to information and offers numerous opportunities for organizations which work actively in the health sector in terms of their efficiency. The system can be integrated with devices defined as wearable technologies. Moreover, all information such as doctor appointments, examinations and drug information can be accessed from anywhere at any time. Patients can also evaluate the service quality through the system. Emergency services can be received by sending location information with 112 emergency button in the smartphone application. Individuals can rapidly access their health information and health services and also share all of his/her information with their medical doctors. The system provides access to contact information not only in national size but also in different geographical areas.

Health services may require instant monitoring of individuals' health data. IoT provides solutions to the problem of receiving instant data, storing and providing effective service in cases requiring intervention. Today, access to such applications is possible not only through websites and special tools but also through different platforms that have become an integral part of human life, from watches to mobile phones.

As a result, it is seen that the increasing awareness about healthy life and increasing numbers of user-friendly tools cause an increase in the use of the applications that become widespread and have increasing service quality in the field of health. It is thought that this development will continue rapidly in the future with tools such as big data, artificial intelligence, RFID technologies, cyber-physical systems within the context of Industry 4.0. This situation will ensure to access to quality health care at the right place and time with low cost and high efficiency.

## 5 The Effects of IoT Usage on the Efficiency in Health Sector

The health sector is one of the sectors highly affected by globalization and technology-based changes. As in other areas, institutions and organizations operating in the field of health care try to be more cost efficient, productive, effective, coordinated and especially, more individual centered. As emphasized before, the fact that having each individual different characteristic makes the health service offered unique. However, the fact that individual health data cannot be collected and stored regularly and health service providers cannot be integrated effectively increases the cost of services and makes access the service difficult. From this point of view, it is very important to reach the right information of individuals at the right place and right time (Turcu and Turcu, 2013; Fernandez and Pallis, 2014). Making right decisions mean applying right interventions to patients. Otherwise, appropriate intervention may take time and may result in deaths.

It is aimed to eliminate time and space limitations by using IoT-based systems in the field of health. IoT creates an integrated communication environment from interconnected devices and platforms by bringing together both virtual and physical worlds. With the appearance of remote digital health-based IoT systems, the transmission of medical data has become a daily routine (Elhoseny et al., 2018). With the application, both healthcare providers and healthcare receivers will take significant time and cost advantages.

In the study conducted by Kulkarni and Sathe (2014), it was stated that the use of IoT in health services is of great importance in terms of improving access to health service and service quality and reducing service costs. The use of IoT-based systems will also create individual health records, reduce the workload of healthcare workers and ensure more efficient and effective time use by all stakeholders.

The participation of individuals, which is one of the characteristics of service production processes, is of great importance in terms of efficiency and effectivity of the system. Since individuals can follow all the data on the system, they can tend to use appropriate services from the first stages. In other words, since they see critical points, they do not tend to receive services when not necessary.

Although the use of IoT in health care provides efficiency and cost advantages, there are also some difficulties in practice. First of all, establishing an appropriate infrastructure is required for the processing of the collected big data. It is important that a strong analytical structure is also provided for effective and cost-efficient data mining and analysis. The system architecture should also be designed correctly. The information obtained from millions of different devices and individuals in different parts of the world needs to be read, combined and brought into a standard form. However, the creation, backup, and security of data warehouses are of great importance (Darshan and Anandakumar, 2015). Although the studies in the literature mentioned about similar points, it was emphasized that there are some points that need to be solved regarding data security of individuals' health information, especially for the protection of personal rights.

In conclusion, effective and efficient use of staff, equipments, materials and other resources is ensured by providing rapid access to information, accurate planning and instant information support in decision-making processes in terms of institutions and employees in the field of health in addition to increasing the quality and satisfaction of individuals.

## 6  Conclusion

Innovation is considered as a popular concept in the new social structure defined as information society. The relationship between developing technology, changing sociocultural structure and innovation is also very effective at this point. Nowadays, the innovation through consensus points is considered as an important competitive tool in many areas.

The rapid increase of the world population, the prolongation of life expectancy, an increase in the value given to people, the acceptance of health field as one of the primary responsibilities of governments and the technological investments of the private sector in health field bring a new dimension to health services. Health services have started to gain a new dimension due to the health is a natural right for every human being and is important to meet the health needs of the society. In this context, health services, which are defined as protecting human health, providing treatment, enabling individuals with disabilities to live without being dependent on anyone and protecting the health level of society, have become a rapidly growing sector.

In recent years, the scope of health services has rapidly become wider and has begun to change the content of health services significantly. The most important reason for the change in the health sector is undoubtedly the developments that have emerged in harmony with the new technologies. Nowadays, the investments made in the field of health under the leadership of the private sector have rapidly come to fruition. In the period defined as the digital age, technology has started to create many opportunities in terms of increasing service efficiency and the reliability of diagnosis and solving the problems experienced in health services. As a result, the use of technology, which offers solutions with the potential to make life easier for people in search of health care, has become rapidly widespread in the field of health.

Different tools have changed the appearance of health care in this period in which data gained great importance from the perspective of Industry 4.0. Rapid access to information by means of IoT connections over the structures such as sensors, Wi-Fi connections, Bluetooth, etc. has made life easier for all stakeholders, especially patients, relatives and healthcare professionals. Rapid access to information also means rapid access to necessary services and can improve the efficiency and quality of health care.

Technology has become an integral part of today's society with its potential to improve the quality of life. The new technologies used in the health sector are indispensable for the development of health services. However, the use of technology in the field of health has become one of the important issues discussed. Nowadays, the technological structure is highly effective on the quality, efficiency and costs of health care. Although the technology-based applications used in the health field will be further developed, the infrastructure opportunities, the difficulties in cost recovery and providing information security are still among the issues that have not been solved in the field of health.

When the current technological development speed is considered, it is not possible to make a distinction between innovative developments and health sector. However, it is foreseen that the development will accelerate with the applications such as artificial intelligence and thus healthcare services will go further. In this context, the increase in the efficiency and quality of the services provided by the technological developments in the field of health will be undeniable. Therefore, it is important to indigenize the technological developments related to data usage in the field of health, to increase the application areas and to rapidly solve the problems related to the delivery of these technology-based services and their costs.

## References

Berwick, D.M. (2003). Disseminating Innovations in Health Care, *JAMA*, 289(15), 1969–1975.

Darshan, K.R. & Anandakumar, K.R. (2015). *A Comprehensive Review on Usage of Internet of Things (IoT) in Healthcare System.* 2015 International Conference on Emerging Research in Electronics, Computer Science and Technology (ICERECT), IEEE, Mandya, India.

Darwish, A. & Hassanien, A.E. (2011). Wearable and Implantable Wireless Sensor Network Solutions for Healthcare Monitoring, *Sensors*, 11(6), 5561–5595.

Elhoseny, M., Ramírez-González, G., Abu-Elnasr, O.M., Shawkat, S.A., Arunkumar, N. & Farouk, A. (2018). Secure Medical Data Transmission Model for IoT-Based Healthcare Systems, *IEEE Access*, 6, 20596–20608.

Farchi, T. & Salge, T.O. (2017). Shaping Innovation in Health Care: A Content Analysis of Innovation Policies in the English NHS, 1948–2015, *Social Science & Medicine*, 192, 143–151.

Fernandez, F. & Pallis, G. (2014). Opportunities and Challenges of the Internet of Things for Healthcare: Systems Engineering Perspective. 2014–4th

International Conference on Wireless Mobile Communication and Healthcare – Transforming Healthcare Through Innovations in Mobile and Wireless Technologies (MOBIHEALTH), IEEE, Athens, Greece.

Gault, F. (2018). Defining and Measuring Innovation in All Sectors of the Economy, *Research Policy*, 47(3), 617–622.

Gope, P. & Hwang, T. (2016). BSN-Care: A secure IoT-Based Modern Healthcare System Using Body Sensor Network, *IEEE Sensors Journal*, 16(5), 1368–1376.

Gubbi, J., Buyya, R., Marusic, S. & Palaniswami, M. (2013). Internet of Things (IoT): A Vision, Architectural Elements, and Future Directions, *Future Generation Computer Systems*, 29(7), 1645–1660.

Herzlinger, R.E. (2006). Why Innovation in Health Care is So Hard, *Harvard Business Review*, 84(5), 58–66.

http://www.health.vic.gov.au/edfactsheets/downloads/turkish-urinary-tract-infections.pdf, (accessed on: 31.01.2019).

http://www.metabolikcerrahi.com/blog/tip-1-diyabet-icin-umut-yapay-pankreas, (accessed on: 31.01.2019).

https://temptraq.healthcare/, (accessed on: 29.01.2019).

https://www.renfrewgroup.com/portfolio/insmart-artificial-pancreas/, (accessed on: 31.01.2019).

https://www.turkdiab.org/diyabet-hakkinda-hersey.asp?lang=TR&id=47, (accessed on: 31.01.2019).

https://www.who.int/topics/innovation/en/, (accessed on: 27.01.2019).

Jimenez, F. & Torres, R. (2015). Building an IoT-Aware Healthcare Monitoring System. 2015–34th International Conference of the Chilean Computer Science Society (SCCC), IEEE, Santiago, Chile.

Kahn, K.B. (2018). Understanding Innovation, *Business Horizons*, 61(3), 453–460.

Kimble, L. & Massoud, M.R. (2017). What Do We Mean by Innovation in Healthcare?, *EMJ Innovations*, 1(1), 89–91.

Kovatchev, B. (2018). Automated Closed-Loop Control of Diabetes: The Artificial Pancreas. *Bioelectronic Medicine*, 4(1), 14.

KPMG. (2018). İlaç Sektörel Bakış, https://assets.kpmg/content/dam/kpmg/tr/pdf/2018/01/sektorel-bakis-2018-ilac.pdf (accessed on: 29.01.2019).

Kulkarni, A. & Sathe, S. (2014). Healthcare Applications of the Internet of Things: A Review, *International Journal of Computer Science and Information Technologies*, 5(5), 6229–6232.

Länsisalmi, H., Kivimäki, M., Aalto, P. & Ruoranen, R. (2006). Innovation in Healthcare: A Systematic Review of Recent Research, *Nurs Sci Q.*, 19(1), 66–72.

OECD. (2005). *Oslo Manual, Guidelines for Collecting and Interpreting Innovation Data*, Third Edition, Proposed guidelines for collecting and interpreting technological innovation data. OECD, Statistical Office of the European Communities, OECD Publishing, Paris.

Omachonu, V.K. & Einspruch, N.G. (2010). Innovation in Healthcare Delivery Systems: A Conceptual Framework, *The Innovation Journal: The Public Sector Innovation Journal*, 15(1), 1–20.

Rosenberg, D., Kadokura, E.A., Bouldin, E.D., Miyawaki, C.E., Higano, C.S. & Hartzler, A.L. (2016). Acceptability of Fitbit for Physical Activity Tracking within Clinical Care among Men with Prostate Cancer. *AMIA Annual Symposium Proceedings*, 2016, 1050–1059.

Turcu, C.E. & Turcu, C.O. (2013). Internet of Things as Key Enabler for Sustainable Healthcare Delivery, *Procedia-Social and Behavioral Sciences*, 73, 251–256.

Tyagi, S., Agarwal, A. & Maheshwari, P. (2016). A Conceptual Framework for IoT-Based Healthcare System Using Cloud Computing. 2016–6th International Conference – Cloud System and Big Data Engineering (Confluence), IEEE, Noida, India.

Varis, M. & Littunen, H. (2010). Types of Innovation, Sources of Information and Performance in Entrepreneurial SMEs, *European Journal of Innovation Management*, 13(2), 128–154.

Varkey, P., Horne, A. & Bennet, K.E. (2008). Innovation in Health Care: A Primer, *American Journal of Medical Quality*, 23(5), 382–388.

Vashi, S., Ram, J., Modi, J., Verma, S. & Prakash, C. (2017). Internet of Things (IoT): A Vision, Architectural Elements, and Security Issues. 2017-International Conference on I-SMAC (IoT in Social, Mobile, Analytics and Cloud) (I-SMAC), IEEE, Palladam, India.

Yeole, A.S. & Kalbande, D.R. (2016). Use of Internet of Things (IoT) in Healthcare: A Survey. WIR '16 Proceedings of the ACM Symposium on Women in Research 2016, Indore, India.

Şirin Özkan

# 15: The Health Professions of the Future

## 1 Introduction

The factors affecting the needs for health professions can be listed as five global changes. The first one is demographic and epidemiological changes such as the aging of populations, urbanization, a more mobile lifestyle and the increase in noncommunicable diseases. Second factor is that people are more educated and more easily access the information. Third factor is that there are ongoing developments in the field of biology and information technologies. Fourth one is that the healthcare costs increase considerably. The fifth factor is that there is an increased recognition of health services as a fundamental human right and general health insurance and the generalization of social equality in health as a result of that. There is a need of redesigning health systems and health professions in accordance with these global changes (Crisp and Chen, 2014).

The roles of health professionals are dynamic. Constantly changing health services, technological developments and new lines of business create new roles or change long-standing roles (Dubois et al., 2006). Sibbald et al. devised a scientific classification on the ways of changing roles of healthcare staff. Although the studies on this subject is not sufficient, most of the forms of change in professional roles gradually occur because some groups assume new roles and others leave them. These gradual changes are rarely defined as innovation as these gradual changes take a long time. As the results of role changes generally occur in different systems and at different times, there are few comparisons between the two different professional groups regarding the realization of roles (Sibbald et al., 2004).

Firstly, the change in health professions occurs with the development of roles without the most common legal definitions. Secondly, the replacement of the roles of a professional group by the roles of another professional group. For example, the studies on the replacement of some roles of physicians with the roles of dieticians showed that the dietitians were more successful compared to the physicians in terms of effective reduction of cholesterol levels of the patients. Thirdly, delegation is the transfer of certain roles to the upper or lower occupational group in the hierarchy between the health profession groups. Fourthly, revision is the creation of new profession groups. For example, today there are specialist nurses in many fields such as diabetes nurse and colostomy care nurse.

In many areas such as quality security, new roles are created for health workers (Dubois et al., 2006). The most demanded occupational groups in all sectors between 2010 and 2014 are system software developers, nurses, market research analysts, marketing specialists, physicians and surgeons, all computer related professions, computer and information systems managers, management and financial analysts (Carnevale et al., 2015). Due to changing living conditions, different health professions are needed in health sector. The health professions which will have increasing importance in the future are examined under 4 major topics as health care, information technologies, genetics, traditional and complementary medicine in addition to the health professions such as nursing, pharmacy, physiotherapy, dietetics are actually needed professions now.

## 2 Professions Related to Providing Health Care

It is estimated that the number of individuals aged 60 and over in the world population will double in 2050 (2.1 billion) compared to their population in 2017 (962 million) (United Nations, 2017). It is expected that the number and quality of health professions that will work in this area related to the aging of the population will increase.

Ireland reduces healthy manpower in hospitals and direct them to primary health care. Therefore, health professionals are expected to develop themselves in a wider multidisciplinary teams, in different working environments and about new working methods. Similarly, new roles and health information technologies are expected to be used effectively for the nursing of elderly population in the social environment in Lithuania, Malta and Finland. In order to develop a standing healthcare process, skills need to be developed through collaboration, teamwork and health information technologies (Hope, 2009). However, there is no appropriate elderly care team and a work plan suitable for everyone. The right team and care plan vary according to the needs of elderly persons. It was determined that the team composed of the professional from different occupational groups increased healthcare quality, life quality and job satisfaction in favorable working conditions (Koopmans et al., 2018).

It is foreseen that the need for occupational groups helping children and young persons for personal care and providing nursing at home in addition to elderly care (Ministry of Health New Zealand, 2014). It is expected that the needs for listed professions will increase in the future compared to now.

**Physiotherapist and Occupational Therapist:** It is foreseen that the need for these professions will increase for the treatment of and increasing physiological problems due to aging immobile lifestyle and office environment and other muscle, joint and bone diseases. Occupational therapists help to treat problems as a result of any illness, accident, congenital disability or aging, to improve existing mental, social or physical abilities of individuals, to maintain their daily life safely. Physiotherapists and occupational therapists often work together to help support people at home (Babatunde et al., 2017).

**Chiropractor:** In chiropractic, which is effective in the treatment of low back pain and hernias, chiropractors determine the axis dysfunction in the body and bring the vertebra as it should be with manipulative therapy. They are very effective in the treatment of non-surgical, rheumatic, fracture or non-tumor-related low back pain. Active muscle oscillation, trigger point therapy, activator technique, mobilization, applied kinesiology, physical therapy methods, massage, dry needling, nutrition counseling and rehabilitation treatments are applied (Vollenweider et al., 2017).

**Respiratory Therapist:** Due to the rapidly increasing asthma and stress-induced breathing problems, it is predicted that the need for this profession making an important contribution to life quality will increase in the future (Zamjbölahn, et al., 2018).

**Massage Therapist:** Nowadays, it is foreseen that there will be more demand for this profession in the future due to the rapid increase in physical problems (Kennedy and Munk, 2017).

**Podologist:** Due to the rapid increase in foot diseases, its importance increases in public health. It is a profession that serves to provide treatment and care services or to take an active role in all foot diseases (Saulite and Andersone, 2017).

**Pharmacist:** The need for a pharmacy profession is expected to increase; this profession is also expected to play new roles. First of all, the number of pharmacists for employment in pharmaceutical companies is expected to increase in the next years. In particular, it is expected that the need to work on the preparation of pharmaceutical synthetic, semi-synthetic or biological originated raw materials, the examination and evaluation of their physical, chemical and biological properties and the production of high-quality medicines and the storage and use of drugs, will increase. The second area where the need will increase is clinical pharmacy. Clinical pharmacists take part in all stages of care from admission of a patient to a hospital until he/she is discharged from this hospital. After discharge, they inform this patient about drug treatment (Yamada and Nabeshima, 2015).

**Home Care/Elderly Care Technician:** It is the field of the profession that covers home health and care services for elderly population or the population in need of nursing. Home care technicians are indispensable for patients and elderly people in need of post-operative care, individuals who continue their treatment at home and those who need short-term aftercare. It is foreseen that these professionals will take more effective occupational roles and specialize in emergency care and crisis intervention in the future (HOPE, 2009).

**Dietician:** Dieticians are expected to play a more active role in health sector in the future because of changing dietary habits, sedentary life, rapidly increasing obesity and the fact that many diseases are caused by overweight (Hickson et al., 2018).

**Social Worker:** Social workers can help people identify their social and personal needs and find the best possible ways to meet them. Every palliative care team needs a social worker or someone fulfilling this role. They speak about individuals' concerns and supports them in times of change and crisis (NASW, 2010).

**Psychiatrist/Psychologist:** As a result of increasing chaos in the world, the mental health of societies deteriorate rapidly. In the meantime, substance abuse also shows an uncontrollable increase. In many countries, primary healthcare services are made more active in order to improve mental health and drug addiction support services for those in need of psychological support, young and elderly people at risk. The need of the primary healthcare services at every stage, especially holistic approach and preventive interventions (Ministry of Health New Zealand, 2014).

**Bereavement Counsellors:** These specialists usually support patients receiving end-of-life care and their relatives. They work in cooperation with the families of persons with widespread sadness, helping them to adapt to their daily life by providing psychological support for their spiritual and emotional concerns (Klasen et al., 2017).

**Music Therapist:** Music therapists are specialized in providing music-based physical, psychological, social and mental support for patients. Music therapy is used as a complementary method in clinics such as neurology, cardiology, oncology and psychiatry clinics and other places in which there are individuals with special needs. It also has an important role in the treatment of alcoholism and substance abuse (Uhlig et al., 2017).

**Speech Therapist:** It is a profession which provides the diagnosis and treatment in the babies, children and adults with sound disorders, swallowing disorders, language disorders, aphasia, delayed speech, motor speech disorders, stuttering, cluttering, pronunciation problems, language and speech problems based on problems such as cleft lip and cleft palate, language and speech disorders due to impaired hearing (Duru et al., 2018).

**Hospitalist:** Hospitalists manage the procedurers related to the follow-up of hospitalisation of patients, the care of them, organisation of their medications, the emergency care services, communication with patients and their relatives, planning the discharge of patients and patient care after discharge. In the hospital, they use both hospital resources efficiently; they can establish a healthy communication with the units in which patients are consulted and their physicians (Başer et al., 2014).

## 3 Health Information Technologies–Related Jobs

Health institutions have to use more technology with each passing day. They undergo a major transformation by including technological advances to all processes in health care. In addition, healthcare institutions spend considerable amount of money to keep up with the innovations in the field of Health Information Technology for Economic and Clinical Health Act (HITECH) and to gain a competitive advantage. It is expected that monitoring and development of public health with information technologies, management of large amounts of data will be more complex and difficult in the future and therefore new professions will be created in this area (Sheikh et al., 2015). The use of artificial intelligence in health information technologies helps patients to arrange their lifestyles, and also provides support for the restructuring of the health system in accordance with the habits and health needs of the society. The biggest concern in this regard is that artificial intelligence will be able to control human life by developing enough to overcome the human brain abilities. However, it can be used advantegously for the community with ethical standards, success and effectiveness criteria, user-friendly and evidence-based applications (Hamet and Tremblay, 2017). On the other hand, some scientists predict that artificial intelligence cannot completely replace health staff in the future, but it will help health staff to make better clinical decisions. Increasing health service data and rapid development of analytical methods of large data necessitate the application of artificial intelligence in health services. Artificial intelligence helps to easily find and take the necessary critical information from massive data set in clinical decision making (Jiang et al., 2017).

One of the technological applications in the health sector is to collect, use and share the information and data required to produce better health services, to perform the production of information by standard methods and to provide the highest level of utilization of the produced information on the HIMS (Çimen, 2016). Many hospitals increasingly demand to offer filmless and paperless health care. Regardless of the physical location of health professionals, the possibility of providing work and family life balance through independent formal reporting and tele-working. In addition, the emblem of access to digitized data causes an increase in the role and effectiveness of a family physician. In the future, all health professionals are expected to improve themselves in using health information technologies (HOPE, 2009).

Some health professions that will be needed more in the health sector in the future are mentioned below.

**Biomedical Engineering:** They carry out the design, development, production, technical operation and maintenance and repair activities of electronic and mechanical devices and systems used in the field of health for diagnosis and treatment. Biomedical Engineering, which constitutes an important bridge between engineering and medicine, gains increasingly more importance in our lives (Bronzino and Peterson, 2015).

**Health Information Manager:** They use scientific analysis methods in diagnosis, treatment, education, communication, data and information gathering, data and information processing, information management and medical decision making in the area of health by using information technologies. A health information manager is responsible for the management of health information technology design, installation, improvement and inspection and the coordination of the department team. In addition, the increase in virtual hospitals and telehealth-based approaches shows that the need for this profession will increase further (Wager et al., 2017).

**Telesurgeon:** These surgeons operate their patients with remote robotic arms and direct the operation from a computer control panel a few meters ahead of the patient and see what they are doing in real time. The surgeons' patients may be in another hospital, in another city or even in another country. Although telesurgery is not common yet, it is predicted that the profession of these surgeons will be much more important in the future (Raison et al., 2015).

**Bioinformatics and Genetics Specialist:** Biotechnology is one of the fastest developing sectors on a global scale. It collects biological data in the areas such as public health, genetics and pharmacy and then analyzes them with complex computer software by using dynamic simulations and mathematical models. Biotechnologists can even develop three-dimensional DNA models in the future (Tsai et al., 2016).

**Medical Robotics Specialist:** In recent years, surgical robots have been directed and used by physicians, but this technology is produced by medical roboticist. They develop numerous intelligent instruments that can be used by healthcare professionals in surgery or in the diagnosis of diseases. They can also develop devices such as mind-controlled prosthetic arm (Yang et al., 2017).

## 4 The Professions Related to Genetics

The discovery of DNA in the mid-twentieth century revolutionized the field of medicine and biology. The determination of the human genome in details by the Human Genome Project and the opening of this big data bank to the use of all scientists started a new era in human health (1000 Genomes Project Consortium, 2015). The main purpose of these studies is to protect humans from diseases with the changes that can be made on DNA, to determine how the body will react to drugs, to determine the weak points of each person and to take precautions. In this way, it is expected that individualized drug production and individualized treatment opportunities will arise. In the future, the studies on genomics, gene chip technology, bioinformatics, new diagnostic technologies, biosensors, drug delivery systems, apoptosis, gene transcription factors, immunotherapy, gene therapy and antisense therapy will become widespread and related technologies will be used more actively in health care. New treatment methods and health disciplines will gain importance in addition to current treatment methods (Akalın, 2015).

**Genetic Consultant:** They work with physicians and other health professionals and help patients in genetic and congenital defects that affect hereditary conditions, patients and their families. There are 2,000 genetic consultants recognized and officially accepted by the ABGC (The American Board of Genetic Counseling). Especially they have a critical role in terms of identifying the problems that can be experienced by analyzing gene maps and conducting research to solve the problems during prenatal period (Sellars and Schaefer, 2018).

**Molecular Biology and Genetics Specialist:** In the last 20 years, important steps have been taken in the fields of molecular biology and gene technology. The professionals can work in many areas such as biotechnology, embryology, DNA analysis, molecular genetics, plant genetics and drug technology. Nowadays, individuals who are predisposed because of their families to the development of colon and breast cancer can be identified by genetic tests; their survival rate and life quality can be prolonged by preventive surgery and/or medical treatment (Bardakçı, 2016).

**Embryologists:** Nowadays, these specialists work in the freezing of embryos and then use of them in IVD. Although it is not yet possible, it is expected that more complex tissues and organs can be frozen and ready for use in the future (Sermon et al., 2016).

**Stem Cell Researcher:** The extensive studies on the use of stem cells in the treatment of Alzheimer's disease, Parkinson's disease, leukemia, cancer and the diseases of nervous system and heart are one of the most important agendas of the world of health. The importance of researchers in this area will increase with the use of stem cells in the treatment (Robinton and Daley, 2012).

Şirin Özkan

## 5 The Professions Related to Traditional and Complementary Medicine

As a result of the insufficiency of modern medicine such as increased treatment costs, chronic diseases and increasing in chronic diseases and cancer prevalence, persons tend to seek complementary and traditional medicine. The interest in traditional medicine increases rapidly in all regions of the world and in industrialized countries. In Europe, North America and other industrialized regions, it was determined that 50%–70 % of the society used at least one of complementary or alternative medicine methods (Doğan and Avcı, 2018).

Complementary medicine covers the practices that are carried out in parallel with traditional medicine, which are supportive, enhance a treatment and alleviate the symptoms and/or side effects of a treatment. Complementary alternative medicine is defined as a broader health area that includes health services, methods, practices, accompanying theories and beliefs that are outside the dominant health system in a certain society (Somer and Vatanoğlu-Lutz, 2017). It is known that meditation, music, light and color therapies have a placebo effect, even though the positive effect of their treatment is not fully proven. In the results of the study on the prevention of nausea and vomiting due to chemotherapy, the most commonly used methods were determined as homeopathy, acupuncture, dietary therapies, herbalism (ginger, etc.) and hypnotherapy (Kutluturkan and Karataş, 2014).

The main purpose of choosing complementary therapies is to improve the quality of life and to alleviate the symptoms. However, these applications may have some side effects. For example, some herbal products change drug metabolism and therefore they may have dangerous side effects (Doğan and Avcı, 2018). For this reason, control mechanisms should be established in terms of the knowledge and education levels of the persons applying these methods and the frequency of the application of these methods by them; it should be ensured that they cooperate with the physicians who conduct the medical treatments when necessary in order to prevent injury and abuse of patients (Ovayolu and Ovayolu, 2013; Somer and Vatanoğlu-Lutz, 2017).

*The Regulations of Traditional and Complementary Medicine Practices* published in Turkey in 2014, some traditional and complementary medicine practices went into operation. According to this, the practices accepted in the regulation are as follows: acupuncture, apitherapy, phytotherapy, hypnosis, leech application, homeopathy, chiropractic, cupping/blood letting, larval application, mesotherapy, prolotherapy, osteopathy, ozone application, reflexology and music therapy (Sağlık Bakanlığı, 2014). It is expected that the demand for these therapists who make this widespreading applications will increase.

# 6 Conclusion

Demographic changes, technological developments, lifestyle changes, increased costs, health sector reform and environmental changes make delivering healthcare services more complex. In order to fulfil the delivery of healthcare services, it is required that the roles of health professionals change and different professionals need to work together effectively and intensively. In the future, new roles and occupational groups are expected to appear in parallel with the rapid changes in the fields of health care, information technologies, genetics, traditional and complementary medicine. Health managers should carry out strategic health human resources planning, training content and legal arrangements in cooperation with the Council of Higher Education in the light of these changes.

# References

1000 Genomes Project Consortium. (2015). A Global Reference for Human Genetic Variation, *Nature*, 526(7571), 68.

Akalın, E. (2015). Vizyon 2023. https://www.tubitak.gov.tr/tubitak_content_files/vizyon2023/si/EK-12.pdf (accessed on 01.02.2019).

Babatunde, F., MacDermid, J. & MacIntyre, N. (2017). Characteristics of Therapeutic Alliance in Musculoskeletal Physiotherapy and Occupational Therapy Practice: A Scoping Review of the Literature, *BMC Health Services Research*, 17(1), 375.

Bardakçı, B. (2016). Makü Fen-Edebiyat Fakültesi, Burdur'da Bilimin Yükselen Sesi, *Ayrıntı Dergisi*, 3(36).

Başer, D.A., Kahveci, R., Döner, P. & Özkara, A. (2014). Dünyada Hospitalist Model Uygulamaları ve Bu Modelin Türkiye'ye Olası Katkıları, *Ankara Medical Journal*, 14(4), 157.

Bronzino, J.D. & Peterson, D.R. (2015). *The Biomedical Engineering Handbook: Four Volume Set*, CRC Press, Florida, USA.

Carnevale, A.P., Jayasundera, T. & Gulish, A. (2015). *Good Jobs Are Back: College Graduates Are First in Line*, Georgetown University, McCourt School of Public Policy, Washington, USA.

Çimen, Ü. (2016). *Solunum Seslerinin Yapay Zekâ Ortamında Sınıflandırılması*, Yayımlanmamış Doktora Tezi, Afyon Kocatepe Üniversitesi Fen Bilimleri Enstitüsü, Afyon.

Crisp, N. & Chen, L. (2014). Global Supply of Health Professionals, *New England Journal of Medicine*, 370(10), 950–957.

Doğan, Ö. & Avcı, A. (2018). Bitkilerle Tedavi ve İlaç Etkileşimleri, *Turkiye Klinikleri Journal of Public Health-Special Topic*, 4(1), 49–54.

Dubois, C.A., McKee, M. & Nolte, E. (2006). *Human Resources for Health in Europe*, European Observatory on Health Systems and Policies Series, Open University Press. Glasgow, UK.

Duru, H. Akgün, E.G. & Maviş, İ. (2018). Public Awareness Levels About the Profession of Speech-Language Therapists in Turkey, *Journal of Language, Speech and Swallowing Research*, 21(1), 55–57.

Hamet, P. & Tremblay, J. (2017). Artificial Intelligence in Medicine, *Metabolism*, 69, 36–40.

Hickson, M., Child, J. & Collinson, A. (2018). Future Dietitian 2025: Informing the Development of a Workforce Strategy for Dietetics, *Journal of Human Nutrition and Dietetics*, 31(1), 23–32.

HOPE. (2009). *Health Professionals in Europe: New Roles, New Skills*, European Hospital and Healthcare Federation. http://www.hope.be/wp-content/uploads/2015/10/HOPE-exchange_2009-synthesis1.pdf (accessed on: 30.03.2019).

Jiang, F., Jiang, Y., Zhi, H., Dong, Y., Li, H., Ma, S. & et al. (2017). Artificial Intelligence in Healthcare: Past, Present and Future, *Stroke and Vascular Neurology*, 2(4), 230–243.

Kennedy, A.B. & Munk, N. (2017). Experienced Practitioners' Beliefs Utilized to Create a Successful Massage Therapist Conceptual Model: A Qualitative Investigation, *International Journal of Therapeutic Massage & Bodywork*, 10(2), 9.

Klasen, M., Bhar, S. S., Ugalde, A. & Hall, C. (2017). Clients' Perspectives on Outcomes and Mechanisms of Bereavement Counselling: A Qualitative Study, *Australian Psychologist*, 52(5), 363–371.

Koopmans, L., Damen, N. & Wagner, C. (2018). Does Diverse Staff and Skill Mix of Teams Impact Quality of Care in Long-Term Elderly Health Care? An Exploratory Case Study, *BMC Health Services Research*, 18(1), 988.

Kutlutürkan, S. & Karataş, T. (2014). Kemoterapiye Bağlı Kusmada Tamamlayıcı Tıp, *Bozok Tıp Dergisi*, 4(3), 63–65.

Ministry of Health New Zealand. (2014). *The Role of the Health Workforce New Zealand*, Wellington: Ministry of Health.

National Association of Social Workers, NASW. (2010). *Social Workers in Hospice and Palliative Care*, NASW Centers for Workforce Studies & Social Work Practice. https://www.socialworkers.org/LinkClick.aspx?fileticket=rq8DPC0g-AM%3D&portalid=0 (accessed on: 30.03.2019)

Ovayolu, Ö. & Ovayolu, N. (2013). Onkolojide Semptom Yönetiminde Kullanılan Kanıt Temelli Tamamlayıcı Yöntemler Ve Etkileri, *ERÜ Sağlık Bilimleri Fakültesi Dergisi*, 1(1), 83–98.

Raison, N., Khan, M.S. & Challacombe, B. (2015). Telemedicine in Surgery: What Are the Opportunities and Hurdles To Realising the Potential?, *Current Urology Reports*, 16(7), 43.

Robinton, D.A. & Daley, G.Q. (2012). The Promise of Induced Pluripotent Stem Cells in Research and Therapy, *Nature*, 481(7381), 295.

Sağlık Bakanlığı. (2014). *Geleneksel ve Tamamlayıcı Tıp Uygulamaları Yönetmeliği*, Resmi Gazete: 27. 10. 2014; Sayı: 29158.

Saulite, M. & Andersone, R. (2017). Development of Career Management Skills of New Podologists for Work in a Multicultural Environment, *Journal of Education Culture and Society*, 8(1), 225–238.

Sellars, E.A. & Schaefer, G.B. (2018). *Genetic Considerations in Infants with Congenital Anomalies*, In Follow-Up for NICU Graduates, Springer, Cham.

Sermon, K., Capalbo, A., Cohen, J., Coonen, E., De Rycke, M., De Vos, A. & et al. (2016). The Why, the How and the When of Pgs 2.0: Current Practices and Expert Opinions of Fertility Specialists, Molecular Biologists, and Embryologists, *Mhr: Basic Science of Reproductive Medicine*, 22(8), 845–857.

Sheikh, A., Sood, H.S. & Bates, D.W. (2015). Leveraging Health Information Technology to Achieve the "Triple Aim" of Healthcare Reform, *Journal of the American Medical Informatics Association*, 22(4), 849–856.

Sibbald, B., Shen, J. & McBride, A. (2004). Changing the Skill-Mix of the Health Care Workforce, *Journal of Health Services Research and Policy*, 9(1), 2838.

Somer, P. & Vatanoğlu-Lutz, E.E. (2017). Geleneksel ve Tamamlayıcı Tıp Uygulamaları Yönetmeliği'nin Hukuki ve Etik Açıdan Değerlendirilmesi, *Anatolian Clinic the Journal of Medical Sciences*, 22(1), 58–65.

Tsai, E., Shakbatyan, R., Evans, J., Rossetti, P., Graham, C., Sharma, H. & et al. (2016). Bioinformatics Workflow for Clinical Whole Genome Sequencing at Partners Healthcare Personalized Medicine, *Journal of Personalized Medicine*, 6(1), 12.

Uhlig, S., Dimitriadis, T., Hakvoort, L. & Scherder, E. (2017). Rap and Singing Are Used by Music Therapists to Enhance Emotional Self-Regulation of Youth: Results of a Survey of Music Therapists in the Netherlands, *The Arts in Psychotherapy*, 53, 44–54.

United Nations, Department of Economic and Social Affairs, Population Division. (2017). *World Population Prospects: The 2017 Revision, Key Findings and Advance Tables*, Working Paper No. ESA/P/WP/248.

Vollenweider, R., Peterson, C.K. & Humphreys, B.K. (2017). Differences in Practice Characteristics between Male and Female Chiropractors in Switzerland, *Journal of Manipulative and Physiological Therapeutics*, 40(6), 434–440.

Wager, K.A., Lee, F.W. & Glaser, J.P. (2017). *Health Care Information Systems: A Practical Approach for Health Care Management*, 3. Edit, John Wiley & Sons. San Francisco, CA.

Yamada, K. & Nabeshima, T. (2015). Pharmacist-Managed Clinics for Patient Education and Counseling in Japan: Current Status and Future Perspectives, *Journal of Pharmaceutical Health Care and Sciences*, 1(1), 2.

Yang, G. Z., Cambias, J., Cleary, K., Daimler, E., Drake, J., Dupont, P. E. & et al. (2017). Medical Robotics-Regulatory, Ethical, and Legal Considerations for Increasing Levels of Autonomy, *Science Robotics*, 2(4), 8638.

Zamjahn, J.B,, Beyer, E.O , Alig, K.L., Mercante, D.E., Carter, K.L. & Gunaldo, T.P. (2018). Increasing Awareness of the Roles, Knowledge, and Skills of Respiratory Therapists through an Interprofessional Education Experience, *Respiratory Care*, 63(5), 510–518.

Mehmet Emin Bilge, Rauf Karasu and Merve Ayşegül
Kulular İbrahim

# 16: Protection of Personal Rights in Healthcare Sector: The Right to Make Choices and the Right to Privacy

## 1 Introduction

Personal rights are one of the basic rights for people. Personal rights can be defined as the rights that enable individuals to develop their independent personalities and reputations in society (Akipek et al., 2002). The right to privacy, the right to protection of personal data and the right to health are within the scope of personal rights. In this study, the effect of eastern and western cultures on medical history was taken into consideration. In this context, we aimed to investigate the regulations in sample countries to set an example for the solution of problems in Turkey affected from both eastern and western cultures. The right to privacy and the right to make choices were examined. In order to investigate Western health law, the United Kingdom was chosen as a sample of developed countries while Japan was selected for Eastern health law. In this context, Japanese law was explained by considering the functionality at first and then English law was analyzed.

## 2 Japan Health Law

### 2.1 The Right to Privacy

In Japanese law, the right to protection of personal data and the right to privacy are regulated by various laws. These will be discussed below:

*In the Context of Penal Code*

The violation of the right to privacy is considered a crime and a prison sentence is foreseen in article 134 of the Criminal Law. According to this, physicians, pharmacists, drug distributors, midwives, lawyers, defendant attorneys, notaries or other persons having such professions are obliged to respect the right to privacy. Here, it is determined that which information should be kept confidential. In such professions, the information that is considered confidential by anyone is confidential information. The disclosure of such confidential information without a legal basis lead to a sanction by imprisonment for up to 6 months or a fine of up to 100,000 Yen (Penal Code, 1907).

It should be noted that there are two types of imprisonment in Japanese penal code. In the imprisonment without working, prisons only serve the sentence of imprisonment and do not work. The other is called imprisonment with working; prisons are imprisoned and have to work in heavy works such as mining and wall construction. Prison sentences are clearly stated as imprisonment with working and imprisonment without working in the provisions of Japanese law. The disclosure of the confidential information of individuals by persons working in listed or similar occupational groups, without any legal basis, are also penalized for the imprisonment with working. In Japan, the penalties of imprisonment with working are applied to more serious crimes. The disclosure of private information in the field of law such as attorney, defense lawyer, notary or in the field of health such as physician, midwife, pharmacist, etc. is sentenced with imprisonment with working. It is important to show that the importance of the protection of personal info and the right to privacy.

## *In the Context of the Act on the Prevention of Infectious Diseases and Medical Care for Patients with Infectious Diseases*

For physicians, the obligation to disclose personal data in certain cases was arranged with Article 12 in the title of 'Notification by Physicians' in the Act on the Prevention of Infectious Diseases and Medical Care for Patients with Infectious Diseases. According to this, infectious diseases are classified and physicians are obliged to notify the name, age, sex and other characteristics determined by the Ministry of Health, Labor and Social Security of persons with infectious diseases to related authorities within 7 days.

There is a disclosure of personal data as an exception to Japanese law, which gives importance to the protection of personal data. Even the disclosure of personal data has been imposed on physicians as an obligation. This is because of public interest. In fact, there is a conflict of interest between the public interest and the protection of personal data. In this way, the conflict of fundamental rights may occur in many cases. The chief point in these situations is how to balance these rights. It is clear that the public interest should outweigh. In order to ensure the healthy living of the society, there is an obligation of informing the authorities about persons with infectious diseases. Here, personal data are disclosed for public welfare.

It should be noted that there is no ordinary explanation; personal data is still protected and disclosed only to related authorities to take necessary measures.

In many European countries, such as the UK, public health organizations are authorized to monitor medical records in order to take early measures against epidemics. It is believed that this permission given to control the diseases actually violates the right to privacy (Gostin, 2005).

Apart from these, Personal Information Protection Commission established in 2016 under the Privacy Act for the protection of personal data in general, works on this issue. On 17 July 2018, Japan official Kumazawa and the European Union official Jourová talked on the telephone and agreed on the final agreement text (Personal Information Protection Commission Japan, 2018) for data sharing between Japan and European countries.

## In the Context of Privacy Act

Protection of privacy and protection of personal data are different phenomena, but they may overlap in some cases. For example, the protection of health information, which is one of the sensitive data of the individuals, is an example of the overlap of the right of protection of personal data and the right to privacy. In Japanese law, the Personal Data Protection Act regulates the sharing of personal data with third parties. The first paragraph of article 23 seeks prior written consent to share personal data. Otherwise, a business operator using personal data is prohibited from sharing personal data with third parties. There are some exceptions about this prohibition. These exceptions are in limited number and are specified in the law. In order to share patients' information with third parties, it is necessary to obtain informed consents from these patients. The cases in which obtaining a consent is not required are listed in a limited number of articles. The fact that Public health and child developmental health are addressed separately can be criticized as public health includes children. However, on the other hand, this can be appreciated as it emphasizes the importance of future generations.

Personal Information Protection Commission was established to ensure that businesses store personal data in accordance with the law and to inspect them about sharing or storing personal data with third parties. This commission is an official institution. Its duty is to ensure that personal data is processed and protected in accordance with the law.

## 2.2 Right to Make Choices

### Patient Consent

According to Japanese law, the action of applying to a healthcare institution is considered to be the general consent. The fact that the action of applying to a healthcare institution is considered to be the general consent is not valid for major treatments. For important treatments, it is necessary to obtain written informed consents from patients after informing them about the treatment and its results as in Turkish law.

It is appropriate to evaluate the application of cancer patients in relation to the obligation of physicians to illuminate patients. Cancer is an important and prevalent health problem in Japan and needs to be solved. Unfortunately, 1 out of every 2 men in Japan has cancer. Early diagnosis of cancer is very important for the protection of patients' right to life (Tejima, 2018). When a patient diagnosed with cancer is informed about the diagnosis, the patient can start treatment early. The right of the patient to start the treatment is taken from the patient when the diagnosis is hidden from the patient. In Japan, the diagnosis is hidden from men diagnosed with cancer, with the concern that they may commit suicide in case they are informed about their disease. In this case, the fact that they had cancer was not shared with the patients who were diagnosed with cancer. This practice aims to prevent patients from committing suicide. There is a conflict of rights here. Patients' right to make choices to end their own life is within the scope of personal rights. On the other hand, the right to life is one of the fundamental rights of every individual.

Individuals are prevented from using their right to end their lives in order to protect the right to life. On the other hand, when it is considered rationally, a person as a patient with untreatable cancer has the right to life which is not same with the right of an individual to live in a normal condition, because his/her life end in a shorter time. In this case, the right to life is violated in order to protect the right to life. When a person is informed about the diagnosis, he/she may continue to live by getting rid of this disease or prolong his/her lifespan by starting the required treatments. When the reality about the diagnosis is hidden from a person, this person does not start cancer treatment and his/her right to live is actually violated. This situation was also discussed in Japan and it was decided that the information about cancer is not hidden from patients, they are informed about their diseases; the opinion that the obligation of physicians to provide information also involves cancer patients, outweighed. This situation affected the practice; the patients diagnosed with cancer started to be informed within the scope of physicians' obligation to inform their patients about their diseases.

## Informed Consent

The informed consent system was adopted in Japanese law at the Japanese Medical Association Bioethics Round Table Conference in 1990. In 1997, the informed consent system was revised in the Health Service Law. According to this, making disclosure to patients was determined as an obligation for physicians.

In Japanese law, informed consent is important for 2 key elements. The first is that the informed consent system gives a person the right to decide on his/her own, thus it ensures that the decision of the person is respected. The other is that the informed consent system ensures that the patient's life, health and happiness are recovered and protected. Informed consent ensures that a physicians respect the decisions of their patients. For example, blood transfusion is not allowed according to a belief. Thus, physician do not conduct blood transfusions without the consent of patients; this situation ensures that patients make decisions about their own. Furthermore, when blood transfusions are conducted without obtaining consents from patients, this situation makes these patients unhappy so they probably reject blood transfusion under normal conditions. Thus, obtaining consents from patients recovers and protects their lives, health and happiness.

There are also exceptional cases in which informed consent is not applied. Informed consent is not required in exceptional cases such as emergency cases or other cases in which other persons are at risk of harm.

## In the Context of Medical Care Act

This issue is described in Article 1–4 of the Medical Treatment Law. Physician, dentist, pharmacist, nurse or other healthcare professionals are obliged to enlighten patients. Accordingly, these persons are obliged to do their utmost to make the appropriate explanation for understanding of it by the patient (Medical Care Act, 1948).

# 3  The UK Health Law

## 3.1  Right to Privacy

### Confidentiality Obligation

While confidentiality obligation has been one of the keystones of medical ethics since the Hippocratic Oath dating back to the 5th century BC, the right to privacy is one of the current concepts in law (De Faria et al., 2014). The protection of privacy constitutes the continuation of confidentiality obligation of physicians, but also covers new topics related to information technologies such as the way of data processing after the collection of data with the developing technology, the conditions in which the data are shared, the way of data update and what to do after reaching the objectives. The answer of the question of which conditions are in the scope the right to privacy varies according to person and time (Woogara, 2001). In summary, the content of the concept of privacy is not fixed. The scope of privacy has expanded and can continue to expand according to new demands in accordance with personal and social needs and technological changes.

## Protection of Personal Data

### In the Context of European Convention on Human Rights

The right to privacy is regulated in Article 7 and the right to protection of personal data in Article 8 of the European Convention on Human Rights. In Article 7 of the new regulation in 2012, with the title of Respect to Private and Family Life, the right to privacy was arranged with the rights of family life and respect to residence and communication (*Official Journal of the European Union*, 2012). The right to privacy is accorded to to everyone as a fundamental right (European Union Delegation to Turkey, 2012). In this way, the right to privacy is secured by the European Convention on Human Rights. Accordingly, it has been stated that the consent of the data holder or the legal basis is required for the processing of related personal data.

The basic principle in the processing of personal data is the presence of the consent of related person. Personal data are collected, processed or shared with third parties under this principle, in other words with the consent of the data owner. In the absence of a consent, the collection, publication and processing of personal data is prohibited. There are exceptions for data sharing. Although a consent is required for such use of the data, there will be different requirements for the continued use of the data after it is collected. When personal data is not up-to-date and the purpose of data collection is over, the data should not be stored. The personal data collected for a specific purpose or shared with third parties must be deleted after achieving this goal (Castellano, 2012).

### In the Context of GDPR (General Data Protection Regulation)

In Article 9 of GDPR, special data types which are not allowed to be processed were determined. These data types are race or ethnicity, political views, religious or philosophical beliefs or union membership, genetic data, biometric data, health-related data, sexual life, sexual orientation (EUR-Lex, 2016). General rule is that health data and other specified situations are not processed, but in some circumstances these data are allowed to be processed. Some of these conditions that may be interested in health law were analyzed in the subheadings below.

## Patient Consent

In line with the statement in the European Convention on Human Rights, the consent of the data owner was accepted as the basic rule in the processing of the data in Article 9 of the GDPR. Obtaining patient consent for processing the data is also important in order not to damage the patient's confidence during the medical treatment process. Because the feeling of trust between the physician and the patient is very important in determining the diagnosis during the treatment and in negotiating the types, risks and benefits of the treatment.

Obtaining the consent of the patient to process the data within the context of privacy protection, also serves to protect the right to make choices of the patient (Braunack-Mayer et al., 2003). The patient's ability to determine who can access his/her own health data or to not give consent when he/she wants to keep the health data confidential is compatible with the patient's right to make choices.

## Nature of Treatment Process

The Article 9/h of the GDPR provides a legal basis for the sharing of patient data due to the nature of the process taking place to provide medical treatment. As it is seen in the widespread practices in medical treatment, sharing the patient data among the healthcare worker group providing treatment services for the patient is made possible. The necessity of processing in terms of providing medical diagnosis, health or social care services or treatment, or the management of health or social care systems and services and sharing of data with each other by health staff during the treatment process are in this Article (Woogara, 2001). The prohibition of processing health data referred to in 1st paragraph is not applied in this condition. Although sharing patient data among health professionals involved in the treatment process is an exemption, it may be considered that there should be a limitation. This limitation is possible with ethics. The limiting criterion for sharing all patient data is the medical ethics (Braunack-Mayer et al., 2003).

## Public Interest

As technological developments increase interventions to individuals' privacy, the demand for the protection of privacy increases and differentiates as the technology develops (Demirsoy et al., 2016). Increased demand for privacy protection also affects the rules for medical treatment and care. Therefore, in the fields of medical ethics and medical law, different opinions develop in order to take necessary steps to protect the privacy of patients who want to benefit from health services. The responsibility of healthcare staff is not limited to providing medical treatment, but also responsible for the protection of fundamental rights such as the right to health, the right to privacy and respect to privacy during the treatment process (Zaybak et al., 2012).

Article 9/i of the GDPR, which specifically states that health data can be processed for the realization of public interest in medicinal products or devices, has brought the exception to the consideration of the public interest in the prohibition of the processing of health data under the right to privacy. It may be required to process the data for public interest such as ensuring the protection against serious cross-border health threats or providing high-quality healthcare services and products. In this case, the processing of health data is made possible (EUR-Lex, 2016). In this article, two different situations as the protection from cross-border threats and the provision of medical technological development have been mentioned in terms of the protection of the public interest. Therefore, it is possible to process the patient's health data in order to eliminate the threats and to provide public interest in the case of cross-border threats.

In addition to them, Article 9/j of the GDPR make possible to process data when processing activity is required for archiving for public interest, scientific or historical research or statistical purposes. Therefore, health data are able to be processed for the researches mentioned in the Article, the data can be processed by subordinating public interest to the right to privacy. In the Article 4 of the GDPR, it is stated that member states can seek additional conditions in the processing of various health data, especially genetic, biometric data (Ministry of the European Union, 2016).

## 3.2 Right to Make Choices

In the United Kingdom, the cases in which the physicians did not adequately informed the patients are considered as a negligence action. This situation allows physicians to be protected in two ways. In a case of negligence, the plaintiff should prove the negligence action which constitutes the basis of the claim and causes harm. For the lawsuits sued against battery, the plaintiff is not required to prove the damage because the action itself is a cause of action. In the negligence action, the plaintiff claimed that he had not been informed; the type of case is important since it would have to prove that he would not give consent for the procedure if he had been informed (Lindley, 2005).

### Relationship between the Physician and the Patient

The physician has a duty of care for the patient (Lindley, 2005). Within the scope of this duty, the physician should inform the patient about the risks

and results of the treatment methods which can be applied with care and cau-
tion during the treatment of the patient, build consensus about the treatment
method by discussing with the patient and obtain the consent of the patient
to be able to apply this treatment method. In other words, the consent of the
patient requires an explanation of the risks, indications and rules of the procedure and the consequences of not performing the recommended surgery and
the negotiatiation of alternative treatments (McManus et al., 2003). When the
physician neglects to inform the patient, the physician may be responsible due to
a wrongful act. After the year of 1931, negligence was recognized as a wrongful
act (Jones, 2000).

The main element under the responsibility of the physicians in Turkish law
is fault. In the determination of a fault, the factors such as whether the physician violates the duty of care, whether the physician fulfills the obligation to
enlighten the patient and whether there is a negligence in the treatment are effective (Hakeri, 2014).

Nowadays, it is emphasized that most of the complaints or legal procedures
are caused by the inability of physicians to communicate properly (Armstrong
et al., 1997). Informing before the surgery as a part of the informed consent procedure does not continue after the operation. The survey conducted on the subject showed that although the written consent form signed by the patients prior
to the surgery provided the fulfillment of the legal requirements, the patients
were not fully aware of the real nature of the treatment (Byrne et al., 1988). On
the other hand, there is also the opinion that the mention of written consent
forms during the dialogue between the patients and the physicians allows the
patients to be better informed before they give informed consents (Armstrong
et al., 1997).

In practice, patients' consents are obtained in writing and on the computer
(Woogara, 2001). The reason for obtaining their consents on the computer is to
ensure that their consents can be seen by different during the treatment process.
Printed consent forms for clinical cases are often also asked for consent to use
their data (European Patients Forum).

## The Case of Bolam v Friern Hospital Management Committee

In English law, duty of care was extended to include health workers through
jurisprudence (Jones, 2000). The standard duty of care in health law within the
scope of duty of care was determined by the case of Bolam v Friern Hospital
Management Committee. In this case, the plaintiff John Hector Bolam sued the
defendant Friern Hospital Management Committee for the harm affecting him

as a result of negligences of it. She had fractures on both side of his pelvis during the treatment (Bolam v Friern Hospital Management Committee, 1957).

Bolam underwent electroconvulsive therapy (ECT) for clinical depression. However, there were differences of opinion about how to minimize the risk of damage caused by convulsions caused by ECT. In this case, manual pressure was not effective and therefore the patient's pelvic bone was broken. Bolam brought the subject to trial and argued that the physician was responsible because the physician did not fulfill the standard care or duty of care during the treatment process; he also argued that the hospital was faulty (Samanta et al., 2003). In this important case, the locus classicus was developed to measure whether the physician fulfills the standard of duty of care (Samanta et al., 2003).

According to Bolam Test, a person who identifies oneself in that profession is responsible for his negligence when this person does not apply the special abilities required for the profession (Mulheron, 2010).

Judge McNair stated that the physician would not be guilty of negligence if he acted in accordance with appropriate procedures which performed by a reasonable physician in this area (Samanta et al., 2003). In other words, the judge emphasized that a physician who acts in accordance with a well accepted procedure does not have the responsibility for negligence even there is an opinion on the contrary. This decision was also approved by the supreme court; it was among the prejudications in law (Samanta et al., 2003). Since 1957, the Bolam test has been applied in the evaluation of professional negligence (Jones, 2000). In conclusion, in English law, when a physician explains a particular risk and this risk is in the same direction of the reasonable professional opinion of the responsible institution, responsibility of negligence do not rise. Furthermore, when any reasonably qualified physician does not mention that risk in the same case, the physician would not be responsible for the negligence (McManus et al., 2003; Earle, 1999). The Bolam test is a physician-focused test. The responsibility is determined by the reasonable average physician. To clarify, a decision is made according to the question of what should a reasonable physician explain to a patient instead of the question of what do reasonable patients expect to be explained to them (Earle, 1999). The Bolam test has been criticized for neglecting patients' opinion and carrying out an evaluation according to physicians when it determines a negligence.

## Prudent Patient Test

The patient should be enlightened for informed consent. However, the framework of this enlightenment has not been clarified yet. Particularly, the limit required for reporting operational risks is discussed. These risks should be explained to a reasonable person who attaches importance to risks in knowing the physician's situation and deciding whether to give up the recommended treatment (Lindley, 2005). Bolam test began to lose its importance over time. Thus, in determining the responsibility, the patient-centered prudent patient test came into use instead of the physician-centered Bolam test. The idea of "the physician knows the best in the Bolam test", which is based on a patriarchal mindset, is left behind. Adults who have sufficient mental capacity are able to make a decision or should make a decision about themselves; their right to do so must be protected by law. Medical physicians are aware of that this right to make choices is not limited by whether others accepted as reasonable (Wong, 2015). It is important to know the risks affecting the decision of the patient to accept or not to accept the treatment. Thus, if the risk occurs, the plaintiff may argue that the fact that the physician neglected to warn him about this risk affects the validity of the consent and that the consent is invalid (Earle, 1999).

The opinion that calls the Bolam test a prudent physician test criticizes the test in which physicians determine the knowledge including common or serious risks should be known by patients (Wong, 2015). In prudent patient test, the explanations are also made by physicians and the limits of these explanations are determined by them. However, the prudent patient test differs from the prudent physician test due to the way of the assessment of the explanation by physicians. In prudent physician test, a physician assesses what to explain according to his or her clinical reasoning. However, in the prudent patient test, physicians are obliged to disclose the information which is important and may affect the evaluation of the patient at the decision-making stage. In other words, the physician who informs the patient in the prudent patient test is obliged to determine the limits of this information according to the information that affects the patient's decision, not according to his/her own clinical information. Patients are not the passive side of medical treatment; they are the active part of the treatment, involve in the process with their own decisions and take responsibility for the results of their decisions. The prudent patient test (Wong, 2015), which is appropriate to the socio-cultural structure of now, ensures the protection of personal rights, especially the right to make choices.

The risks, outcomes and alternative methods that may affect patients' decisions are presented to patients; patients make their own decisions. Therefore, physicians have no responsibility about the problems in the post-treatment period.

# 4 Conclusion

Personal rights are fundamental rights as a result of being a person. The subject was shaped according to jurisprudence in the UK with anglo-saxon system. In Japan Law which is considered to be compatible with German Law based continental European legal system, there are fundamental cases and these legal precedents are taken as basis in some cases. In the processing of personal data within the framework of health law, the consent of the data holder is the main criterion in the treatment for both samples. However, the exceptions were arranged differently.

In Turkish law, the rights of privacy and the protection of personal data have newly developed with the legalization process of 2016. In the health sector, it is necessary that both the legal regulations for health data with the characteristics of sensitive personal data and putting this data into practice should be qualified. It is necessary to make informing health staff about personal rights and providing the necessary environment to them for self-improvement obligatory. Thus, the satisfaction of health workers will increase and the problems in the health sector will decrease. In our country, not only the European Union directives but also practices in other developed countries should be investigated and taken into account when making legal arrangements. On the other hand, national laws on the protection of personal data are not sufficient as the internet removes the state boundaries (Kulular İbrahim, 2015). Access to personal data from different countries is possible. Therefore, international regulations are necessary for the protection of personal rights.

This study was funded by the Scientific Research Projects Commission of Social Sciences University of Ankara (SSUA). Project Code: SBA-2017-139

# References

Akipek, J. & Akinturk, T. (2002). *Introductory Rules of the Turkish Civil Law – Law of Persons*, Istanbul, Beta.

Armstrong, A. P., Cole, A.A. & Page, R.E. (1997). Informed Consent: Are We Doing Enough?, *British Journal of Plastic Surgery*, 50, 637–640.

Avrupa Birliği Bakanlığı. (2016). *Avrupa Birliği Genel Veri Koruma Tüzüğü* (GDPR). 1–88. 4.5.2016 Tarih ve L 119 sayılı Avrupa Birliği Resmi Gazetesi. https://www.kisiselverilerinkorunmasi.org/wp-content/uploads/2017/09/GDPR-T%C3%BCrk%C3%A7e-%C3%87eviri-AB-Bakanl%C4%B1%C4%9F%C4%B1.pdf (accessed on: 10.01.2019)

Avrupa Birliği Türkiye Delegasyonu. (2012). Avrupa Birliği Temel Haklar Bildirgesi. https://www.avrupa.info.tr/tr/avrupa-birligi-temel-haklar-bildirgesi-708 (accessed on: 21.01.2019)

Bolam v Friern Hospital Management Committee, 1956 B. No. 507 (Queen's Bench Division Şubat 26, 1957). https://lexlaw.co.uk/wp-content/uploads/2018/02/Bolam.pdf (accessed on: 01.01.2019)

Braunack-Mayer, A.J. & Mulligan, E.C. (2003). Sharing Patient Information between Professionals: Confidentiality and Ethics, *The Medical Journal of Australia (MJA)*, 178(6), 277–279.

Byrne, D.J., Napier, A. & Cuschieri, A. (1988). How Informed is Signed Consent?, *British Medical Journal*, 296(6625), 839, 840.

Castellano, P.S. (2012). The Right to be Forgotten under European Law: A Constitutional Debate, *Lex Electronica*, 16(2), 1–30.

De Faria, P.L. & Cordeiro, J.V. (2014). Health Data Privacy and Confidentiality Rights: Crisis or Redemption?, *Revista Portuguesa de Saúde Pública*, 32(2), 123–133.

Demirsoy, N. & Kirimlioglu, N. (2016). Protection of Privacy and Confidentiality as a Patient Right: Physicians' and Nurses' Viewpoints, *Biomedical Research*, 27(4), 1437–1448.

Earle, M. (1999). The Future of Informed Consent in British Common Law, European *Journal of Health Law*, 6, 235–248.

EUR-Lex. (2016). General Data Protection Regulation. Regulation (EU) 2016/679 of the European Parliament and of the Council of 27 April 2016 on the Protection of Natural Persons with regard to the Processing of Personal Data and on the Free Movement of Such Data. https://eur-lex.europa.eu/legal-content/EN/TXT/?qid=1528874672298&uri=CELEX%3A32016R0679 (accessed on: 19.01.2019)

European Patients Forum. (n.d.). *The new EU Regulation on the Protection of Personal Data: What Does It Mean for Patients?*, Brussels.

Gostin, L.O. (2005). Law and the Public's Health, *Issues in Science and Technology*, 21(3), Issues in Science and Technology: https://issues.org/gostin/ (accessed on: 31.01.2019)

Hakeri, H. (2014). Tıp Hukukunda Malpraktis Komplikasyon Ayrımı, *Toraks Cerrahisi Bülteni*, 5(1), 23–28.

Jones, J.W. (2000). The Healthcare Professional and the Bolam Test, *British Dental Journal*, 188(5), 237–240.

Kulular Ibrahim, M.A. (2015) *Protection of Privacy and Personal Data in the Absence of "The Code": The Case of Turkey*, LLM Thesis, London.

Lindley, R. (2005). *Informed Consent and the Ghost of Bolam*, In M. Brazier, & M. Lobjoit (Eds.), *Protecting the Vulnerable: Autonomy and Consent in Health Care*, Routledge. New York, USA.

McManus, P.L. & Wheatley, K.E. (2003). Consent and Complications: Risk Disclosure Varies Widely Between Individual Surgeons. *Annals of the Royal College of Surgeons of England*, 85(2), 79–82.

Medical Care Act. (1948) Act No. 205. Retrieved from Japanese Law Translation. http://www.japaneselawtranslation.go.jp/law/detail/?id=2199&vm=04&re=02 (accessed on: 21.01.2019)

Mulheron, R. (2010). *Medical Negligence: Non-Patient and Third Party Claims*, Routledge.

Official Journal of the European Union. (2012). Charter of Fundamental Rights of the European Union. https://eur-lex.europa.eu/legal-content/EN/TXT/?uri=celex:12012P/TXT (accessed on: 20.01.2019)

Penal Code. (1907). Act No. 45. Retrieved from Japanese Law Translation. http://www.japaneselawtranslation.go.jp/law/detail/?id=1960&re=02&vm=04 (accessed on: 21.01.2019)

Personal Information Protection Commission Japan. (2018). https://www.ppc.go.jp/en/aboutus/roles/international/cooperation/20180717/ (accessed on: 12.12.2018)

Samanta, A. & Samanta, J. (2003). Legal Standard of Care: A Shift from the Traditional Bolam Test. Clinical Medicine, *Journal of the Royal College of Physicians*, 3(5), 443–446.

Tejima, Y. (2018). *Medical Law Introductory*, Shima, ARMA.

Wong, D.S. (2015). An Important Update on Medical Consent, *Hong Kong Medical Journal*, 21(4), 376–377.

Woogara, J. (2001). Human Rights and Patient's Privacy in UK Hospitals, *Nursing Ethics*, 8(3), 234–246.

Zaybak, A., Eşer, İ. & Gunay Ismailoglu, E. (2012). Bir Üniversite Hastanesinde Hastaların Hasta Haklarını Kullanma Tutumunun İncelenmesi, *Florence Nightingale Hemşirelik Dergisi*, 20(2), 104–111.

# Section 4: New Approaches in Other Health Sciences

Özgü İnal and Berna Tunçer

# 17: Telerehabilitation

## 1 Introduction

Telerehabilitation (TR) is an important sub-discipline of telemedicine and is a new method for remotely providing and monitoring of rehabilitation services. The use of TR has become more widespread with the increasing speed and development of communication and information technologies. It is accepted that TR has the potential to reduce global health disparities, especially in access to rehabilitation as an important advantage; the lack of adequate technological systems or inadequate use of technological systems in rural areas are defined as the limitations of TR applications. A common idea in literature is that the TR will be an effective application comparable to conventional rehabilitation service by increasing TR technologies and applications. This section aims to summarize the concept of TR, its advantages, limitations and areas of use by taking into account the current literature.

## 2 What Is Telerehabilitation?

In the literature, the words of telehealth, telemedicine and telerehabilitation are used interchangeably; this situation results in confusion. Telehealth is the most comprehensive term and includes both telemedicine and telerehabilitation concepts (Cason, 2009; Rogante et al., 2015). TR as one of the important areas of telemedicine, is a rehabilitation method which remotely provides service to clients by rehabilitation professionals (e.g. physicians, physiotherapists, occupational therapists, speech and language therapists and other rehabilitation team members) via telehealth technologies (Peretti et al., 2017). According to the American Occupational Therapy Association (AOTA), TR is defined as the application of counseling, prevention, and diagnosis and treatment services through duplex interactive telecommunication technology (Wakeford et al., 2005). Although telecommunication technologies are diverse, some of them are remote telemonitoring systems, video and telephone conference systems.

## 3 Why Telerehabilitation?

The World Health Organization focuses on the ability of individuals to function effectively in their environment (Weinstein et al., 2008; Kuipers et al., 2009). The

210 Ínal and Tunçer

literature supports the natural environment model of TR. The evidences have suggested that the implementation of rehabilitation services and interventions in natural setting, rather than in clinical setting increase the effect of treatments (Piron et al., 2008; Kumar and Cohn, 2012).

Rehabilitation should begin immediately after the reduction of functional capacity or an injury and end with a successful return to home. The inadequacy of rehabilitation often decreases the level of independence and life quality of individuals. Nowadays, many patients cannot get enough rehabilitation service or begin rehabilitation programs early enough because of different reasons (living in rural areas, cost, transportation problems due to long distances, lack of adequate health personnel in some regions, lack of health insurance of individuals).

Patients need to be simultaneously followed up by different health disciplines such as physiotherapists, occupational therapists, speech and language therapists, especially for the diseases requiring long-term rehabilitation, such as stroke. This situation results in high cost and repeated application to hospitals for individuals. Another issue is the general aging of the population and the limited resources allocated to public health. The development of new rehabilitation models and practices seems to be necessary in order to cope with the needs related to healthcare services. When all of these situations are considered, the use of TR has become more common with the development of communication technologies. The advantages of TR are as follows:

- Ensuring ease of service access and time saving for persons in distant places and with limited access to rehabilitation services
- Ensuring fairness in access to health services
- Ensuring continuity of rehabilitation
- Increasing patients' compliance and motivation
- Shortening of hospitalization period
- Cost effectiveness (Burger, 2016; Shenoy and Shenoy, 2018)

## 4 Telerehabilitation Types

As technology plays an important role in TR, it is important to take technology and availability into consideration. There are many kinds of technologies such as text-based, audio-based, vision-based, virtual reality based, web-based and wireless integrated systems. However, selecting a remote rehabilitation system requires more than one decision factor. The factors such as budget, being suitable for the purpose, technical support structure, ease of use should be considered in the selection of appropriate technology. Although very complex technological systems can be associated with high cost and learning capacity, this situation may also cause these systems cannot be used.

# 5 Application Areas of Telerehabilitation

## 5.1 Neurological Rehabilitation

Stroke is a clinical condition that requires long-term rehabilitation and should be followed up simultaneously by different health disciplines. Patients should continue their treatment regularly after discharge. This results in high costs and repeated hospital visits for individuals and caregivers. However, individuals with stroke may have limited access to stroke services after discharge because of many different reasons (inadequate healthcare personnel, transport difficulties, etc.). In this case, alternative service delivery models that are accessible, modifiable and equally therapeutic should be used (Butler et al., 2014; Burger, 2016). In the literature, the studies on the efficacy of TR in individuals with stroke are generally promising.

According to the results of a systematic review and meta-analysis, there is limited, moderate evidence that TR practice has the same effect as conventional rehabilitation in improving daily living activities and motor functions in patients with stroke (Chen et al., 2015).

In a study in which 8 patients with chronic aphasia after stroke underwent speech therapy–based telerehabilitation program (iAphasia), the participants received telespeech therapy for 4 weeks. The status before and after treatment were compared. A significant improvement in language functions was determined after treatment. The recovery continued at 1 month follow-up. Overall, the level of satisfaction of individuals with iAphasia was high. Although the results of the study suggested that this application is an effective and feasible treatment method for patients with chronic aphasia; it was also stated that follow-up studies with more individuals and control groups are needed (Choi et al., 2016).

In a pilot study with the patients with stroke, a total of 9 sessions of TR were administered 3 sessions per week for 3 weeks. According to the findings of the study, it was found that the balance levels of the individuals improved after the treatment. However, there was no difference in their life quality and mental status. In this study, it was stated that the routine use of TR was beneficial because it supported functionality in stroke patients. However, it was also stated that the necessary technological equipment for TR application was not sufficient in rural areas where the study is performed (Hüzmeli et al., 2017).

In a systematic review on the efficacy of TR interventions on motor recovery and depression in stroke patients, the results of the studies were generally associated with significant improvements in depression in the motor recovery and intervention groups. However, only 8 of the 22 studies reported significant differences between the intervention and control groups in favor of the TR group, while the other studies reported no significant difference (Sarfo et al., 2018).

In a systematic review and meta-analysis on the efficacy of TR in post-stroke patients, it was stated that TR can be a suitable alternative to conventional rehabilitation, especially in those living in remote and rural areas. It was stated that further studies are needed to evaluate the life and cost effectiveness with the ongoing developments within the scope of TR (Tchero et al., 2018).

TR studies on multiple sclerosis (MS) are limited but encouraging results have been obtained. However, given the methodological and design features, there is limited evidence of the effect of TR on improving functional activities and life quality in individuals with MS (Khan et al., 2015).

In a study using virtual reality system and applying TR program, it was shown that the balance and postural control levels of the individuals with MS improved (Gutiérrez et al., 2013).

In two different systematic reviews (Khan et al., 2015; Rintala et al., 2018), it was stated that TR applications may be effective in increasing physical activity but there is a need for more mounting evidence.

In a randomized, prospective study designed to demonstrate the feasibility of TR and to compare its efficacy with conventional therapy in patients with MS with ambulatory insufficiency, 30 participants were included in one of three different 8 weeks long intervention programs. Group 1 (control) – customized unsupervised home-based exercise program 5 days a week; Group 2 – remote PT supervised via audio/visual real-time telecommunication twice a week; Group 3 – in person physical therapy at the medical facility twice a week. In the study, it was found that TR had a comparable effect with conventional physiotherapy in terms of the outcomes reported by the patients and the objective outcome measures of gait and balance (Fjeldstad-Pardo et al., 2018).

In a multicenter, single-blind, randomized controlled study on the virtual reality application via TR for postural instability in the patients with Parkinson's disease, home-based virtual reality balance training was shown to reduce postural instability in these patients. In this multicenter study, 76 patients with Parkinson's disease were randomly divided into two groups for receiving 21 sessions of 50 minutes of virtual reality-TR at home, or sensory integration balance training in the clinic for 7 weeks. Nintendo Wii Fit system was used in the virtual reality-TR group while postural stability exercises were applied in sensory integration balance training group. The patients were evaluated before, after the treatment and in 1 month follow-up. The results demonstrated that virtual reality may be an alternative to sensory integration balance training in clinical practice to reduce postural instability in parkinson's patients (Gandolfi et al., 2017).

Twenty patients with Parkinson's disease participated in a study using a video conferencing system to investigate the efficacy and feasibility of vocal TR in the patients with Parkinson's disease by using the extended version of Lee Silverman® method. The patients were evaluated by video conferencing before and after the treatment. The results of the study showed that TR has the potential to improve the voice quality of these patients. In addition, all patients reported higher satisfaction with TR application compared to face-to-face rehabilitation (Dias et al., 2016).

According to the results of a systematic review evaluating the applicability and effectiveness of traumatic brain injury, telephone-based and Internet-based interventions, 4 of 5 randomized controlled trials reported positive effects after intervention. However, the duration of these effects has not been shown or studied by these studies. Only 3 Internet-based interventions focusing on activity were found. The evidence for the effectiveness of these applications in individuals with traumatic brain injury is generally not clear. In this study, it was emphasized that the fact that future studies on the comparison of clinical and cost effectiveness of face-to-face therapy and different TR applications will make contributions to the literature (Ownsworth et al., 2018).

In a multicenter, prospective, parallel-designed, single-blind study investigating the application of TR in the patients with severe traumatic brain injury, patients were randomly divided into two groups as TR (Group 1) or conventional rehabilitation training (Group 2). TR was implemented through an advanced video conferencing system. In both groups, each treatment (cognitive or motor or both of them according to patients' functional status) continued for approximately 1 hour per day and 5 days per week for 12 weeks. The clinical evaluations were performed blindly before and after the treatments. The results of the study showed that this application was not as effective as conventional rehabilitation in terms of the functional recovery capacity and psychological well-being of the patients, caregiver burden and health costs when TR was compared with standard functional rehabilitation therapies (Calabrò et al., 2018).

Web-based cognitive rehabilitation for dementia has been shown to be beneficial in improving cognitive performance as well as psychological well-being in demented individuals living at home (De Luca et al., 2016).

In a pilot study conducted with the patients with Alzheimer's disease, the effects of lexical-semantic stimulation by telecommunication technology were compared with those of cognitive rehabilitation. Twenty five patients with very early stage Alzheimer's disease were divided into three groups: Alzheimer's staging was performed according to the Mini-Mental State Test. First group received lexical-semantic stimulation TR, second group received lexical-semantic stimulation face-to-face rehabilitation and third group received control conditional cognitive rehabilitation. As a result of the study, it was found that telecommunication technology was applicable in cognitive rehabilitation and increased cognitive performance in the elderly patients with neurodegenerative cognitive impairment (Jelcic et al., 2014).

## 5.2 Dysphagia Rehabilitation

Although the increasing use of TR in the fields of physiotherapy and occupational therapy, the studies on the applications related to swallowing disorders are still limited but promising.

One hundred patients (25 non-dysphagic, 25 mild, 25 moderate and 25 severe dysphagic) were included in a study investigating their clinician perceptions about dysphagia severity, clinical decision-making for the safety of oral intake or swallowing assessment via TR. The patients were evaluated using the telehealth system and the methodology reported in previous studies; the clinicians performed online and face-to-face synchronously structured clinical swallowing assessment for each evaluation. In each of the four groups, an acceptable level of agreement was observed among clinicians at a level of 90 % in terms of three primary outcome measures (oral/non-oral intake and decisions on safe foods and drinks) and the items of clinical swallowing assessment.

The clinicians stated that they could establish a good relationship with most of the patients in all groups. However, a small but an important part of the clinicians disagreed in terms of making the best use of their skills in evaluating the use of the TR system in the severe dysphagic group. In the study, it was found that TR was comparable to face-to-face assessments, regardless of the severity of dysphagia, in terms of clinical swallowing assessment and clinical decisions as a consequence of it. The clinicians pointed out some difficulties that occurred during the evaluation in the severe dysphagia group (Ward et al., 2014).

In a systematic review investigating the efficacy of TR in the dysphagic patients (Nordio et al., 2018), although there were recent TR studies on this subject, it was stated that only a single suitable study was found according to inclusion criteria (Wall et al., 2017). In conclusion, there is no clear evidence for the efficacy of TR in dysphagia rehabilitation in this review article.

## 5.3 Spinal Cord Injury (SCI) Rehabilitation

There is some evidence that telecommunications is effective in reducing pain and sleep problems in patients with SCI (Dorstyn et al., 2013).

In a study investigating the effectiveness of home exercise/TR program in 16 SCI patients using manual wheelchairs and with shoulder pain and subacromial impingement symptoms, it was reported that the exercise program applied via TR is a promising method for the treatment of shoulder pain in individuals with SCI and using manual wheelchairs (Van Staaten et al., 2014).

## 5.4 Oncologic Rehabilitation

In a study conducted with the patients with head and neck cancer, their suitability for TR was evaluated by investigating the computer literacy of them and how their health controls were performed were investigated. It was consequently found that the computer literacy of the individuals with head and neck cancer was high; this situation may be a factor supporting TR-based rehabilitation protocols. It has been thought that TR may provide positive support to the treatment proceses by increasing self-management during the treatment process (Cartmill et al., 2016).

In a randomized controlled trial of patients with glioma, the feasibility of TR-based home exercise program was investigated. The follow-up period was evaluated as 6 months. As a result of the study, it was stated that TR-based home exercise application was applicable in the patients with stable glioma. The cardiorespiratory capacity of the patients improved as a result of the treatment (Gehring et al., 2018).

In a study investigating the efficacy of TR-based control compared to usual care control to improve functional capacity in the breast cancer patients, the individuals were divided into two groups. One group was treated with TR-based exercise approaches for 8 weeks while the other group was evaluated as control group and usual care was applied. Evaluations were made three times at the beginning, immediately after the first session and 6 months later. The 6-minute walk test, Auditory Consonant Trigrams and Trail Making Test were used in the evaluation. The results of the study have supported the efficacy of the telehealth system to achieve improvements and maintain them after 6 months of follow-up in terms of functional and cognitive performance in breast cancer patients (Galiano-Castillo et al., 2017).

## 5.5 Cardiopulmonary Rehabilitation

In a randomized controlled study, the feasibility and efficacy of the TR-based home program in the elderly individuals with chronic obstructive pulmonary disease (COPD) and chronic heart failure (CHF) were investigated. In this study, the patients were followed up for 4 months. Their exercise tolerance was evaluated with a 6-min walk test and it was stated as the primary assessment criterion. Secondary assessment criteria included duration (hospitalization and death), dyspnea assessment, physical activity assessment, disability assessment and quality of life assessment. In the TR-based home program, cardiorespiratory parameters were monitored remotely, telephone interviews were made with the nurse weekly and the exercise program was monitored weekly by the physiotherapist. The 4-month long TR-based home program was found to be feasible and effective in the elderly patients with COPD and CHF (Bernocchi et al., 2017).

In a study investigating the current status smartphone-based cardiac TR application in heart patients and their needs, it was stated that there was a high level of use and interest in mobile health technology in the patients with heart failure and heart transplantation. It has been stated that the smart phone-based cardiac TR program should be arranged in accordance with different diagnoses and developed for the requested areas (Kim et al., 2018).

Kinect-based home exercise software program was developed for the tele pulmonary rehabilitation in COPD patients. The exercises prepared by the Turkish Thoracic Society were modeled in the developed software system and it was recorded whether the patients performed the specified number of related exercises and the necessary instructions for performing the exercise were presented to patients through the software. The related exercises were consequently regularly carried out by the patients with a fun way by improving the patients' movements in a 3D model and 3D environment (Çatal et al., 2014).

In a systematic review investigating the efficacy of TR in cardiopulmonary diseases, the studies conducted between the years of 1990 and 2013 were searched from four electronic databases in total. Inclusion criteria were stated as the application of home-based TR, having at least two exercise sessions, being randomized controlled trials and reporting physical or functional outcomes in the adult patients with coronary heart disease, chronic heart failure and chronic respiratory disease. A total of 11 studies were included. According to the results, although TR is promising in patients with cardiopulmonary disease, evidence is still limited (Hwang et al., 2015).

## 5.6 Pediatric Rehabilitation

In the literature, the studies on the effectiveness of TR in pediatric diseases are generally promising. In a study evaluating the applicability of computer-based cognitive education at home for pediatric patients with brain damage,

32 adolescents aged 11–16 years with a diagnosis of congenital or acquired brain damage (traumatic or non-traumatic) were included. Five days a week for 8 weeks and 40 sessions of total therapy were applied. As a result, it has been reported that TR is an applicable treatment method in adolescents with brain damage (Corti et al., 2018).

In a study evaluating the efficacy of home-based TR in the patients with hemiparesis, it was reported that TR was a feasible and effective treatment method in the patients with hemiparesis (Valdés et al., 2018).

In a randomized controlled study evaluating the efficacy of the web-based TR method in the children and adolescents with unilateral cerebral palsy, it was stated that web-based TR improved motor activity, visual perception and physical capacity in these patients but these results were not statistically significant (M Piovesena et al., 2017).

In a randomized controlled study evaluating the efficacy of caregiver-directed home-based intensive bimanual training in the children with unilateral spastic cerebral palsy, home-based activities were administered to 24 children for 2 hours a day, 5 day a week for 9 weeks, for a total of 90 hours. The caregivers were trained and the process was followed with TR method. Home-based TR method has been consequently reported to offer a family-centered approach to increase the effectiveness of the treatment (Ferre et al., 2017).

## 5.7 Orthopedic Rehabilitation

In a study evaluating the effectiveness of patient follow-up with TR in chronic low back pain, 3 women with chronic low back pain were followed up for 12 months in total. The daily pain levels of them and their adherence to the home exercise program was followed up by recording with mobile phone after conventional face-to-face treatment. TR sessions supported with voice and video were implemented at 1st, 3rd, 6th and 12th months. It was consequently stated that the application of TR in patients with chronic low back pain may be a useful application for both evaluation and continuity of treatment (Peterson, 2018).

In a randomized controlled study examining the effect of TR on physical activity after total knee arthroplasty, a total of 100 patients underwent unilateral arthroplasty and aged between 50–85 years were included in the study (Kline et al., 2018).

In a study on TR in shoulder pain, the validity and reliability of the musculoskeletal system evaluations were evaluated. All measurements for physical evaluation parameters were found to be statistically significant and consistent (Steele et al., 2012).

# 6 Conclusion

In recent years, the increasing use of TR in the field of health care has given pos-itive results in terms of access of individuals living in rural and remote areas to health services and a couple of healthcare professionals, patient motivation, trans-portation, cost-effectiveness and patient and care-giver. TR is a developing field. There is currently no standard procedure or protocol for TR applications; most of the studies have been implemented as pilot studies. As stated in many studies in the literature, the effectiveness of TR applications in different patient groups should be investigated with randomized controlled studies. Thus, the evidences of the potential benefits of TR for both patients and healthcare systems will be pro-vided. In conclusion, the best technologies should be combined with the most ef-fective rehabilitation therapies for the success of TR and effective service delivery.

## References

Bernocchi, P., Vitacca, M., La Rovere, M.T., Volterrani, M., Galli, T., Baratti, D. & et al. (2017). Home-Based Telerehabilitation in Older Patients with Chronic Obstructive Pulmonary Disease and Heart Failure: A Randomised Controlled Trial, *Age and Ageing*, 47(1), 82–88.

Burger, H. (2016). Telerehabilitation, *Fizikalna Rehabilitacijska Medicina*, 28(1–2), 41–46.

Butler, A.J., Bay, C., Wu, D., Richards, K.M. & Buchanan, S. (2014). Expanding Tele-rehabilitation of Stroke through In-home Robot, *International Journal of Physical Medicine and Rehabilitation*, 2, 1–11.

Calabrò, R.S., Bramanti, A., Garzon, M., Celesti, A., Russo, M., Portaro, S. & et al. (2018). Telerehabilitation in Individuals with Severe Acquired Brain Injury: Rationale, Study Design, and Methodology, *Medicine*, 97(50), 1–6.

Cartmill, B., Wall, L.R., Ward, E.C., Hill, A.J. & Porceddu, S.V. (2016). Computer Literacy and Health Locus of Control as Determinants for Readiness and Acceptability of Telepractice in a Head and Neck Cancer Population, *International Journal of Telerehabilitation*, 8(2), 49.

Cason, J. (2009). A Pilot Telerehabilitation Program: Delivering Early Intervention Services to Rural Families, *International Journal of Telerehabilitation*, 1(1), 29.

Çatal, Ç., Serbetçloglu, E. & Alper, H. (2014). KOAH Hastalarinda Tele Pulmoner Rehabilitasyon İçin Kinect Temelli Ev Egzersiz Yazılımı, *UYMS*, 96–101.

Chen, J., Jin, W., Zhang, X.X., Xu, W., Liu, X.N. & Ren, C.C. (2015). Telerehabilitation Approaches for Stroke Patients: Systematic Review and

Meta-analysis of Randomized Controlled Trials, *Journal of Stroke and Cerebrovascular Diseases*, 24(12), 2660–2668.

Choi, Y.H., Park, H.K. & Paik, N.J. (2016). A Telerehabilitation Approach for Chronic Aphasia Following Stroke, *Telemedicine and e-Health*, 22(5), 434–440.

Corti, C., Poggi, G., Romaniello, R., Strazzer, S., Urgesi, C., Borgatti, R. & Bardoni, A. (2018). Feasibility of a Home-Based Computerized Cognitive Training for Pediatric Patients with Congenital or Acquired Brain Damage: An Explorative Study, *PloS One*, 13(6), e0199001.

De Luca, R., Bramanti, A., De Cola, M.C., Leonardi, S., Torrisi, M., Aragona, B. & et al. (2016). Cognitive Training for Patients with Dementia Living in a Sicilian Nursing Home: A Novel Web-Based Approach, *Neurological Sciences*, 37(10), 1685–1691.

Dias, A.E., Limongi, J.C.P., Barbosa, E.R. & Hsing, W.T. (2016). Voice Telerehabilitation in Parkinson's Disease, *In Codas*, 28(2), 176–181.

Dorstyn, D., Mathias, J. & Denson, L. (2013). Applications of Telecounselling in Spinal Cord Injury Rehabilitation: A Systematic Review with Effect Sizes, *Clinical Rehabilitation*, 27(12), 1072–1083.

Ferre, C.L., Brandão, M., Surana, B., Dew, A.P., Moreau, N.G. & Gordon, A.M. (2017). Caregiver-Directed Home-Based İntensive Bimanual Training in Young Children with Unilateral Spastic Cerebral Palsy: A Randomized Trial, *Developmental Medicine & Child Neurology*, 59(5), 497–504.

Fjeldstad-Pardo, C., Thiessen, A. & Pardo, G. (2018). Telerehabilitation in Multiple Sclerosis: Results of a Randomized Feasibility and Efficacy Pilot Study, *International Journal of Telerehabilitation*, 10(2), 55–60.

Galiano-Castillo, N., Arroyo-Morales, M., Lozano-Lozano, M., Fernández-Lao, C., Martín-Martín, L., Del-Moral-Ávila, R. & Cantarero-Villanueva, I. (2017). Effect of an Internet-Based Telehealth System on Functional Capacity and Cognition in Breast Cancer Survivors: A Secondary Analysis of a Randomized Controlled Trial, *Supportive Care in Cancer*, 25(11), 3551–3559.

Gandolfi, M., Geroin, C., Dimitrova, E., Boldrini, P., Waldner, A., Bonadiman, S. & et al. (2017). Virtual Reality Telerehabilitation for Postural Instability in Parkinson's Disease: A Multicenter, Single-Blind, Randomized, Controlled Trial, *BioMed Research International*, 2017, 1–11.

Gehring, K., Kloek, C.J., Aaronson, N.K., Janssen, K.W., Jones, L.W., Sitskoorn, M.M. & Stuiver, M. M. (2018). Feasibility of a Home-Based Exercise Intervention with Remote Guidance for Patients with Stable Grade Iı and Iıı Gliomas: A Pilot Randomized Controlled Trial, *Clinical Rehabilitation*, 32(3), 352–366.

Gutiérrez, R.O., Galán del Río, F., Cano de la Cuerda, R., Diego, A., Isabel, M., González, R.A. & Page, J.C.M. (2013). A Telerehabilitation Program by Virtual Reality-Video Games Improves Balance and Postural Control in Multiple Sclerosis Patients, *NeuroRehabilitation*, 33(4), 545–554.

Hüzmeli, E.D., Duman, T. & Yıldırım, H. (2017). Türkiye'de İnmeli Hastalarda Telerehabilitasyonun Etkinliği: Pilot Çalışma, *Turkish Journal of Neurology*, 23, 21–25.

Hwang, R., Bruning, J., Morris, N., Mandrusiak, A. & Russell, T. (2015). A Systematic Review of the Effects of Telerehabilitation in Patients with Cardiopulmonary Diseases, *Journal of Cardiopulmonary Rehabilitation and Prevention*, 35(6), 380–389.

Jelcic, N., Agostini, M., Meneghello, F., Bussè, C., Parise, S., Galano, A. & et al. (2014). Feasibility and Efficacy of Cognitive Telerehabilitation in Early Alzheimer's Disease: A Pilot Study, *Clinical Interventions in Aging*, 9, 1605.

Khan, F., Amatya, B., Kesselring, J. & Galea, M. (2015). Telerehabilitation for Persons with Multiple Sclerosis, *The Cochrane Library*, 9(4), CD010508.

Kim, J.S., Yun, D., Kim, H.J., Ryu, H.Y., Oh, J. & Kang, S.M. (2018). Need Assessment for Smartphone-Based Cardiac Telerehabilitation, *Healthcare Informatics Research*, 24(4), 283–291.

Kline, P.W., Melanson, E.L., Sullivan, W.J., Blatchford, P.J., Miller, M.J., Stevens-Lapsley, J.E. & Christiansen, C.L. (2018). Improving Physical Activity Through Adjunct Telerehabilitation Following Total Knee Arthroplasty: Randomized Controlled Trial Protocol, *Physical Therapy*, 99(1), 37–45.

Kuipers, P., Foster, M., Smith, S. & Fleming, J. (2009). Using ICF-Environment Factors to Enhance the Continuum of Outpatient ABI Rehabilitation: An Exploratory Study, *Disability and Rehabilitation*, 31(2), 144–151.

Kumar, S. & Cohn, E.R. (Eds.). (2012). Telerehabilitation, Springer Science & Business Media, Londan, UK.

Nordio, S., Innocenti, T., Agostini, M., Meneghello, F. & Battel, I. (2018). The Efficacy of Telerehabilitation in Dysphagic Patients: A Systematic Review, *Acta Otorhinolaryngologica Italica*, 38(2), 79.

Ownsworth, T., Arnautovska, U., Beadle, E., Shum, D.H. & Moyle, W. (2018). Efficacy of Telerehabilitation for Adults with Traumatic Brain Injury: A Systematic Review, *The Journal of Head Trauma Rehabilitation*, 33(4), 33–46.

Peretti, A., Amenta, F., Tayebati, S.K., Nittari, G. & Mahdi, S.S. (2017). Telerehabilitation: Review of the State-of-the-Art and Areas of Application, *JMIR Rehabilitation and Assistive Technologies*, 4(2), 1–7.

Peterson, S. (2018). Telerehabilitation Booster Sessions and Remote Patient Monitoring in the Management of Chronic Low Back Pain: A Case Series, *Physiotherapy Theory and Practice*, 34(5), 393–402.

Piovesana, A., Ross, S., Lloyd, O., Whittingham, K., Ziviani, J., Ware, R.S. & Boyd, R.N. (2017). Randomized Controlled Trial of a Web-Based Multi-Modal Therapy Program for Executive Functioning in Children and Adolescents with Unilateral Cerebral Palsy, *Disability and Rehabilitation*, 39(20), 2021–2028.

Piron, L., Turolla, A., Tonin, P., Piccione, F., Lain, L. & Dam, M. (2008). Satisfaction with Care in Post-Stroke Patients Undergoing a Telerehabilitation Programme at Home, *Journal of Telemedicine and Telecare*, 14(5), 257–260.

Rintala, A., Päivärinne, V., Hakala, S., Paltamaa, J., Heinonen, A., Karvanen, J. & Sjögren, T. (2018). Effectiveness of Technology-Based Distance Physical Rehabilitation Interventions for Improving Physical Functioning in Stroke: A Systematic Review and Meta-Analysis of Randomized Controlled Trials, *Archives of Physical Medicine and Rehabilitation*, 40(4), 373–387.

Rogante, M., Kairy, D., Giacomozzi, C. & Grigioni, M. (2015). A Quality Assessment of Systematic Reviews on Telerehabilitation: What Does the Evidence Tell Us?, *Annali dell'Instituto Superiore di Sanità*, 51(1), 11–18.

Sarfo, F.S., Ulasavets, U., Opare-Sem, O.K. & Ovbiagele, B. (2018). Tele-Rehabilitation after Stroke: An Updated Systematic Review of the Literature, *Journal of Stroke and Cerebrovascular Diseases*, 27(9), 2306–2318.

Shenoy, M.P. & Shenoy, P.D. (2018). Identifying the Challenges and Cost-Effectiveness of Telerehabilitation: A Narrative Review, *Journal of Clinical & Diagnostic Research*, 12(12), 1–4.

Steele, L., Lade, H., McKenzie, S. & Russell, T.G. (2012). Assessment and Diagnosis of Musculoskeletal Shoulder Disorders over the Internet, *International Journal of Telemedicine and Applications*, 20, 1–8.

Tchero, H., Teguo, M.T., Lannuzel, A. & Rusch, E. (2018). Telerehabilitation for Stroke Survivors: Systematic Review and Meta-analysis, *Journal of Medical Internet Research*, 20(10), e10867.

Valdés, B.A., Glegg, S.M., Lambert-Shirzad, N., Schneider, A.N., Marr, J., Bernard, R. & et al. (2018). Application of Commercial Games for Home-Based Rehabilitation for People with Hemiparesis: Challenges and Lessons Learned, *Games for Health Journal*, 7(3), 197–207.

Van Straaten, M.G., Cloud, B.A., Morrow, M.M., Ludewig, P.M. & Zhao, K.D. (2014). Effectiveness of Home Exercise on Pain, Function, and Strength of Manual Wheelchair Users with Spinal Cord Injury: A High-Dose Shoulder Program with Telerehabilitation, *Archives of Physical Medicine and Rehabilitation*, 95(10), 1810–1817.

Wakeford, L., Wittman, P.P., White, M.W. & Schmeler, M.R. (2005). Telerehabilitation Position Paper, *The American Journal of Occupational*

*Therapy: Official Publication of the American Occupational Therapy Association*, 59(6), 656–660.

Wall, L.R., Ward, E.C., Cartmill, B., Hill, A.J. & Porceddu, S.V. (2017). Adherence to a Prophylactic Swallowing Therapy Program during (Chemo) Radiotherapy: Impact of Service-Delivery Model and Patient Factors, *Dysphagia*, 32(2), 279–292.

Ward, E.C., Burns, C.L., Theodoros, D.G. & Russell, T.G. (2014). Impact of Dysphagia Severity on Clinical Decision Making via Telerehabilitation, *Telemedicine and e-Health*, 20(4), 296–303.

Weinstein, R.S., Lopez, A.M., Krupinski, E.A., Beinar, S.J., Hocomb, M., McNeely, R.A. & et al. (2008). Integrating Telemedicine and Telehealth: Putting in All Together, (ed. Latifi, R.), *Current Principles and Practices of Telemedicine and E-Health*, IOS Press, Amsterdam.

Hamiyet Yüce

# 18: Basic Body Awareness Therapy (B-BAT)

## 1 Introduction

In today's medicine, it is very important to accept human beings as an integrated part of the physical, psychological and social environments and also as a whole. In this bio-psychosocial approach, physiotherapists focus not only on biological and physical aspects of the patients, but also on their psychosocial aspects. Body awareness therapy is related to wide range of professional fields such as physiotherapy, psychiatry, medical and psychotherapy. Body awareness knowledge is a general concept for the use and experience of the body, which represents body consciousness, body management and in-depth body experience (Roxendal, 1985). Basic body awareness therapy is a common name for a series of body-oriented physiotherapeutic approaches that use a holistic perspective in physiotherapy applications towards awareness about body function behavior, its interaction with himself and others, how the body is used (Gyllensten, 2001).

Body-oriented therapies address the boundaries between conscious and unconscious existence where the focus is based on bodily experience and non-verbal behavior (Roxendal, 1985). Compared with other body-oriented or mindfulness therapies, there is a systematic training of ego at the physical level that originates from certain body functions, intention and self-observation at the mental level (Hedlund and Gyllensten, 2010). In physiotherapy content, body awareness is defined in two ways: (1) body experience (dimension of experience) and (2) actions and behavior in movement and activities (dimension of movement). In the dimension of experience, body awareness therapy emphasizes subjective body experiences. In the dimension of movement, body awareness therapy aims to normalize the posture, balance, breathing, muscle tension or stiffness that can be observed and experienced in a movement pattern (Gyllensten et al., 2010).

The aim of body awareness therapy is to increase sensory-motor awareness, dysfunctional movement patterns, perception of habits and movement control by increasing grounding, stability at the centerline, centering, breathing and flow (Gyllensten et al., 1999). In this way, individuals awareness of themselves, their environment, other people and the world as a whole increase by strengthening their bodies (Gyllensten et al., 2010). This health effect provides opportunities to individuals to increase their creativity and make their own choices in life.

## 2 Development of Basic Body Awareness Therapy

Basic Body Awareness Therapy (B-BAT) is the common name of several physiotherapeutic approaches for the body which use a holistic perspective in physiotherapy. The B-BAT was inspired from western movement traditions such as Feldenkrais, Alexander technique and European movement traditions (Grindler and Silver). Body-oriented psychotherapy (Reich and Lowen) also affected the B-BAT. From the east, Zen meditation and Tai-Chi Chuan (Tai Chi) are important sources of influence. The B-BAT was developed from Tai Chi's starting exercises and therefore it tends to follow the same principles. French psychotherapist and actor Jacques Dropsy synthesized the traditions mentioned above and published two books explaining the method. Dropsy called the movement system as "Psychotoni" or "Basic Movements".

Swedish physiotherapist Gertrud Roxendal met with Jacques Dropsy, a French psychoanalyst and movement instructor in the early 1970s. She deemed Dropsy's movement practice significant and integrated it into the physiotherapy practice and curriculum under the name of basic body awareness therapy (Basal Kroppskännedom). She also developed Body Awareness Scale (BAS), which was target Basic Body Awareness Therapy and measured grounding, posture, coordination, breathing and flow. She used the B-BAT method and the BAS in the treatment of schizophrenia patients and published her results with a thesis at the University of Gothenburg Medical Faculty (Roxendal, 1985).

Then, the method was used in long-lasting pain rehabilitation, mostly in psychiatric physiotherapy. Roxendal developed the concept of body ego in the 1990s. The concept of body ego was first used by Freud in 1923; Roxendal described it as a bodily appearance of the inseparable unit of mind/body and being human (Gyllensten, 2001). Grounding, vertical balance in the center line, centering in movements, coordination from torso and solar plexus area, breathing, flow and awareness are seen as important aspects of body ego trained in the BAT (Gyllensten, 2001; Hedlund and Gyllensten, 2010).

## 3 Theories of Basic Body Awareness Therapy (According to J. Dropsy)

Basic Body Awareness Therapy is based on Jacques Dropsy's theories. These theories are as follows:

### 3.1 Theories about Movements

*Dynamic postural balance* is essential for movement quality. It is stimulated by placing the weight slightly forward in front of feet. The ability to trust the ground in carrying the body weight is also trained in this content. When dynamic postural balance is found, the body is experienced as weightless. One of his main theories is the organization of the muscular system in three layers, from its deepest layer to superficial muscle layer. The deepest layer, which is close to the bones, consists of antigravity muscles that have the function of protecting the body in a stable but in an elastic upright position against gravity. The next layer consists of the muscles associated with breathing function. The superficial layer of voluntary muscles is associated with the ability to direct voluntary movements. When the body is well balanced, the three layers work very well with respect to the natural basic functions. When the body is not balanced, the superficial muscle layer, which is only intended to direct movements, is used to hold the body upright against gravity. According to Dropsy, voluntary muscles cannot do this. Muscle cramps or pain and other musculoskeletal problems burst later. Respiration will not become well functional and be experienced as blocked or restricted. The movements are often uncoordinated; much more of effort is made even when making a small movement.

The quality of coordination in movements also follows three main ways of coordination in torso. They all consist of the area around the thoracic vertebra 12 region at the back and the center of movement in the solar plexus region at the front. Three basic coordination: a) Coordination of flexion/extension around the center of movement in the solar plexus region; this coordination, breathing coordination and emotional, instructive life are highly interrelated. The coordination in the center is shown in the peripheral movement of the extremities. b) Rotation around the vertical axis; This is the coordination of rotation with a spiral and twisting movement of the body around the vertical axis from the feet to the head. We can observe how the whole body rotates in the same direction as a whole. In rotation around the central axis, hip and shoulders move to the right or left side simultaneously. c) Torso rotation and counter-rotation coordination (walking coordination); Upper and lower part of body rotate in the opposite direction. In the search for coordination lines, the relationship between rotation and counter-rotation around the central region can be observed. These three coordination of the torso are considered to be the source of all possible actions which start in the torso center in other words diaphragm region. These coordination ways in the torso are the drivers of all other coordination in the body, including the arms and legs. The coordinations are closely related to respiratory and psychological functions (Gyllensten, 2001; Skjaerven et al., 2003).

## 3.2 Theories about Breathing

Theories about breathing play a fundamental role in the movement model. Breathing has a pair of innervations that are both voluntary and automatic stimulation. According to Dropsy, this means that breathing is a part of conscious and unconscious life, and acts as a bridge between these two aspects of life. Breathing can be somehow controlled by our conscious. We can breathe fast or slow if we want to. Unconscious factors also affect breathing. These factors may suppress the feelings or individuals may expend energy to adapt the situations such as stress and anxiety. This situation may cause tension in respiratory muscles. When breathing is inhibited, diaphragm retaining and short breath can cause symptoms such as disorders ftom stomach-to-heart and decreased vitality (Gyllensten, 2001).

## 3.3 The Theory of Three-Fold Contact Problem

Dropsy states that psychological problems are seen in three dimensions: the relationship with the body and self, relationship with other people and relationship with reality perception. In this theory, Dropsy suggested that the problems in getting in contact with one's own body indicate a problem in getting in contact with others and the perception of reality or vice versa. According to this theory, the lack of awareness is expressed in the body and can be seen as non-functionality in other the movements with lack of dynamism, flow, rhythm and integrity. The clinical studies on three-fold contact problem showed that it is beneficial (Gyllensten, 2001; Gard, 2005; Skjaerven et al., 2010).

## 4 Body Functions

### 4.1 Daily Movements and Function

Functional skills in daily movements depends on stability in function, coordination, breathing, self-awareness and awareness of others and making contacts. This situation is consistent with the theories of Dropsy about balance, freedom and awareness. According to the World Confederation for Physiotherapists (WCPT), movement and functional skills are the main fields of physiotherapists and are of great importance for individuals' health-related life quality and physical, psychological, emotional and social well-being.

## 4.2 Balance and Posture

In order to maintain a balanced sitting and standing posture, a harmony between the upward and downward forces is required. The base of the balanced posture is the feet. In order to achieve dynamic balance, the weight of body should be placed in the middle of the feet and in front of the ankles. In this way, a dynamic and balanced posture is formed upwards along the balance line. This dynamic posture requires freedom in the knees and hips and thus balanced curvatures form in the spine with lumbar lordosis, thoracic kyphosis and cervical lordosis. A good posture should not contain any effort, be comfortable and provide the basis for functional movements. Balance and posture are closely linked to each other and cannot occur separately (Gyllensten et al., 2018).

**Standing Function:** A good contact between the soles of the feet and the floor gives a feeling of increase in safety, stability, balance and it makes the movements free. In the B-BAT, this is called as grounding. It is accepted as an aspect of optimal postural stability and is very important for daily functions. Grounding exercises are paid attention to movements and actively emphasized. Another training in B-BAT is the applications of staying within the stability limits. Stability limits are the areas in which the body can maintain stability without changing the support surface. This means that the soles of the feet remain in contact with the floor as the whole body moves backward and forward.

**Sitting Function:** Finding the internal stability in sitting is based on sitting in which gravity and correction functions balance each other. When relaxed balance is found, the superficial muscles gradually relax and the deep postural muscles such as multifidus and rotators, transversus abdominus and pelvic floor muscles are activated. In an unstable sitting posture, the person is assisted by being instructed to place his or her feet firmly on the floor and to consciously hold the sitting bones against the chair in the BAT.

**Lying Function:** There is minimal postural activity in lying; it is the easiest position to find relaxation. Lying on the ground and resting naturally provides a good recovery for a while. In B-BAT movements, the relationship with the ground is applied. For example, the relationship with the ground is consciously considered. An example of this is the ability to be carried by the floor and to leave it up to the gravity.

**Walking Function:** The way of walking reflects both universal rules and individual characteristics. A person is easily recognized from a distance with his/her walking style. Walking is affected by both internal and external factors; the functional walking pattern is easily impaired. The aim of the BAT is to find a functional stable gait with walking along the longitudinal axis that is called as the balance line. Making contact with postural stability requires effective walking. This balance line is not static and stiff, but it is dynamic; it gives a constant feeling and is also a flexible reference point. When the balance line is provided appropriately, walking becomes easy. In BBAT, walking trainings individuals' attention is directed to walking perception and different walking patterns. The exercises are done in relation with time (slow/fast, slower/faster), space-related (circle/straight/free), direction-related (forward, backward) and in coordination with others within the group (Roxendal, 1985; Gyllensten et al., 2018).

### 4.3 Breathing

Breathing is partly conscious and partly unconscious and people usually don't notice how they breathe. Breathing adapts to body movements and changes the degree of activity. It is prevented or stimulated by different feelings and emotions. Mental trauma or diseases often cause persistent disorders related to breathing (Roxendal, 1985). When a peaceful state of mind is reached, breathing becomes easier and there is no tension in the body. Free breathing provides freedom, efficiency and harmony in movements, and also comes into contact with internal needs and desires. When only the voluntary skeletal muscles in the torso, arms and legs are balanced and relaxed, the breathing wave may spread towards the periphery. The interaction between inhaling and exhaling is like a continuous tide consisting of a series of rhythmic contraction and relaxation. Breathing exercises are often initiated by directing the individual's attention to how breathing works alone. Then breathing is consciously integrated with movements and the training continues. The aim is to change one's habits of holding breath and tense up while doing movement or activity. In the BAT, breath relieving is also made by using of some sounds. Training with sounds functions by decreasing the muscular tension around the thorax and diaphragm by increasing the energy experience. Doing the exercises with breath and voice easily evoke emotional reactions. Therefore, it should be performed with great care and professionalism (Roxendal, 1985; Gyllensten, 2001; Gyllensten et al., 2018).

### 4.4 Rhythm

Human life and movements are subject to constant rhythmic changes like those of other living things. Physiologically dominant rhythms include heartbeat, breathing and menstrual cycles, and have an evident connection with psychic life. Each individual is considered to have his or her own basic rhythm that changes in different life situations. This personal basic rhythm fits other external rhythms. The sense of rhythm is trained in different ways. Breathing determines the rhythm which fits movements. Rhythm is another aspect of centering. Well-coordinated and harmonious movement can be seen as a result of rhythmic change between tension and relaxation (Roxendal, 1985; Gyllensten et al., 2018).

## 4.5 Coordination/Center of Movement

The freedom in motor function depends on the ability of the body to effectively control of movements as well as the integration of breathing, balanced posture. This is achieved by contact with the center of movement. The center of movement is of great importance both for good functional coordination and for using of force and freedom in movements. When the movements are centered, they become fluent, circular or spiral, i.e., three-dimensional. The experience that is obtained from mevements is feeling the movement easily and free. The coordination depends on the balance between the center and the periphery. Muscle tensions in the waist, diaphragm or abdominal muscles can cause stress and stiffness in the area around the center of movement. The movement pattern may then become fragmented, rough and less coordinated. When the movements are centered and integrated, it is experienced and expressed as a smooth wave motion in which the least force is required and the whole body is in a connection. The stability in the longitudinal axis or balance line is also important for coordinating and centralizing the movement (Gyllensten et al., 2018).

## 4.6 Intention and Integrity

Both intention and integrity are important for the quality of movement. When performing B-BAT movements, intentions and images are often used to create meaning from a function or situation imagined. This involves imagining of "pushing something away" that results in stretching the legs or "sea waves" that cause rising of arms when the legs are fixed to the ground by an individual. Therefore, attention is focused on the task of movement, not on local muscle work. In the B-BAT, intention and purpose are defined by different images and aphorisms. Intention and purpose in movement define the quality of the movement and give clarity to the movement. Internal movements experienced as sensations and emotions are important in the B-BAT. The expression of "one eye in and one eye out" used in the B-BAT means to be in contact with both oneself and external contextual goals/world in movements and actions (Gyllensten et al., 2018).

## 4.7 Body Awareness and Relationship with Oneself

It has been shown that there is an interaction between increasing body awareness and improving ability to contact with oneself, others and environment.

Therefore, it is important that an individual should train own body awareness regularly. Body awareness is constanly updated sensory information about our ability to use our body and the information constantly provided by the motor system. Increasing body awareness means self-experimentation and self-contact by – internal perspective – which means strengthening the identity of the individual. The training on the ability of body awareness is started by focusing on the body parts that are in contact with the ground while lying on the floor. Patients are encouraged to experience everything as they are, without trying to change or evaluating them in practice (Gyllensten et al., 2018).

## 4.8 The Movement Quality Model_(MQM)

The phenomenon of movement quality is frequently used in the BAT, in which patients' attention is directed to how the movements are performed under the supervision of a physiotherapist. Movement quality can be defined as the way in which movements are associated with space, time and energy. The different aspects of movements and the quality of movement in connection with the B-BAT were expressed by Skjaerven et al. They focused on the movement quality related to different factors that are four existence dimensions: the physical, physiological, psychological/relational and existential perspectives of movement (Skjaerven et al., 2003; Skjaerven et al., 2008; Skjaerven and Gard, 2018) (Fig. 18.1).

**Physical Perspective:** It addresses the physical or anatomical body and shows the skeleton, muscles, tendons, ligaments, arteries, nerves, etc. It is associated with a biomechanical perspective and shows a spatial view of human movement. It includes two aspects: 1) Postural stability and 2) Movements characteristics of the path and shape in movement. Postural stability and balance are important prerequisites for the quality of movement at this level. Three basic coordination are parts of this perspective.

**Physiological Perspective:** It is associated with a physiological perspective that shows the appearance of time in human movements. It includes two aspects: 1) Free breathing and centering; and 2) Flow, elasticity and rhythm characteristics of movement. These qualities depend on muscle tension, balance and free breathing. Free breathing gives fluency to movement; it is like incoming and outgoing waves and is expressed as flow in movement. When flow, elasticity and rhythm are integrated, there will be an aliveness in movements.

**Psycho-Social and Cultural Perspective:** It is related to the psycho-social and cultural perspective and shows the use of energy. It includes two main aspects: 1) Awareness and 2) Emotional, cognitive, intentional and socio-cultural

| Movement Quality as Biomechanical | Movement Quality as Physiological |
|---|---|
| -Related to space | -Related to time |
| Element: Alignment ve postural stability | Element: Breathing and centering |
| Aspects: Form and path | Aspects: Flow, elasticity, rytyhm |

| Movement quality as a general and integrated phenomenon |
|---|

| Movement as Psycho-socio-cultural | Movement Quality as Existential |
|---|---|
| -Related to energy | -Related to the individual |
| Element: Awareness | Element: Self-awareness |
| Aspects: Intention, emotion, socio-cultural | Aspects: Personal characteristics, unity. |

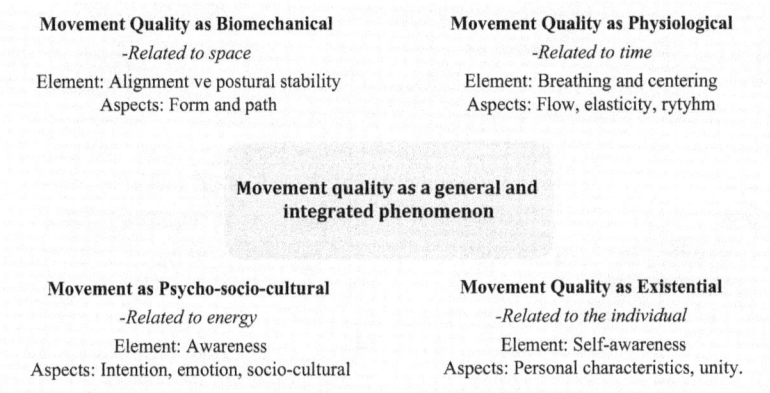

**Fig. 18.1:** Movement Quality Model (Skjaerven and Gard, 2018)

perspectives. This quality of movement or the expression of movement depends on attention and intention. Awareness is important in movement quality and is a prerequisite. If you are avaliable in your body, this situation will be expressed in movement quality. If you are not available in your body, you will incautiously move by using your automatic pilot.

**Existential Perspective:** It is associated with an existential perspective, and it also demonstrates personal and wholeness aspects. It includes two aspectss: 1) Self awareness and 2) Personal and integrity perspectives expressed in the move- ment. This existential dimension focuses on clearness of the movement and the experience of self-awareness with "I" uniquenes. It addresses a conscious person who has the experience of being "here and now" as in reflecting oneself. It is important to be in contact with the body and perceive the body as a whole thus a sense of integrity develops.

# 5 Basic Body Awareness Therapy in Clinical Practice

The B-BAT focuses on the basic movement functions associated with pos- ture, coordination, natural breathing and awareness, which are essential in movement quality, self-expression, interaction with others and in performing daily life movements (Gard, 2005). When doing movements, it is impor- tant for the person to direct his attention on both what he/she does and experiences in the movements, and this stimulates awareness and movement performance. B-BAT consists of stillness and simple exercises in movements.

B-BAT movements represent daily movements such as lying, sitting, standing, walking, relational movements and massage (touching). The therapy environment does not require any equipment other than floor, mat and stool. Physiotherapist requests from patients to wear clothing that allows to breathe freely and to move easily in it. Physiotherapist acts as a guide by bringing daily life and needs in the therapy environment. The B-BAT method can be applied both as individual therapy and group exercise. In general, patients perform simple movement together with their physiotherapist. Physiotherapist encourages the patients to perform postural control, balance, comfortable breathing and coordination more appropriately by using both his/her own body and words to guide the patients (Gard, 2005; Skjaerven and Mattson, 2018). This personal experience that is based on body is both verbalized by patients and approved as a reflection tool by physiotherapists (Hedlund and Gyllensten, 2010). Brief reflective speeches provide support to participants for learning and developing an insight about their own movement experiences (Roxendal, 1985).

In the application of body awareness therapy method, each therapy program consists of three parts:

• Relaxation: Body scan is passive relaxation or journey in the body. In lying exercises include breathing and sound working, opening-closing exercises, stretching and relaxation.
• Sitting and standing exercises include grounding, the relationship between the balance line and the body, flow and stability in daily movements.
• Massage: Massage applied on clothes involves bodily contact and affects the massage receivers and who apply massage. In terms of holistic approach, massage is not touching a body or tissue, but touching a person. Such a perspective helps to integrate, not distribute individuals who receive massage. In group practices, participants apply message to each other.

## 6  Observation and Evaluation in Body Awareness Therapy

Some reliable and valid assessment tools have been developed to assess body awareness and movement quality. Physiotherapeutic assessment focusing on the movement quality has been reported as a useful measure to understand the clinical needs of the individual and to develop an effective rehabilitation program (Bergström et al., 2014). Body Awareness Scale (BAS) and Body Awareness Rating Scale (BARS) are examples of body awareness assessment tools used in evidence-based studies.

## 6.1 Body Awareness Scale Movement Quality and Experience (BAS MQ-E)

The BAS MQ-E was inspired by the Body Awareness Scale (BAS), BAS-Health (Roxendal, 1985) and the international function classification (ICF). The BAS MQ-E consists of movement test, a short questionnaire and a short interview form. Movement test is structured and it includes daily movements. Movement test are assessed for balance, stability, coordination, breathing and ability of relationship with one's own body and others. The questionnaire includes 9 questions about pain, muscle tension symptoms, ability to do daily activities, exercise habits, body experiences such as appearance and relationship with breathing. Quality interviews focus on patients' experiences of stability, movement coordination, breathing, the ability of standing up and being present (Probst, 2018).

## 6.2 Body Awareness Rating Scale-Movement Quality and Experience (BARS-MQE)

It is originated from psychiatry and was most recently developed by Skjaerven and Sundal. The BARS-MQE consists of two parts: 1) Evaluating of patients' movement quality by physiotherapists and 2) A phenomenological interview on the patient's explanations during the movement experience (Probst, 2018).

# 7 Evidence-Based Studies Evaluating Body Awareness Therapy

The B-BAT has been found to be useful in various diseases such as long-lasting musculoskeletal pain, fibromyalgia, rheumatic diseases, schizophrenia, eating disorders, personality disorder and irritable bowel syndrome.

## 7.1 The BAT in Chronic Pain and Musculoskeletal Disorders

The principles of movement are increasingly applied in somatic health care, including the care of patients with rheumatology and hip arthrosis. Compared to traditional physiotherapy in patients with chronic musculoskeletal system disorders, the BAT with cognitive and relaxation therapy have a positive effect on quality of life (Grahn et al., 1998); The BAT and Feldenkrais method have been reported to be more effective (Malmgren-Olsson et al., 2001), particularly in terms of increased general health and improved movement harmony (Kendall et al., 2001; Mannerkorpi and Arndorw, 2004). In the studies on fibromyalgia, the patients expressed positive experiences in the process of learning. Health-related life quality and treatment efficacy have increased with the discovery of new movement strategies (Mannerkorpi and Gard, 2003; Gard, 2005).

Improvement in movement quality and decrease in vegetative disorder experience were observed with the BAT (Gustafsson et al., 2004). It has been reported that the BAT may be an effective intervention for pain, movement quality and anxiety in fibromyalgia patients followed up at 12 and 24 weeks (Bravo et al., 2018). In a randomized clinical trial, the BAT compared to exercise therapy provided more recovery on physical function in chronic Whiplash Syndrome (Seferiadis et al., 2016). In chronic rheumatic diseases, touching the body with the B-BAT can help patients to discover and develop their own resources for a more functional movement quality in daily life (Olsen and Skjaerven, 2016); it also strengthens physical functions and coping strategies (Sundén et al., 2013); the planning of patient education after the therapy may provide permanent benefits that will positively affect daily life functions (Strand et al., 2016; Olsen et al., 2017).

## 7.2 The BAT in Mental Health and Psychiatric Patients

The BAT was reported to be effective in patients with schizophrenia, somatoform, mood and personality disorder in short-term and long-term. A first randomized, prospective study on the BAT showed significant improvement in movement quality, body image, anxiety and interest in the patients with schizophrenia (Roxendal, 1985). Another randomized controlled trial conducted with the psychiatric patients, the B-BAT showed improvements in psychiatric symptoms, body and movement attitudes (Gyllensten et al., 2003a). With BAT, positive results were obtained in personal participation, awareness and use of body signs and movement control. As the patients' awareness of body signs develop and their bodies strengthened in movement, their self-confidence increased (Gyllensten et al., 2003b). It was concluded that BBAT the regulation of emotions, body awareness and self-esteem, clearer thinking and social abilities were affected, moreover BBAT was also an effective intervention in long-term psychiatric care in the patients with somatic symptoms (Gyllensten et al., 2009; Hedlund and Gyllensten, 2010). In a study conducted with the patients with moderate psychiatric disorders and pain, it was shown that patients experienced reintegration of their bodies and created new meanings for their bodies (Johnsen and Råheim, 2010).

Body Awareness Group Therapy (BAGT) as the main component in the treatment program of the patients with personality disorders was showed in two studies. It was concluded that the BAT promotes psychological growth and personal development via "harmonizing-accommodating" (Skatteboe et al., 1989). Other study was showed that the patients with personality disorders had more contact with both their emotions and their physical senses; they also focused more attention. The major change in function and symptoms was found as significantly high (Leirvåg et al., 2010). In the patients with irritable bowel syndrome, the BAT was shown to both reduced somatic complaints and psychological symptoms and normalized tension; it was also showed that improved body awareness had a positive effect on the ability to take care of their own resources (Eriksson et al., 2002; Eriksson et al., 2007).

The BAT was shown to have a positive effect on depression, anxiety and post-traumatic stress disorder (Danielsson and Rosberg, 2015; Madsen et al., 2016). It was showed that the patients with major depression were more aware of their bodies as a means of attachment to life and their inner senses and emotions were more regulated. Depression-related symptoms were decreased by improving motivation towards behavior change (Danielsson and Rosberg, 2015). Traumatized refugees have been positively affected by B-BAT; they largely experienced the movements to transfer in daily life (Madsen et al., 2016). In another study showed that Body Awareness Scale Movement Quality Evaluation (BAS MQ-E) is an applicable and benefical measurement tool of the movement function, somatic complaints and subjective body experiences in the patients with post-traumatic stress disorder (Nyboe et al., 2017).

The results in patients with eating disorders related to body and body image have special importance. The studies showed that the B-BAT is beneficial in providing a realistic body image with positive effects on distorted body image (Wallin et al., 2000; Thörnborg and Mattson, 2010; Catalon-Matamoros et al., 2011). It was emphasized that family therapy and the BAT have a positive effect on impaired body perception in young adolescents with eating disorders (Wallin et al., 2000); In the individuals with eating disorders, Basic Body Awareness can be a therapeutic tool in establishing a realistic body image (Thönborg and Mattson, 2010). Moreover it can improve eating attitude and thus it can help to reduce the severity of eating disorders (Catalan-Matamoros et al., 2011). The results showed that the BAT is useful in creating a more realistic body image.

# 8  The Training of Physiotherapist in Body Awareness Therapy

Becoming a certificated body awareness therapist requires a five-stage training program – the Swedish example – (www.ibk.nu). The program consists of theoretical, practical and clinical training by taking into account of the treatment experience and process of physiotherapist. Students do their homeworks by attending in a one week training session for 5 times. The first two levels focus on developing body awareness and understanding the process with an internal perspective. In working with patients with the theoretical framework and historical development of body awareness also focus on how goals and motivational aspects will be verbailzed. At the third level, students are trained on the body awareness scale. They write the report about on the role of the therapist in the BAT and the process of treating patients as individual and group with the BAT method in the fourth and fifth level training. Students also read about 2000 pages of literature related to the subject which is seriously evaluated from a clinical perspective. All reports are evaluated by a teacher who approves and gives feedback (Hedlund and Gyllensten, 2010). Training on the B-BAT method is given as a post-graduate certificate program at institutes or universities in different countries. After this training, students become certificated specialist therapists of the B-BAT method. While other professionals such as psychologists, social workers are accepted to the first level training, five levels of training are only for graduate physiotherapists. The training of a therapist consists of 25 weeks during 4–5 years. In the last 30 years, quality improvement, professional development and research have been started by the International Association of Teachers in Basic Body Awareness Therapy – IATBBAT (Skjaerven and Mattson, 2018). The teachers group comes together by organizing annual seminars to study on method development and quality issues. Nowadays, Sweden, Norway, Denmark, Finland, Estonia, Iceland, the Faroe Islands, England, Holland, Switzerland, Austria, Spain and Turkey constitute teachers network (http://www.iatbbat.com).

## 9 Conclusion

Basic Body Awareness Therapy (B-BAT) is a treatment method that is used in physiotherapy and rehabilitation to provide physical and emotional balance. In the B-BAT, western therapeutic methods and daily movements inspired from Tai Chi are used to improve balance, stability and movement quality. The method includes biomedical, physiological, psycho-socio-cultural and existential perspectives. The B-BAT is used in mental healthcare and psychiatric physiotherapy, pain rehabilitation, primary health care, preventive health services and the protection and promotion of health. There is a need for clinical evaluation, research and clinical review besides to the opinions patients and the society about B-BAT.

## References

Bergström, M., Ejelöv, M., Mattsson, M. & Stalnacke, B.M. (2014). One-Year Follow-Up of Body Awareness and Perceived Health after Participating in a Multimodal Pain Rehabilitation Programme – A Pilot Study, *European Journal of Physiotherapy*, 16(4), 246–254.

Bravo, C., Skjaerven, L.H., Espart, A., Sein-Echaluce, L.G. & Catalan-Matamoros, D. (2018). Basic Body Awareness Therapy in Patients Suffering from Fibromyalgia: A Randomized Clinical Trial, *Physotherapy Theory and Practice*, 3, 1–11.

Catalon-Matamoros, D., Skjaveren, L.H., Labajos-Manzanares, M.T., Arboleas, M.S. & Sánchez-Guerrero, E. (2011). A Pilot Study on the Effect of Basic Body Awareness Therapy in Patients with Eating Disorders: A Randomized Controlled Trial, *Clinical Rehabilitation*, 25, 617–626.

Danielsson, L. & Rosberg, S. (2015). Opening Toward Life: Experiences of Basic Body Awareness Therapy in Persons with Major Depression, *International Journal of Qualitative Studies in Health and Well-being*, 7, 10.

Eriksson, E., Nordwall, V., Kurlberg, G., Rydholm, H. & Eriksson, A. (2002). Effects of Body Awareness Therapy in Patients with Irritable Bowel Syndrome. *Advances in Physiotherapy*, 4, 125–135.

Eriksson, E.M., Moller, I.E., Soderberg, R.H., Eriksson, H.T. & Kurlberg, G.K. (2007). Body Awareness Therapy: A New Strategy for Relief of Symptoms in Irritable Bowel Syndrome Patients. *World Journal of Gastroenterology*, 13, 3206–3214.

Gard, G. (2005). Body Awareness Therapy for Patients with Fibromyalgia and Chronic Pain. *Disability and Rehabilitation*, 27, 725–728.

Grahn, B., Ekdahl, C. & Borgqvist, L. (1998). Effects of a Multidisciplinary Rehabilitation Programme on Health-Related Quality of Life in Patients with Prolonged Musculoskeletal Disorders; A 6-Month Follow-Up of a Prospective Controlled Study, *Disability and Rehabilitation*, 20, 285–297.

Gustafsson, M., Ekholm, J. & Ohman, A. (2004). From Shame to Respect: Musculoskeletal Pain Patients' Experience of a Rehabilitation Programme, A Quality Study, *Journal of Rehabilitation Medicine*, 36(3), 97–103.

Gyllensten, A.L. (2001). *Basic Body Awareness Therapy*. Thesis. Lund University, Department of Physiotherapy, Sweden.

Gyllensten, A.L., Ekdahl, C. & Hansson, L. (1999). Validity of The Body Awareness Scale-Health (BAS-H), *Scandinavian Journal of Caring Sciences*, 13(4), 217–226.

Gyllensten, A.L., Ekdahl, C. & Hansson, L. (2009). Long-Term Effectiveness of Basic Body Awareness Therapy in Psychiatric Outpatient Care. A Randomized Controlled Study, *Advances in Physiotherapy*, 11(1), 2–12.

Gyllensten, A.L., Hansson, L. & Ekdahl, C. (2003a). Outcome of Basic Body Awareness Therapy. A Randomized Controlled Study of Patients in Psychiatric Outpatient Care, *Advances in Physiotherapy*, 5, 179–190.

Gyllensten, A.L., Hansson, L. & Ekdahl, C. (2003b). Patient Experiences of Basic Body Awareness Therapy and the Relationship with the Physiotherapist, *Journal of Bodywork and Movement Therapies*, 7(3), 173–183.

Gyllensten, A.L., Skär, L., Miller, M. & Gard, G. (2010). Embodied Identity – A Deeper Understanding of Body Awareness, *Physiotherapy Theory and Practice*, 26(7), 439–446.

Gyllensten, A.L., Skoglund, K. & Wulf, I. (2018). *Basic Body Awareness Therapy. Embodied Identity*. Vulkan, Stockholm.

Hedlund, L. & Gyllensten, A.L. (2010). The Experiences of Basic Body Awareness Therapy in Patients with Schizophrenia, *Journal of Bodywork and Movement Therapies*, 14(3), 245–254.

http://www.iatbhat.com, (accessed on 23.05.2019).

http://www.ibk.nu/, (accessed on 23.05.2019).

Johnsen, R.W. & Råheim, M. (2010). Feeling More in Balance and Grounded in One's Own Body and Life. Focus Group Interviews on Experiences with Basic Body Awareness Therapy in Psychiatric Healthcare, *Advances in Physiotherapy*, 12(3), 166–174.

Kendall, S.A., Brolin-Magnusson, K., Sören, B., Gerdle, B. & Henriksson, K.G. (2001). A Pilot Study of Body Awareness Programs in the Treatment of Fibromyalgia Syndrome, *Arthritis Care & Research*, 15, 304–311.

Leirvåg, H., Pederson, G. & Karterud, S. (2010). Long-Term Continuation Treatment after Short-Term Day Treatment of Female Patients with Severe Personality Disorders: Body Awareness Group Therapy Versus Psychodynamic Group Therapy, *Nordic Journal of Psychiatry*, 64(3), 153–157.

Madsen, T.S., Carlsson, J., Nordbrandt, M. & Jensen, J.A. (2016). Refugee Experiences of Individual Basic Body Awareness Therapy and Level of Transference into Life. An Interview Study, *Journal of Bodywork and Movement Therapy*, 20(2), 243–251.

Malmgren-Olsson, E.B., Armelius, B.A. & Armelius, K. (2001). A Comparative Outcome Study of Body Awareness Therapy, Feldenkrais, and Conventional Physiotherapy for Patients with Nonspecific Musculoskeletal Disorders: Changes in Psychological Symptoms, Pain, and Self-Image, *Physiotherapy Theory and Practice*, 17, 77–95.

Mannerkorpi, K. & Arndorw, M. (2004). Efficiancy and Feasibility of Combination of Body Awareness Therapy and Qigong in Patients with Fibromyalgia: A Pilot Study, *Journal of Rehabilitation Medicine*, 36(6), 279–281.

Mannerkorpi, K. & Gard, G. (2003). Physiotherapy Group Treatment for Patients with Fibromyalgia – An Embodied Learning Process, *Disability and Rehabilitation*, 25, 1372–1380.

Nyboe, L., Bentholm, A. & Gyllensten, A.L. (2017). Bodily Symptoms in Patients with Post Traumatic Stress Disorder: A Comparative Study of Traumatized Refugees, Danish War Veterans, and Healthy Controls, *Journal of Bodywork & Movement Therapies*, 21, 523–527.

Olsen, A.L. & Skjaerven, L.H. (2016). Patients Suffering from Rheumatic Disease Describing Own Experiences From Participating in Basic Body Awareness Group Therapy: A Qualitative Pilot Study, *Physiotherapy Theory and Practice*, 32(2), 98–106.

Olsen, A.L., Strand, L.I., Skjaerven, L.H., Sundal, M.A. & Magnussen, L.H. (2017). Patient Education and Basic Body Awareness Therapy in Hip Osteoarthritis – A Qualitative Study of Patients' Movement Learning Experiences, *Disability and Rehabilitation*, 39(16), 1631–1638.

Probst, M. (2018). Observation and Evaluation Tools within Physiotherapy in Mental Health, (Eds. Probst, M., Skjaerven, L.H.), *Physiotherapy in Mental Health and Psychiatry. A Scientific and Clinical Based Approaches*, (98–119), Elsevier. Poland.

Roxendal, G. (1985). *Body Awareness Therapy and the Body Awareness Scale, Treatment and Evaluation in Psychiatric Physiotherapy* (Doctoral degree), University of Göteborg. Department of Psychiatry, Göteborg.

Seferiadis, A., Ohlin, P., Billhult, A. & Gunnarsson, R. (2016). Basic Body Awareness Therapy or Exercise Therapy for the Treatment of Chronic Whiplash Associated Disorders: A Randomized Comparative Clinical Trial, *Journal Disability and Rehabilitation*, 30, 442–451.

Skatteboe, U.B., Friis, S., Kvamsdal, H.M. & Vaglum, P. (1989). Body Awareness Group Therapy for Patients with Personality Disorders, *Psychoterapy Psychosomatics*, 51(1), 11–17.

Skjaerven, L.H. & Gard, G. (2018). Perspectives on Human movement, the Phenomenon of Movement Quality and How to Promote Movement Quality through Movement Awareness as Physiotherapy in Mental Health, (Eds. Probst, M., Skjaerven, L.H.), P*hysiotherapy in Mental Health and Psychiatry. A Scientific and Clinical Based Approaches*, (23–31), Elsevier. Poland.

Skjaerven, L.H. & Mattson, M. (2018). Basic Body Awareness Therapy (BBAT): A Movement Awareness Learning Modality in Physiotherapy, Promoting Movement Quality, (Eds. Probst, M., Skjaerven, L.H.), *Physiotherapy in Mental Health and Psychiatry. A Scientific and Clinical Based Approaches*, (59–68), Elsevier. Poland.

Skjaerven, L.H., Gard, G. & Kristoffersen, K. (2003). Basic Elements and Dimensions to the Phenomenon of Quality of Movement – A Case Study, *Journal of Bodywork and Movement Therapies*, 7(4), 251–260.

Skjaerven, L.H., Kristoffersen, K. & Gard, G. (2008). An Eye for Movement Quality: A Phenomenological Study of Movement Quality Reflecting a Group of Physiotherapists' Understanding of the Phenomenon, *Physiotherapy Theory and Practice*, 24(1), 13–27.

Skjaerven, L.H., Kristoffersen, K. & Gard, G. (2010). How Can Movement Quality Be Promoted in Clinical Practice? A Phenomenological Study of Physical Therapist Experts, *Physical Therapy*, 90, 1479–1492.

Strand, L. I., Olsen, A.L., Nygard, H., Furnes, O., Magnussen, L.H., Lygren, H. & et al. (2016). Basic Body Awareness Therapy and Patient Education in Hip Osteoarthritis: A Multiple Case Study, *European Journal of Physiotherapy*, 18(2), 116–125.

Sundén, A., Ekdahl, C., Magnusson, S.P., Johnsson, B., & Gyllensten, A.L. (2013). Physical Function and Self-efficacy – Important Aspects of Health-Related Quality of Life in Individuals with Hip Osteoarthritis, *European Journal of Physiotherapy*, 15, 151–159.

Thörnborg, U. & Mattson, M. (2010). Rating Body Awareness in Person Suffering from Eating Disorders – A Cross Sectional Study, *Advance in Physiotherapy*, 12(1), 24–34.

Wallin, U., Kronvall, P. & Majewski, M.L. (2000). Body Awareness Therapy in Teenage Anorexia Nervosa: Outcome after Two Years, *European Eating Disorders Review*, 8, 19–30.

Yeliz Şahin and Mesut Sancar

# 19: New Generation Pharmacy

## 1 Introduction: The Past and Present of Pharmacy

Even though pharmacy had a history dated back to old times and had practice areas as a part of medical science, the oldest written evidence that plants
have been used in the preparation of medicines was found in a Sumerian clay
tablet (Petrovska, 2012). The pharmacy profession continued to develop in the
ancient Mesopotamia, Egypt, Hittite, Indian, Chinese, Roman, Greek, and Islam
in middle ages, Medieval Europe and Renaissance periods. (http://e-kutuphane.
teb.org.tr/pdf/mised/ekim01/3.pdf).

Pharmaceutical sciences are considered as one of the most complex and
sophisticated efforts of mankind, which forms the basis of the discovery, development, production and use of medications. Eight service areas have been
defined by the International Pharmaceutical Federation (FIP) within the scope
of the advanced practices of the pharmacy profession (FIP, 2012):

- Academic pharmacy
- Clinical biology
- Community pharmacy
- Health and medicines information
- Hospital pharmacy
- Industrial pharmacy
- Military and emergency pharmacy
- Social and administrative pharmacy

In the last century, pharmacy has gained different perspectives and new
approaches to keep up with the changing world like other professions. In parallel with the rapid changes in the health sector, pharmacy has continued its
professional development with the areas such as clinical pharmacy, pharmaceutical care, medication therapy management, pharmaceutical biotechnology,
pharmacogenetics, targeted therapy, and personalized medicine with a common
goal of improving treatment outcomes. It is an undeniable fact that all these
developments are reflected in pharmacy curricula and open new horizons for
pharmacists who will work in the academic field. It is expected that the importance of the accreditation of pharmacy programs will increase in the future as a
result of the use of new educational technologies.

## 2 Patient-Oriented Pharmacy

Patient-oriented concepts presented as new facets of the pharmacy profession in the report prepared by the World Health Organization (WHO) and the International Pharmaceutical Federation (FIP) (Wiedenmayer et al., 2006) are clinical pharmacy, pharmaceutical care, good pharmacy practice, evidence-based pharmacy, chronic patient care, self-care and pharmacovigilance. As mentioned in this report, the pharmacy practices have changed from the product-oriented traditional role of pharmacy to patient care over the past 40 years; the role of pharmacists have evolved from the persons who prepare and dispense medicines to the persons who produce services and information in patient care.

When we look at the historical background of patient-oriented concepts, we see that the first developments started with those in clinical pharmacy about 50 years ago. The American College of Clinical Pharmacy (ACCP) has defined clinical pharmacy as a pharmacy field that deals with the science and practice of rational use of medicines in all areas of pharmacy; it has been also defined as a health science for providing patient care through the prevention and treatment of diseases and maintenance of health through optimizing drug treatments by pharmacists by the same institution. Clinical pharmacy is a service not only provided in hospitals, but also in community pharmacies, nursing homes, home care services, clinics and in all other areas of medication (http://www.accp.com/about/clinicalPharmacyDefined.aspx). Many studies showed that such patient-oriented services reduce costs in healthcare system, improve therapeutic outcomes and increase patient satisfaction. According to the report of the Joint Commission of Pharmacy Practitioners (JCPP) on pharmaceutical services in the United States in 2015, it was stated that pharmacists are healthcare professionals who are responsible for providing the necessary patient care to achieve optimal pharmacotherapy outcomes. It was also stated that most pharmacists are expected to be clinical pharmacists providing advanced patient care services in the future (https://www.accp.com/docs/positions/misc/JCPPVisionStatement.pdf).

Another concept frequently referred to in patient-oriented pharmacy practice is pharmaceutical care. Pharmaceutical care was firstly defined by Hepler and Strand as the professional responsibility of pharmacists in achieving therapeutic outcomes that improve patient's quality of life (Hepler and Strand, 1990). In 2004, Hepler (2004) discussed it in an article and it was emphasized that clinical pharmacy and pharmaceutical care are complementary concepts. Also, the necessity of clinical pharmacy as a condition for the presence of pharmaceutical care was mentioned.

The Good Pharmacy Practices Guide, which was updated by WHO and FIP in 2011 also indicated similar patient-focused roles of pharmacists (GPP, 2011). According to this manual, the 4 main roles of pharmacists are:

- Traditional roles
- Effective medication therapy management
- Maintaining and improving professional performance
- Making contribution to improve public health and healthcare system

One of the concepts that has been on the agenda in the United States in recent years is Medication Therapy Management (MTM) which also substitutes pharmaceutical care. This concept, which was defined by an agreed declaration of 11 pharmaceutical organizations in the United States in 2004 (American Pharmacists Association, 2008), is considered as a different service or group of services that optimize therapeutic outcomes for individual patients. All patients using prescription and non-prescription medicines, herbal products and food supplements have the right to potentially benefit from medication therapy management services, particularly when they have problems with a medicine. The MTM service model encourages patients to take a more active role in the management of their medications. The services are provided on the basis of the cooperation of pharmacists with physicians and other health professionals to improve the use of medicines in accordance with evidence-based guidelines. One of the most important factors making medication therapy management different is that it focuses on patient care in which all drug therapy are evaluated collectively instead of evaluating a single drug used by a patient. It is possible for patients to get support from these clinics, especially for monitoring blood pressure, blood glucose, INR, body weight and peak flow rate parameters. While being similar with pharmaceutical care in terms of its definition and scope, however, MTM services are considered as the management of all patient-oriented services (patient education, disease management and pharmaceutical care), which must be provided by pharmacists and are considered to be guided by the pharmaceutical care philosophy (McGivney et al., 2007).

# 3 The Place of Informatics in the Future of Pharmacy

It is accepted that informatics plays an important role in order to carry out all the patient-oriented pharmaceutical services mentioned above based on evidences and in the light of the current literature. In 2007, the American Society of Health System Pharmacists (ASHP) published a report describing the pharmacist's role in informatics. In this report, this subspecialty of pharmacy practices was defined as the use and integration of data, information, technology, automation in the process of medication use in order to improve health outcomes (Ma et al., 2015). One of the concepts defined in the field of informatics in recent years is big data; it is described as the developing use of complex data that can be collected very quickly. Its aim is to improve treatment alternatives and to individualize them (Erickson, 2014). Health information technology uses big data to capture different information flows and translates them into applicable information. Pharmacy is also prepared to take the advantage of big data to help patients' drug safety, to improve outcomes and to reduce costs. The main areas in which big data can be used in pharmacy were stated as risk management, decision process, clinical guidelines, drug safety, drug formulary management, hospitals, community pharmacies, adherence, drug reconciliation, individualized therapy and epidemiological models (Ma et al., 2015).

Onc of the areas in which the big data is used is drug reconciliation as mentioned above. Drug reconciliation is a technique for detecting conflicts in medications prescribed in different clinics or at different times, in order to gain knowledge and to prevent medication errors. In other words, making the most accurate and as complete as possible list of the drugs used by a patient and the process of comparing this list with the medication in this patient's records or drug orders (Boockvar, 2004). The confusion about drug regimens is one of the major causes of adverse drug events during hospital stay and after discharge. The Joint Commission for Accreditation of Healthcare Organizations (JCAHO) noticed this problem. In its report in 2004, it asked from all accredited institutions to develop a consensus process for the lists made with a complete and accurate drug history of patients until 2006 (the Joint Commission, 2006).

In pharmacy, one of the areas where informatics is widely used is drug consultation service. In 2016, the American Council on Pharmaceutical Education (ACPE) revised its standards for faculties of pharmacy and stated that pharmacy graduates should be prepared to contribute directly to patient-centered care, to work within professional teams, to use evidence-based information, to improve quality and to use informatics. Drug information centers, which have become widespread since 1960s, have begun to close in recent years. This change does not mean that drug information is not important. Drug information was firstly provided by telephone in a physical environment; people have started to costlessly access this information by using their smart phones or computers as a result of developing information technology. In a center or hospital, it was possible for clinical pharmacists, who are drug information specialists, to provide service without a physical drug information center (Carter, 2016).

Artificial intelligence is expected to be included in many areas of our life and pharmacy in the future, although it is not yet in every field. The American Society of Health System Pharmacists (ASHP) announced an inter-disciplinary committee meeting on the date of 5 March 2019 to examine the effects of artificial intelligence on health and pharmacy practices. The 20-membered Commission on Goals has aimed to receive the contributions of leaders having key positions in medicine, nursing, pharmacy, informatics, technology and health policy. The Commission plans to discuss how to integrate artificial intelligence into health services to improve patient outcomes, including how to use electronic medical records and electronic drug information sources (https://www.ashp.org/news/2019/03/04/ashp-commission-to-look-at-impact-of-artificial-intelligence-on-healthcare-pharmacy).

It is known that robotic systems are used in some areas such as hospital/pharmacy medication dispensing systems and drug preparation units in pharmacy profession. Although there are some studies showing that medication errors have been reduced by using robotic systems such as medication dispensing systems, these systems have not reached a very widespread use due to high costs and insufficient level of evidence (Rodriguez-Gonzalez et al., 2019). Robotic systems are known to have an increasing use in the preparation of chemotherapy protocols.

One of the areas where new technologies can be used more extensively in the future would be monitoring of adherence through drug boxes or systems with sensor technology. It is aimed to increase adherence with the help of a sensor, especially in inhaler type devices in which adherence is known as very low. However, it has been stated that it is not possible to use it all over the world because of the current costs but it can be suggested for certain patient groups (Hew and Reddel, 2019).

## 4 Pharmacy and Pharmacogenetics

The profession of pharmacy has provided valuable services such as therapeutic drug monitoring (e.g., pharmacokinetics), drug management and pharmacotherapy for a long time. Similarly, pharmacists try to adapt pharmacogenomics data to clinical practice in different practice environments. The practice-based leadership and professional role of pharmacists in pharmacogenomics has become more apparent by increasing number of pharmacists involved in clinical pharmacogenomics (Roederer et al., 2017).

The inter-personal variability of responses to treatments is largely due to genetic differences in drug metabolism, drug transporter and drug target proteins, as well as disease-associated proteins. Pharmacogenetics is a branch of science that investigates genetic variations that lead to differences in the responses of individuals to drugs. The term of pharmacogenetics is often used interchangeably with the term of pharmacogenomics. Pharmacogenetic studies examine differences in a single gene affecting the response to a drug; pharmacogenomics studies investigate all genes that may affect the activity and safety of a drug (Cavallari and Lam, 2008).

There is a clear consensus among national pharmaceutical organizations on the importance of the pharmacist to use pharmacogenomics information in patient care. In 2011, the American Pharmacists Association (APhA) published a notice that promotes the integration of pharmacogenomics with pharmaceutical applications through Medication Therapy Management (MTM) (Roederer et al., 2017). The American Society of Health-Systems Pharmacists (ASHP) also published a report on the role of pharmacists in clinical pharmacogenomics, as in other areas of profession (ASHP, 2015). According to this report, pharmacists have the responsibility to ensure the appropriate use of pharmacogenomics tests, to interpret the results of clinical pharmacogenomics tests and to educate other pharmacists, health professionals, patients and the public about pharmacogenomics. In order to fulfill these responsibilities, it has been emphasized that pharmacists should be well-supported for pharmacogenomics. The most important proof of the fact that these responsibilities are going to increase is that more and more approval is given to the drugs containing pharmacogenomics information in the prescription information by the FDA each day. According to a study conducted by ASHP, pharmacogenomics tests were performed in 7 % of the hospitals. In a survey on the future of pharmacy covering 2015–2019, 79 % of the participants expected to have a pharmacy-based pharmacogenomics service in at least 1 academic medical center in their regions in the next 5 years (Roederer et al., 2017).

Pharmacists are expected to play an important role in the development of individualized therapies with all pharmaceutical developments. Personalized medicine is expected to develop with the use of pharmacogenomics information in drug prescribing, the regulation of drug treatments according to phenotypic data and the use of pharmacometric modeling to individualize drug doses. It is important to consider clinical care for the next 10 years and for a longer time (Dong et al., 2018).

## 5 Biotechnology, Nanotechnology and Their Place in Pharmacy

Pharmaceutical biotechnology was emerged as one of the most important disciplines for drug discovery and development. Pharmaceutical biotechnology was limited to the fermentation and production of recombinant therapeutic proteins in the past; this definition has been updated and redefined nowadays by The European Association of Pharma Biotechnology (EAPB) as all the technologies required for production, manufacturing and registration of biotechnological products (Kayser and Warzecha, 2012). Population increase in the world, the spread of cancer and neurological diseases have necessitated the development of new treatment models and new pharmaceutical product designs in the future. Accordingly, pharmacy had to improve itself like other medical sciences (Azadi et al., 2015).

Advances in protein science, genetic and molecular biology provide new opportunities for the production of specific recombinant proteins for better disease management and the development of more specific effective drugs. In the future, it is expected that the design of engineered proteins become even more complex. Synthetic biology techniques that allow in silico de novo protein design and provide better designed integrated production processes can be used (Kayser et al., 2012). In the future, pharmaceutical industry is expected to make larger investments in biotechnological products because pharmaceutical biotechnology is a relatively new and growing field in which biotechnology principles are applied to develop new drugs. Most of the therapeutic drugs in the current market (such as antibodies, nucleic acid products and vaccines) are bioformulations (Mallela, 2010).

Nanotechnology is defined as science, engineering and technology carried out on a nanoscale (about 1 to 100 nanometers). Nanoscience and nanotechnology is the investigation and use of extremely small things and can be reflected in all other fields of science, such as chemistry, biology, physics, materials science and engineering (https://www.nano.gov/nanotech-101/what/definition). Systems and structures based on this technology aim to improve the quality of human life. Nowadays, researchers have a significant approach to the production and use of smaller particles in drug delivery systems. By this time, many drug delivery systems based on nanotechnology have taken their places in the global pharmaceutical market (Azadi et al., 2015). It is expected that nanoparticles will be replaced by picoparticles in the future.

One of the most recent developments in pharmaceutical science and pharmacy are smart drug delivery systems. Smart nanocarriers are the systems designed for carrying tissue-specific targeted delivery drugs, having the ability of sustained or triggered drug release, and to develop safer and more effective therapeutic agents for co-delivery of synergistic drug combinations. These advances in drug transport systems aim to reduce side effects, to extend half-life and to improve pharmacokinetic properties (Unsoy and Gunduz, 2018).

It is known that smart drug delivery systems are used successfully, especially in cancer treatment. There is a need for advanced diagnostic methods due to the increased incidence of cancer. Although surgical, radiotherapy and chemotherapy are well-known conventional methods for cancer treatment, the use of new, improved and reliable drug delivery methods (nano-drugs, DNA origami, nanoparticles and exosomes) make contributions to the reduction of side effects related to cancer treatment (Kesari et al., 2018). One of the new drug classes targeting cancer cells is antibody-drug conjugates (ADC). It has been estimated that only about one percent of ADCs can enter cancer cells; however, it has been considered that even this small amount is more effective than traditional cancer treatments (Hayat and Sahebkar, 2019).

## 6 Preventive Health Care, Vaccines and Pharmacists

Preventive healthcare services are known as the measures that try to eliminate or reduce diseases, accidents and related complications. Preventive healthcare services are considered as a part of primary care services in many countries due to lower costs, ease of implementation and reducing effect on the burden on hospital admissions compared to therapeutic services. In recent years, pharmacists directly focusing on patient care have a greater role in primary healthcare and treatment management. According to the Brazil Report of International Pharmaceutical Federation (FIP) in 2006, it was stated that pharmacists have an important place in healthcare teams and they are the most accessible members of healthcare facility for community. Therefore, they have an important position in the early detection of chronic diseases and in the determination of the unhealthy lifestyles (FIP, 2006). Preventive healthcare services is one of the subheadings of the item of making contribution to the improvement of public health and healthcare system which is one of the 4 main roles of the pharmacists in the Good Pharmacy Practice Guideline (GPP, 2011). Pharmacists, who are good health advisers, can inform the community about the risks of diseases and the measures which should be taken against them; pharmacists can determine individuals at risk and refer them to doctors for early diagnosis and treatment and thus contribute to preventive health. It is possible to find some studies showing that these kinds of contributions are also economically beneficial (Crawford, 2005; ASHP, 2008; Zadeh, 2015).

According to the World Health Organization (WHO), over 60 % of deaths worldwide are caused by non-communicable diseases (NCDs). The FIP Working Group on Non-communicable Diseases conducted a survey of all FIP member organizations and published an overview of the role of pharmacists in NCDs.

This paper not only encourages pharmacists worldwide in NCD management by combining practice and examples, but also presenting proper actions to take on this subject, such as:

- Prevention and screening activities
- Patient referral when appropriate
- Pharmacist-led, patient-centred NCD management

Researches show that pharmacists have significant role on the management of NCDs especially by being the most accessible healthcare facility, therefore being able to focus on prevention and early detection.

In a paper published by the American Public Health Association (APHA) in 2006, the main roles of the pharmacist in public health are listed as follows (APHA, 2006):

- Consultancy on the lifestyle changes that directly affect health outcomes
- Screening of diabetes, cholesterol and osteoporosis
- Vaccination
- Pain control
- Health education
- Self-treatment in asthma, hypertension and HIV (Human Immunodeficiency Virus) infection
- Smoking cessation
- Protection against alcohol and drug addiction
- Birth control

When preventive health services are mentioned, protective measures against infectious diseases are often considered. It is recognized that pharmacists have an important role in identifying risk groups for vaccination and in informing the community, especially those advocating for anti-vaccine defenses in recent years. There are several things which are considered among the primary responsibilities of pharmacists (Grabenstein and Bonasso, 1999), such as:

- Recommendation of pneumococcal and influenza vaccines (especially for patients over age 65 or with a known chronic disease or immunocompromised patients),
- Periodic checking of immunization registrations of patients,
- Storage, transfer and delivery of vaccines under appropriate conditions like in any other medicines.

Pharmacists in some countries of the world are known to have the authority to vaccinate at pharmacies. In particular, various organizations in the United States published recommendations on the need for the pharmacist to take an active role in the future, in addition to their current role in vaccination programs (Bach and Goad, 2015).

## 7 Rational Management of Pharmaceutical Waste

Patients can sometimes pollute the environment by throwing away unused medicines into household garbages or by pouring them into the toilet or sink. Active pharmaceutical ingredients which may have harmful effects on aquatic species and ecosystems have been detected on the surface, in soil and in drinking water (Bekker et al., 2018).

According to the results of different studies, it has been understood that in many parts of the World, people do not have enough knowledge about the destruction of drugs and its effects on the environment. In many countries, it has been stated that the most common disposal methods (throwing away solid drugs into garbages and pouring liquid drugs into sinks or toilets) are harmful to the environment; pharmacies are not very willing to take back medicines; there is no standard waste protocol available (Tong et al., 2011). Therefore, the efforts for reducing drug waste and unwanted economic and environmental burden are very important. Pharmacists are in a position to contribute to reduce drug waste as key players in the drug supply chain (Bekker et al., 2018). In the future, pharmaceutical science and pharmacy profession are expected to develop methods and policies for rational disposal of drugs.

## 8 Conclusion

The profession and science of pharmacy, which reaches into the depths of history, have made valuable contributions to the protection and improvement of health and the treatment of diseases throughout human history. As described in this chapter, there is a better patient care philosophy at the center of all new developments in the field of pharmacy. The greatest change in the profession over the last century has been its evolution from a traditional compounding role to patient-oriented roles. This period, known as clinical pharmacy, is expected to occupy the agenda of the profession in the near future.

Clinical pharmacy services and direct patient care have a promising future in many countries. Clinical pharmacists are now more specialized for specific services or complex care. These advancements have ensured the further development of clinical pharmacy services in many countries (Carter, 2016). The pharmacy profession absorbed science and technology into new updated pharmaceutical science extensions, and it will continue to make significant contributions to healthcare as a profession open for development in the next century.

# References

American Pharmacists Association; National Association of Chain Drug Stores Foundation. (2008). Medication Therapy Management in Pharmacy Practice: Core Elements of an MTM Service Model, Version 2, *J Am Pharm Assoc*, 48(3), 341–53.

APHA. (2006). The Role of the Pharmacist in Public Health, Policy Statements and Advocacy https://www.apha.org/policies-and-advocacy/public-health-policy-statements/policy-database/2014/07/07/13/05/the-role-of-the-pharmacist-in-public-health (accessed on: 22.04.2019).

ASHP-American Society of Health-System Pharmacists. (2008). ASHP Statement on the Role of Health-System Pharmacists in Public Health, *Am J Health-Syst Pharm*, 65, 462–7.

ASHP-American Society of Health-System Pharmacists (2015). ASHP Statement on the Pharmacist's Role in Clinical Pharmacogenomics, *Am J Health-Syst Pharm*, 72, 579–81.

Azadi, A., Morowvat, M.H., Sakhteman, A. & Mohagheghzadeh, A. (2015). Pharmacy or Pharmanbic: Thinking about 50 Years Ahead of Pharmacy, *Trends Pharmaceut Sci*, 1(4), 191–8.

Bach, A.T. & Goad, J.A. (2015). The Role of Community Pharmacy-Based Vaccination in the USA: Current Practice and Future Directions, *Integr Pharm Res Pract*, 4, 67–77.

Bekker, C.L., Gardarsdottir, H., Egberts, A.C.G., Bouvy, M.L. & van den Bemt, B.J.F. (2018). Pharmacists' Activities to Reduce Medication Waste: An International Survey, *Pharmacy (Basel)*, 6(3), pii: E94.

Boockvar, K., Fishman, E., Kyriacou, C.K., Monias, A., Gavi, S. & Cortes, T. (2004). Adverse Events due to Discontinuations in Drug Use and Dose Changes in Patients Transferred Between Acute and Long-Term Care Facilities, *Arch Intern Med*, 164, 545–50.

Carter, B.L. (2016). Evolution of Clinical Pharmacy in the USA and Future Directions for Patient Care, *Drugs Aging*, 33(3), 169–77.

Cavallari, L.H., Lam, Y.W.F. (2008). Pharmacogenetics. (eds: Dipiro J.T. et al.), *Pharmacotherapy A Pathophysiologic Approach*, 7th, McGraw Hill, China.

Crawford, S.Y. (2005). Pharmacists' Roles in Health Promotion and Disease Prevention. *Am J Pharmaceut Educ*, 69(4), Article 73.

Dong, O.M., Howard, R.M., Church, R., Cottrell, M., Forrest, A., Innocenti, F., et al. (2018). Challenges and Solutions for Future Pharmacy Practice in the Era of Precision Medicine, *Am J Pharmaceut Educ*, 82(6), 6652.

Erickson, A.K. (2014). Pharmacy: Harnessing the Power of Big Data, *Pharm Today*, 20(11), 8.

FIP https://www.fip.org/pharmacy_practice (accessed on: 27.03.2019).

FIP. (2006). Statement of Policy the Role of the Pharmacist in the Prevention and Treatment of Chronic Disease. https://www.fip.org/www/uploads/database_file.php?id=274&table_id (accessed on: 27.03.2019).

FIP. (2012). Impact of Pharmaceutical Sciences on Healthcare. International Pharmaceutical Federation. https://fip.org/files/fip/Pharmaceutical_Sciences/PSMO_Guide_PPT_August_2014.ppt (accessed on: 22.04.2019).

GPP. (2011). Good Pharmacy Practice (GPP) Guidelines, FIP/WHO

Grabenstein, J.D. & Bonasso, J. (1999). Health-System Pharmacists' Role in Immunizing Adults Against Pneumococcal Disease and Influenza, *Am J Health Syst Pharm*, 56(17 Suppl 2), 3–22.

Hayat, S.M.G. & Sahebkar, A. (2019). Antibody-Drug Conjugates: Smart Weapons against Cancer. *Archives of Medical Science*. https://doi.org/10.5114/aoms.2019.83020 (accessed on: 22.04.2019).

Hepler, C.D. (2004). Clinical Pharmacy, Pharmaceutical Care, and the Quality of Drug Therapy, *Rev Pharmacother*, 24, 1491–8.

Hepler, C.D. & Strand, L.M. (1990). Opportunities and Responsibilities in Pharmaceutical Care, *Am J Hosp Pharm*, 47, 533–43.

Hew, M. & Reddel, H.K. (2019). Integrated Adherence Monitoring for Inhaler Medications, *JAMA*, 321(11), 1045–6.

http://e-kutuphane.teb.org.tr/pdf/mised/ekim01/3.pdf (accessed on: 27.03.2019).

http://www.accp.com/about/clinicalPharmacyDefined.aspx (accessed on: 27.03.2019).

https://www.accp.com/docs/positions/misc/JCPPVisionStatement.pdf (accessed on: 27.03.2019).

https://www.ashp.org/news/2019/03/04/ashp-commission-to-look-at-impact-of-artificial-intelligence-on-healthcare-pharmacy (accessed on: 27.03.2019).

https://www.nano.gov/nanotech-101/what/definition (accessed on: 27.03.2019).

Kayser, O. & Warzecha, H. (2012). *Pharmaceutical Biotechnology: Drug Discovery and Clinical Applications*. Wiley-Blackwell, Wiley-VCH Verlag & Co. KGaA. Weinheim, Germany.

Kesari, K.K., Jamal, Q.M.S., Siddiqui, M.H. & Arif, J.M. (2018). Networking of Smart Drugs: A Chem-Bioinformatic Approach to Cancer Treatment. (ed.

Roy, K.) *Multi-Target Drug Design Using Chem-Bioinformatic Approaches. Methods in Pharmacology and Toxicology.* Humana Press, New York.

Ma, C., Smith, H.W., Chu, C. & Juarez, D.T. (2015). Big Data in Pharmacy Practice Current Use, Challenges, and The future, *Integr Pharm Res Pract*, 4, 91–9.

Mallela, K. (2010). Pharmaceutical Biotechnology – Concepts and Applications, *Hum Genomics*, 4(3), 218–9.

McGivney, M.S., Meyer, S.M., Duncan-Hewitt, W., Hall, D.L., Goode, J.V. & Smith, R.B. (2007). Medication Therapy Management: Its Relationship to Patient Counseling, Disease Management, and Pharmaceutical Care, *Am Pharm Assoc*, 47, 620–8.

Petrovska, B.B. (2012). Historical Review of Medicinal Plants' Usage, *Pharmacogn Rev*, 6(11), 1–5.

Rodriguez-Gonzalez, C.G., Herranz-Alonso, A., Escudero-Vilaplana, V., Ais-Larisgoitia, M.A., Iglesias-Peinad, I. & Sanjurjo-Saez, M. (2019). Robotic Dispensing Improves Patient Safety, Inventory Management, and Staff Satisfaction in an Outpatient Hospital Pharmacy, *J Eval Clin Pract*, 25, 28–35.

Roederer, M.W., Kuo, G.M., Kisor, D.F., Frye, R.F., Hoffman, J.M., Jenkins, J. & Weitzel, K.W. (2017). Pharmacogenomics Competencies in Pharmacy Practice: A Blueprint for Change, *J Am Pharm Assoc*, 57(1), 120–5.

The Joint Commission. (2006). *Sentinel Event Alert*, 35. https://www.jointcommission.org/assets/1/18/SEA_35.PDF (accessed on: 28.03.2019).

Tong, A.Y.C., Peake, B.M. & Braund, R. (2011). Disposal Practices for Unused Medications around the World, *Environ Int*, 37, 292–8.

Unsoy, G. & Gunduz, U. (2018). Smart Drug Delivery Systems in Cancer Therapy, *Curr Drug Targets*, 19(3), 202–12.

Wiedenmayer, K., Summers, R.S., Mackie, C.A., Gous, A.G.S. & Everard, M. (2006). *Developing Pharmacy Practice: A Focus on Patient Care: Handbook.* World Health Organization, Geneva.

Zadeh, P.S. (2015). Pharmacists on the Frontline of Preventive Healthcare Services. https://www.drugtopics.com/community-practice/pharmacists-frontline-preventive-healthcare-services (accessed on: 28.03.2019).

İnci Adalı

# 20: New Approaches in Audiology

## 1 Introduction

It is not possible for the health field to stay out of the trend line in our rapidly changing and developing world with technological progress. Audiology Science has a special position in the human-oriented health sciences, which use technological equipment in its works and aims to benefit from the developments at the highest level. Smartphone-based application, artificial intelligence and virtual reality stand out among the current applications that are studied and developed in our brunch of science where technology is used extensively during both the examination and diagnosis phase and the treatment rehabilitation phase.

## 2 New Approaches in Audiology

### 2.1 Hearing Evaluation with Smart Phone Applications

Measuring the hearing health with conventional hearing test methods cause time loss and an economic burden for the patient. While trying to develop this process, studies are being carried out to place smartphone based audiometric measurement methods alongside existing methods. In a hearing screening study, 162 children (324 ears) aged between 5 and 7 years were tested (Swanepoel et al., 2014). For this study, the Sennheiser HD 202 headphones were adapted and used with 4 android phones. Hearing screening was performed using narrowband noise in the 30–75 dB SPL sound range. The control group consisted of 15 subjects with an age range of 18–22 years and normal hearing limits. During the study, care was taken to calibrate the audiometer and android phones used for control. As a result of this study, no significant difference was found between the android phone application and the traditional audiometric method. It can be concluded that the measurements made with the smartphone application can be compared with the results of traditional methods, if the correct calibration is performed.

In another study of smartphone-based audiometric measurement as an alternative to traditional audiometric measurement in primary care, 64 samples were subjected to a hearing test on an android phone without a silent cabin, and air conduction threshold was measured in a clinic that provided primary care. Then, audiometric measurements were applied to this group by conventional method in the silent cabin. In conclusion, the results of the audiometric measurements performed without a cabin in the 1st stage medical service showed that there was no significant difference when compared with the results of the audiometric measurements performed by conventional method and smartphone based audiometric measurement methods. However, it should be kept in mind that smartphone-based audiometric measurements are based on air conduction and should be studied with careful calibrations (Sandström et al., 2016).

In another study conducted in 2017, 95 subjects were tested. 30 subjects were approximately 59 years old adult with bilateral hearing loss, and 65 adolescent subjects consisted of 4 with mild hearing loss and 61 with normal hearing. For smartphone-based threshold audiometry, the air conduction threshold was measured by calibrated on-ear headphones and subsequently by conventional audiometric method. Comparisons have been made between the thresholds and the duration of the test performed by both test procedures. No significant difference was found between the two groups of hearing thresholds and test times in the adult group. In the adolescent group, a difference of <10 dB (With a rate of 79.3 %) was found between the threshold values at 1 KHz, but the conventional test time was found to be shorter than the smartphone test period at this frequency and this difference was found to be significant (van Tonder, 2017). In this study, it was concluded that smartphone-based audiometric measurement with calibrated on-ear headphones is a cost-effective option for the detection of air conduction thresholds. This technique, which is supported by new studies, is especially preferred in developing countries and residential areas which are difficult to reach (Yousuf Hussein, 2016).

## 2.2 The Ambient Volume Measurements with Smartphone Applications

Another issue that is open to development is the studies on the environmental conditions we are in. The negative effects of the noise level in our environment on human health cannot be denied. This fact encourages researchers to work to measure the ambient sound level in the easiest, cheapest and most accurate way. This search has brought the work done with smart phones that have been formatted in recent years into spotlight. Another application that uses smartphones in audiology is the measurement of ambient sound levels. The ambient volume is measured by the "Sound Level Meter" (SLM). Application programs have been developed to customize smartphones to measure ambient sound level (SLMA: Sound Level Meter Application). With the fact that them being cheap and easy to use, and by equipping them with this program and measuring the built-in microphone calibration by increasing the sensitivity of smart phones, research is being conducted to find the answer to the question: "can smart phones be preferred as devices that measure and monitor the ambient noise level?". In 2018, a study was conducted by Serpanos et al. and it is found that more accurate measurements were made when the ambient sound level was above 40–50 dB (Serpanos). A single iOS-based smartphone was used in the study. With this device, non-calibrated and calibrated media measurements were made at 1000 Hz, and additionally "narrowband noise" (NBN) and "White noise" (WN) were applied. The results of SLM and SLMA measurements were compared. Deviations –independent from the calibration – were found in room noise level measurements below 50 dB. In this study, it was concluded that the use of NBN and WN would be appropriate for the detection of low ambient noise levels below 50 dB with this technique, but even with calibration, it could be assumed that the measurement results could have a margin of error below this level. It was also emphasized that these results should not be generalized for all types of smartphones at the end of the study, and that research with SLMAs using the next generation smartphone should be continued (Serpanos, 2018). While on one hand, the practices are continuing; on the other hand, the use of the applications is also becoming widespread.

From the point of the fact that the noise adversely affects human health, and worsens the course of chronic diseases such as hypertension and cardiopulmonary diseases, the researchers carried out some studies in the direction of measuring the ambient sound level easily, cheaply and accurately and monitoring it for a long time. For this purpose, it is aimed to monitor the environmental noise and to develop measures to the effects that threaten human health. One of the studies carried out in this sense was carried out between January 2014 and January 2016 in the Abuja Municipality (Ibekwe, 2016). In this long-term study, noise measurement was made by dividing the residential area into 12 different regions such as residents, workplace and market. In addition to SLM, smartphones –which were appliqued by various software, were used in the study. Noise measurements were measured at different points in all regions and at different times of day and night. The values were compared with the "ambient noise safety level standard value" of the World Health Organization (WHO). As a result of the study, it was emphasized that day and night noise levels are above the WHO recommended values; and studies should be conducted to raise awareness and solution.

Another study was conducted in 2014 (Kardous, 2014). The iOS app was evaluated using more than 130 smartphones and tablets for ambient sound measurement. The study showed that some iOS applications could be used with professional environment volume measurements with a ± 2 dB margin.

An interesting study was conducted by Huth et al. (2014) to measure noise exposures in movie theaters (8). For this study, an SPL meter software program was installed on 6 smartphones, the phones were calibrated for use in ambient noise measurement, and an extra SPL meter was added to the system. Two different films (one action film and one children's film) were selected, and on different days, 6 different measurements were made at 10 different points. Compared to SPL meter measurements, it has been observed that smart phone measurements have high accuracy. It was determined that the number of spectators did not affect the noise level, the sound level was higher in the action films than the others and the sound level decreased as it moved away from the stage. As a result of the study, it is considered that the noise level in the cinema halls does not exceed the safe exposure limit and smart phones can be an alternative to SPL meter with a suitable software and good calibration.

While there are many studies on the use of smartphones in ambient noise measurement; In 2014, Nast et al. have examined the "utility/accuracy" values of these applications (Nast, 2014). They stated that SLM devices require training for the correct use and mobile technology is sufficient to measure the ambient sound level using software-installed smartphones. In this study, the ambient sound measurement values – obtained by mobile technology – were compared with the calibrated SLM. In most of the applications, error was detected at high sound levels, while it was noted that the error margin remained within ± 5 dB in measurements with SLM. This finding supports the other studies that concluded that "ambient measurements with smartphone software give the most accurate level around 40–50 dB". It is possible to reach the following conclusions based on the examples we have quoted in this study: The ambient sound level should be measured and monitored with systematic methods. In this process, the use of a calibrated smartphone with an amplified microphone can be an easily accessible, inexpensive, and more preferable equipment with an accurate measurement.

## 2.3 Pairing of Hearing Aids with Smartphones and Other Devices

Audiology Science may recommend hearing aids for the treatment of the individual with hearing loss. Today's hearing aids are designed to restore the sound quality to the patient while restoring the hearing comfort to the patient with its digital features, and to this end, advanced technological equipment are installed on the hearing aids. This allows the hearing aid to be paired with a smartphone or any other digital-capable device with its Bluetooth feature.

The Federal Communications Commission (FCC) accepts Hearing Aid Compatibility (HAC) requirements for digital wireless phones. This means, most smartphone devices are compatible with a range of hearing aid models within the FCC requirements for HAC. These compliance studies follow the ANSI (American National Standards Institute) standard requirements. The "ANSI-C63.19-2007" standards have 2 types of ratings for digital phones: M and T ratings. M-grade is for acoustic coupling while T-rating is for inductive coupling. Each of these values are scaled from 1 to 4. The highest degree of compatibility is 4. M/T rating of the hearing aid is examined to evaluate the compatibility degree of the hearing aid to the digital telephone. According to the FCC rules, a digital telephone is considered compatible with the hearing aid if it has M3 or M4 for acoustic coupling and if it has T3 or T4 rating for the inductive coupling. However, in view of the fact that clinical experience is healthier, researchers suggest that it would be more beneficial if the user of the hearing aid or cochlear implant would test the phone to be evaluated in different locations, and in various settings (support.apple.com/tr-tr/HT202186).

The integration of mobile technology and hearing aids provides daily comfort to the user. In this way, the user can talk comfortably with digital phones, use the bluetooth equipment in the device to enable the "hands-free" function to listen to the music or "stream" to watch the TV, or to use the digital phone as a "hearing aid remote". Said bluetooth functions are referred to as "Bluetooth protocols". Bluetooth protocols such as hands-free, air stream and low energy are included in the agenda to provide the user with the ease of using hearing comfort in their daily life. For example, with the hands-free function, the user can speak hands free with the digital phone at a distance of approximetely 14 meters. They can watch TV and listen to music with a connector plugged into a TV or music system. They can use Facetime and GPS. In addition, the use of the smartphone as a "hearing aid remote" provides great comfort to the user. With this application called "touch control", the user can make changes in terms of volume and direction selectivity by using mobile phone and can reach maximum compliance with the device.

It is possible to take advantage of the richness of the software in accordance with the height of the M/T scaling of the compatibility of hearing aids with smartphones (FCC). For example, a device producer provides an "urgent call service" to older users by installing a software to the hearing aid that can detect a "fall" (to the ground). With the same method it is possible to detect heart rate, rhythm disturbances and send a warning to a selected recipient. Another device company combines device data in a "cloud" environment, allowing its experts to organize (new and present) devices in the direction of the user's preferences and satisfaction. The Artificial Intelligence works are continuously renewed with such software and contribute to the user's hearing comfort as well as their vital comfort (www.phonak.com/tr/tr/hearing-aids/uygulamalar.html).

## 2.4 Artificial Intelligence in Audiology

Artificial Intelligence (AI) is an area of information processing science where programs are created to apply multidimensional, intelligent solutions to complex problems. One of the most common practices is to process large amounts of information and try to achieve the goals set out in the framework of rules. It should be remembered that the formation of AI is directed by the human brain and rules set by it. AI studies developing in the field of audiology are mostly in the field of hearing aids, and with the use of digital technology in the devices, the studies on this subject are increasing day by day. With AI studies, it is sought to provide the highest level of hearing comfort in the direction of the user's needs and preferences. The key to this work is software development and algorithms (Algorithm is a procedure consisting of a series of algebraic formulas and/or logical steps to calculate or determine a particular task). The software-enriched hearing aid makes a multi-dimensional assessment of the sound environment the user enters, and converts the amplification strategy into the most appropriate form for speech perception. Noise, general sound level, direction of speech, wind sound (if any), etc. are detected. By means of software, the clearest speech signal is detected, direction perception is created, optimal S/N (signal/noise) ratio is captured and noise management and frequency compression are created, and as a result, most appropriate sound perception for the user is formed. As the environment changes, the device's settings are updated for optimal use. In other words; audiological solutions are searched by algorithms to the chaos of the auditory environment.

AI studies attract the attention of researchers. A group of experts from Columbia University's Engineering Faculty, with the help of AI in hearing aids, have reported that they are working to analyze brain activities and conduct research that is relevant to them to understand what sounds are more relevant to the user. According to the study, the cognitive hearing aid produced is programmed to read the user's brain activities and to distinguish the original sounds according to their preferences from the background sounds of the noisy environment (www.digitaltrends.com/cool-tech/cognitive-hearing-aid-columbia).

Current hearing aids are based on user specific living conditions and listening selectivity. The strategy in the use of hearing aids is to amplify incoming voice information and send it to the upper center. However, while providing this integrated software and product design, smart gain, frequency selectivity and binaural synchronization are targeted. In other words, the hearing aid is programmed to ensure maximum compliance in the ambient change. With this gain, the user continues his social life without having to worry about distinguishing sound when the environment changes and without having to manually change the program.

In order to restore the hearing comfort of modern hearing aids to the user, many improvement studies have been made based on social environments. Here, in 2018, a neuro-technological study conducted by Anderson et al. should be mentioned: In this study, the user entering the noisy environment selectively/ primarily chooses the sounds coming from the direction in which they look through a multi-channel microphone assembly. This device, called Cochlearity, consists of an improved multichannel microphone system and is mounted on a point or perching above the eyes (eg on glasses), and is adapted to an android device. With this improved device, the user primarily perceives the sounds in the direction in which he/she is looking (Anderson et al., 2018).

AI work samples can be diversified in the hearing aid. However, laboratory studies for AI use in audiology are open to improvements and algorithm studies continue intensively.

In audiology, AI studies have been performed in the clinical field for the diagnosis of some diseases such as Meniere's disease. In this study; along with the genetic coding study, the neural network was monitored and a decision diagram was established (Juhola et al., 2001).

In a study conducted by Rajkumar et al., in 2018, devices for the greater satisfaction of hearing aid users have been effectively programmed. The aim of the study is to improve the device availability by developing an intelligent software (Software Intelligent System-SIS). During the application of SIS, device parameters such as gain control, frequency compression ratio are automatically predicted and the test signals are generated by means of the standard hardware and software algorithm in the computer system. The proposed system has been studied with data from 243 people in the Chennai City Government General Hospital in India. As a result, 221 people were satisfied with the gain values proposed by SIS and their satisfaction rate was 91 %. As a result of the study, it was found that the proposed system reduces the time spent by audiologists to test hearing aids by 75 %. Therefore, it is concluded that the proposed software (SIS: Software Intelligent System) can be used to recommend hearing instrument parameters to provide optimal solutions to hearing aid users (Rajkumar et al., 2017).

The findings suggest that the proposed SIS can be used to perform audiological screening tests and to recommend hearing aid gain values to hearing impaired individuals. This result confirms that SIS may assist audiologists in routine hearing screening studies or when the hearing aid needs to be programmed quickly (Rajkumar et al., 2018).

## 2.5 The Reflection of Development in Power Supply Technology on Hearing Aids

While studies are continued in order to increase the benefit of hearing aids to the users the batteries that are the power supply of the devices continue to be the subject of research/development. Zinc-Air batteries, which are used in most of the hearing aids nowadays, are "disposable" batteries. Despite their many disadvantages, they have been in use for a long time. For example, reasons such as the inadequate battery life of conventional batteries, economic cost, the need to change frequently, the difficulty of changing the battery in elderly patients, durability and (them being a) risky waste in terms of environmental pollution lead researchers to new battery forms and concentrated them on rechargeable battery studies (Lay Ekuakille et al., 2008). The results are positive and improvement studies are continuing.

Among many types of rechargeable batteries, Ag-Zn (Silver-Zinc) and Li-ion (Lithium-Ion) batteries are leading the way. Ag-Zn batteries work with high capacity and with a battery life of 1 year. The full charge time is 4 hours, providing 16 hours of continuous audio transmission after full charge. However, the battery life is 1 year, with each year requiring a battery replacement. Li-ion batteries are the most technologically advanced batteries: among the most rechargeable batteries, Li-ion batteries, the lightest of the kind, are used in smartphones, laptops, smart watches, tablet computers and cameras. They are the longest used batteries with the fastest charging time. They can be charged for many times and at desired times, and their hearing performance is not affected. A Li-ion battery that got charged 1-night in the charging unit can provide 24 hours of uninterrupted audio streaming, 3 hours with 15 minutes of charging, and 12 hours of audio streaming with 1-hour charging. Battery life is up to 7 years. In other words, the same battery can be used for 7 years. If the battery cover of the hearing aids with a rechargeable battery is removed and the integrated battery design of the cabinet is used, there will be no corrosion of the battery charge contacts as well as the user's ease of use. Hearing aids that carry integrated battery to the cabinet are charged on the desktop charging plate. In addition, the user can also carry a mini-charger if desired. In addition, a lighted indicator can be placed in the system to see the charging status.

The superiority of the use of rechargeable Li-ion batteries for replacing Zinc-Air/Disposible batteries can be summarized as follows:

- Fast-charging option
- Freedom to charge at any time and for any length of time
- Long battery life (~7 years)

- Battery durability
- 24 hours long audio streaming with just 3-hours of charging
- Performance increase
- Ease of use (to use a desktop charging plate for integrated battery charging)

## 2.6 Use of Virtual Reality (VR) in Audiology

Virtual Reality/Virtual Reality studies are most useful in the field of balance pathology in the audiology and studies in this field are ongoing.

Regardless of the circumstances, the protection of balance is an absolute necessity for people. In our space, the sense of balance requires the synthesis of data from the visual, vestibular and deep sense (proprioceptive and somatosensory) systems. All the cues from these systems are oriented to create the sense of balance and are integrated by the Central Nervous System (CNS) with different strategies. The question of how the CNS synthesizes all data and makes cognitive conclusions about the balance strategies continues to be the research subject of biomedical specialists. It is interesting to note that in the absence or conflict of one or more data, the CNS adapts to the new situation and gives less weight to conflicting data. The focus of this study is to review the integration of the CNS with the sensory data, and the strategies that the researchers put forward to explain these. In this study, the different approaches to balance used by young and older adults are compared. With age, not only the locomotor system, but also the vision and vestibular system are disrupted. Therefore, elderly individuals have to use their impaired sensory data as much as possible to preserve their postural stability. In this study, the research is being done to evaluate the effectiveness of balance training and rehabilitation given by using virtual reality in changing the strategies of head and eye movement, and to determine the role of responses in the balance. Virtual reality rehabilitation studies are discussed not only in the elderly, but also in movement disorder and occupational impairment. Due to its relatively low cost, there is a wide research area in the studies of balance rehabilitation and education (Virk and McConville, 2006).

Virtual Reality is a new technology that simulates a 3D virtual world on a computer with simulation and enables users to produce visual, auditory and tactile feedback for complete immersion. Users can interact with objects in a 3D visual field without limitation. Nowadays, this visual media simulation is the main point for the use of virtual reality education in balance disorders and rehabilitation. Nowadays, Virtual Reality (VR) education is frequently used in balance disorder and rehabilitation, but also in the treatment of some neurological diseases. According to this study, while patients receive VR training, prefrontal, parietal cortical areas and some motor cortical networks are activated. These activations may play a role in the reconstruction of some neurons in the cerebral cortex. Again, according to this study, evidence from clinical trials suggests that VR training improves the neurological function of patients with some neurological disorders such as spinal cord injury and cerebral palsy. As a result of the study, it is emphasized that these findings indicate that VR training can stimulate the cerebral cortex and improve the adaptive capacity of the patients, thus facilitating the enhancement of the function of the cortex with vestibular control (Mao et al., 2014).

VR provides hope in the implementation of health services. In practicing vestibular rehabilitation, it is a fun and engaging process for patients, which positively affects their use (Rose, Nam and Chen, 2018). In this article, 18 studies are reviewed for performance and results after using VR for rehabilitation purposes. The aim is to see the effect and results of VR immersion applied, to increase the patient's enjoyment of VR application and to ensure that the application is adopted, and therefore to define the relationship between these two, and to investigate the effect of tactile feedback on the use of VR in the immersion. Performance metrics such as postural stability, navigation effect, and joint elasticity showed different relationships with immersion. Since the data is limited, there is no firm conclusion between fun and dependence. In the study, however, the observation of patient enjoyment from the application and the desire to participate were noted. In addition, it was concluded that the use of tactile devices such as immersion gloves and control devices was evaluated as both strong and weak in terms of motion accuracy. This result confirms that studies should be enriched.

In a study conducted by Yeh et al. (2014), they argue that vestibular rehabilitation is effective in improving balance control. During the study, they organized simple and repetitive movements of vestibular rehabilitation exercises such as Cawthorne-Cooksey Exercises with training protocols and implemented these protocols with VR support. The aim of the study was to investigate the effectiveness of 3D VR system for vestibular rehabilitation. As a result of the study, it is emphasized that VR-supported rehabilitation exercises play a positive role in improving balance control in patients with vestibular dysfunction.

In patients with peripheral vestibular dysfunction, there are studies suggesting that VR studies specialized with visual stimuli produce positive results in terms of vestibular rehabilitation. For example, Yeh et al. (2014), Pavlou et al. (2012), and Gascuel et al. (2012) suggested that VR studies enriched with visual enhancements affect visual vertigo symptoms. In a pilot study conducted by Pavlou et al., 3 groups were formed as static, dynamic and static + dynamic from participants with peripheral vestibular dysfunction. Participants were given 3D/ VR exercises in accordance with the exercise protocol established for 4 weeks,

2 days a week. This protocol was supported by the exercise program given home. At the end of the process, the response of the subjects to the treatment was evaluated by taking the symptoms and psychological conditions into consideration. It was concluded that dynamic VR training/exercise programs supported by 3D are positive contributions to vestibular rehabilitation programs for patients with peripheral vestibular disorders.

In conclusion, the applicability of these studies to the patients of all ages with the applications in the field of VR training with 3D for balance rehabilitation is widening the scope of the studies. However, standardization of training protocols is required, and for this, a larger number of patients should be followed up for longer periods of time to establish working sequences.

Studies are under way to assess the effectiveness of vestibular rehabilitation training with Virtual Reality and to define the role of responses in treatment.

# 3 Conclusion

Audiology science is not only about the presence, nature and depth of human hearing loss. If there is a disability, it provides solutions for diagnosis and treatment methods, while providing rehabilitation methods, so that the user can continue his/her academic and social life.

It uses all the possibilities of the technology in order for the hearing aid user to have maximum compliance with the hearing aid. Studies in this direction are diversifying and developing in parallel with the increasing technological acceleration worldwide.

In addition to hearing loss, the balance problem is tried to be rehabilitated by technological methods. Positive results are obtained and VR training studies are in progress.

Another area of interest of audiology is the determination of ambient sound level and taking preventive medicinal measures against noise risk. Studies on the search for the most accurate and most useful method are in progress while measuring ambient sound.

New technological experiences in audiology are pleasing, but this issue is open to improvements and should be enriched with time-based studies. As in all health sciences, Audiology Science aims to utilize technological developments at the highest level and use these accesses for human health.

# References

Anderson, M.H., Yazel, B.W., Stickle, M.P.F., Espinosa Inguez, F.D., Gutierrez, N.S., Slaney, M. & et al. (2018). Towards Mobile Gaze-Directed

Beamforming: A Novel Neuro-Technology for Hearing Loss, *Conf Proc IEEE Eng Med Biol Soc*, 2018, 5806–5809.

Gascuel, J.D., Payno, H., Schmerber, S. & Martin, O. (2012). Immersive Virtual Environment for Visuo-Vestibular Therapy: Preliminary Results, *Stud Health Technol Inform*, 181, 187–91.

https://support.apple.com/tr-tr/HT202186, (accessed on: 26.04.2019).

https://www.digitaltrends.com/cool-tech/cognitive-hearing-aid-columbia/, (accessed on: 27.04.2019).

https://www.phonak.com/tr/tr/hearing-aids/uygulamalar.html, (accessed on: 26.04.2019).

Huth, M.E., Popelka, G.R. & Blevins, N.H. (2014). Comprehensive Measures of Sound Exposures in Cinemas Using Smartphones, *Ear Hear*, 35(6), 680–6.

Ibekwe, T., Folorunso, D., Ebuta, A., Amodu, J., Nwegbu, M., Mairami, Z. & et al. (2016). Evaluation of the Environmental Noise Levels in Abuja Municipality Using Mobile Phones, *Ann Ib Postgrad Med*, 14(2), 58–64.

Juhola, M., Viikki, K., Laurikkala, J., Auramo, Y., Kentala, E. & Pyykkö, I. (2001). Application of Artificial Intelligence in Audiology, *Scand Audiol Suppl*, 52, 97–9.

Kardous, C.A. & Shaw, P.B. (2014). Evaluation of Smartphone Sound Measurement Applications, *J Acoust Soc Am*, 135(4), 186–92.

Lay-Ekuakille, A., Vendramin, G. & Trotta, A. (2008). Design of an Energy Harvesting Conditioning Unit for Hearing Aids, *Conf Proc IEEE Eng Med Biol Soc*, 2008, 2310–3.

Mao, Y., Chen, P., Li, L. & Huang, D. (2014). Virtual Reality Training Improves Balance Function, *Neural Regen Res*, 9(17), 1628–34.

Nast, D.R., Speer, W.S., Le Prell, C.G. (2014). Sound Level Measurements Using Smartphone "Apps": Useful or Inaccurate?, *Noise Health*, 16(72), 251–6.

Pavlou, M., Kanegaonkar, R.G., Swapp, D., Bamiou, D.E., Slater, M. & Luxon, L.M. (2012). The Effect of Virtual Reality on Visual Vertigo Symptoms in Patients with Peripheral Vestibular Dysfunction: A Pilot Study, *J Vestib Res*, 22(5-6), 273–81.

Rajkumar, S., Muttan, S., Sapthagirivasan, V., Jaya, V. & Vignesh, S.S. (2018). Development of Improved Software Intelligent System for Audiological Solutions, *J Med Syst*, 42(7), 127.

Rajkumar, S., Muttan, S., Sapthagirivasan, V., Jaya, V. & Vignesh, S.S. (2017). Software Intelligent System for Effective Solutions for Hearing Impaired Subjects, *Int J Med Inform*, 97, 152–162.

Rose, T., Nam, C.S. & Chen, K.B. (2018). Immersion of Virtual Reality for Rehabilitation-Review, *Appl Ergon*, 69, 153–161.

Sandström, J., Swanepoel de, W., Carel Myburgh, H. & Laurent, C. (2016). Smartphone Threshold Audiometry in underserved Primary Health-Care Contexts, *Int J Audiol*, 55(4), 232–8.

Serpanos, Y.C., Renne, B., Schoepflin, J.R. & Davis, D. (2018). The Accuracy of Smartphone Sound Level Meter Applications with and without Calibration, *Am J Speech Lang Pathol*, 27(4), 1319–28.

Swanepoel de, W., Myburgh, H.C., Howe, D.M., Mahomed, F. & Eikelboom, R.H. (2014). Smartphone Hearings Creening with Integrated Quality Controland Data Management, *Int J Audiol*, 53(12), 841–9.

Van Tonder, J., Swanepoel, W., Mahomed-Asmail, F., Myburgh, H. & Eikelboom, R.H. (2017). Automated Smartphone Threshold Audiometry: Validity and Time Efficiency, *J Am Acad Audiol*, 28(3), 200–8.

Virk, S. & McConville, K.M. (2006). Virtual Reality Application in Improving Postural Control and Minimizing Falls, *Conf Proc IEEE Eng Med Biol Soc*, 1, 2694–7.

Yeh, S.C., Chen, S., Wang, P.C., Su, M.C., Chang, C.H. & Tsai, P.Y. (2014). Interactive 3-Dimensional Virtual Reality Rehabilitation for Patients with Chronic Imbalance and Vestibular Dysfunction, *Technol Health Care*, 22(6), 915–21.

Yousuf Hussein, S., WetSwanepoel, D., Biagio de Jager, L., Myburgh, H.C., Eikelboom, R.H & Hugo, J. (2016) Smartphone Hearing Screening in Mhealth Assisted Community-Based Primary Care, *J Telemed Telecare*, 22(7), 405–12.

# List of Figures

# List of Tables

www.ingramcontent.com/pod-product-compliance
Lightning Source LLC
Chambersburg PA
CBHW060240220326
41598CB00027B/3992